Progress in Oncology 2001

Edited by

Vincent T. DeVita, Jr.
Yale Cancer Center
New Haven, Connecticut

Samuel Hellman
Department of Radiation Oncology
University of Chicago
Chicago, Illinois

Steven A. Rosenberg
National Cancer Institute
National Institutes of Health
Bethesda, Maryland

JONES AND BARTLETT PUBLISHERS
Sudbury, Massachusetts
BOSTON　　TORONTO　　LONDON　　SINGAPORE

World Headquarters
Jones and Bartlett Publishers
40 Tall Pine Drive
Sudbury, MA 01776
info@jbpub.com
www.jbpub.com

Jones and Bartlett Publishers Canada
2406 Nikanna Road
Mississauga, ON L5C 2W6
CANADA

Jones and Bartlett Publishers International
Barb House, Barb Mews
London W6 7PA
UK

Copyright © 2001 by Jones and Bartlett Publishers, Inc.

All rights reserved. No part of the material protected by this copyright notice may be reproduced or utilized in any form, electronic or mechanical, including photocopying, recording, or by any information storage and retrieval system, without written permission from the copyright owner.

Library of Congress Cataloging-in-Publication Data

Progress in oncology / edited by Vincent T. DeVita, Jr., Samuel Hellman, Steven A. Rosenberg.
    p. ; cm.
Includes bibliographical references and index.
ISBN 0-7637-1589-1
    1. Cancer. 2. Cancer–Treatment. I. DeVita, Vincent T. II. Hellman, Samuel. III. Rosenberg, Steven A.
    [DNLM: 1. Neoplasm–therapy. 2. Neoplasms–diagnosis. QZ 266 P9649 2001]
RC261 .P74 2001
616.99'4–dc21

                                                    2001025720

Production Credits:
Acquisitions Editor: Christopher Davis
Production Editor: Elizabeth Platt
Interior Design: Anne Spencer
Editorial Asitant: Thomas Prindle
Page Layout: Modern Graphics, Inc.
Cover Design: Anne Spencer
Cover Image: Dennis Kunkel, © Dennis Kunkel Microscopy
Printing and Binding: Malloy Lithographing
Cover Printer: Malloy Lithographing

Printed in the United States of America
05 04 03 02 01   10 9 8 7 6 5 4 3 2 1

Contents

List of Contributors   v

Part 1: Basic Science

Chapter 1	Gene Analysis Using DNA Microarrays Cloud P. Paweletz, Verena E. Bechsel, and Lance A. Liotta	1
Chapter 2	Progress in the Molecular Diagnostics of Cancer Eva Musulen and José C. Costa	16
Chapter 3	Dendritic Cells and Cancer Immunization Karolina A. Palucka and Jacques Banchereau	29
Chapter 4	Rolling Circle Amplification Technology: Potential Applications in Cancer Research and Clinical Oncology John H. Leamon, Stefan Hamann, José C. Costa, David C. Ward, and Paul M. Lizardi	46
Chapter 5	Influencing the Apoptotic Mechanism in Cancer Treatment Rebecca L. Elstrom and Craig B. Thompson	72

Part 2: Clinical Applications

Chapter 6	Genetic Susceptibility to Tobacco Carcinogenesis Margaret R. Spitz, Xifeng Wu, and Qingyi Wei	91
Chapter 7	Thalidomide for Cancer Therapy Bart Barlogie, Guido Tricot, Elias Anaissie, and Hartmut Goldschmidt	117
Chapter 8	Oxaliplatin in the Treatment of Patients with Advanced Colorectal Cancer Carmen J. Allegra	139
Chapter 9	Chemoradiation for Patients with Cervical Cancer Franco Muggia, Silvia Formenti, and John Curtin	168
Chapter 10	Tyrosine Kinase Inhibitors in the Treatment of Chronic Myelogenous Leukemia Brian J. Druker	191

Chapter 11	Rituximab for the Treatment of Patients with B-Cell Non-Hodgkin's Lymphoma *David G. Maloney and Peter W. McLaughlin*	204
Chapter 12	Graft versus Tumor Reactions: Mobilizing Allografting as a Treatment for Cancer *Bimalangshu R. Dey and Thomas R. Spitzer*	228
Chapter 13	Radiofrequency Ablation for the Treatment of Liver Metastases *T. S. Ravikumar and Ronald Kaleya*	258

Part 3: Current Controversies

Chapter 14.1	Treatment of Prostate Cancer: Surgery *James A. Eastham and Peter T. Scardino*	278
Chapter 14.2	Treatment of Prostate Cancer: External Beam-Radiotherapy *Steven A. Leibel, Zvi Fuks, Michael J. Zelefsky, and C. Clifton Ling*	313
Chapter 14.3	Treatment of Prostate Cancer: Brachytherapy *Irving D. Kaplan and Edward J. Holupka*	335

| Subject Index | 347 |
| Index of Tables | 360 |

List of Contributors

Carmen J. Allegra, MD
National Cancer Institute, National Institutes of Health, Bethesda, MD

Elias Anaissie, MD
The Myeloma and Transplantation Research Center/Arkansas Cancer Research Center at the University of Arkansas for Medical Sciences, Little Rock, Arkansas

Jacques Banchereau, PhD
Baylor Institute for Immunology Research, Dallas, Texas

Bart Barlogie, MD, PhD
The Myeloma and Transplantation Research Center/Arkansas Cancer Research Center at the University of Arkansas for Medical Sciences, Little Rock, Arkansas

Verena E. Bichsel, MD
Division of Therapeutic Proteins/Center for Biologic Evaluation and Research, Food and Drug Administration, and Laboratory of Pathology, National Cancer Institute, National Institutes of Health, Bethesda, Maryland

José C. Costa, MD
Department of Pathology and Yale Cancer Center, Yale University School of Medicine, New Haven, Connecticut

John Curtin, MD
Department of Obstetrics and Gynecology, New York University Medical Center, New York, New York

Bimalangshu R. Dey, MD
Bone Marrow Transplant Program, Massachusetts General Hospital, Harvard Medical School, Boston, Massachusetts

Brian J. Druker, MD
Leukemia Program, Oregon Health Sciences University, Portland, Oregon

James A. Eastham, MD
Department of Urology, Memorial Sloan-Kettering Cancer Center, New York, New York

Rebecca L. Elstrom, MD
Abramson Family Cancer Research Institute, University of Pennsylvania, Philadelphia, Pennsylvania

Silvia Formenti, MD
Department of Radiation Oncology, New York University Medical Center, New York, New York

Zvi Fuks, MD
Department of Radiation Oncology, Memorial Sloan-Kettering Cancer Center, New York, New York

Hartmut Goldschmidt, MD
The Myeloma and Transplantation Research Center/Arkansas Cancer Research Center at the University of Arkansas for Medical Sciences, Little Rock, Arkansas

Stefan Hamann, PhD
Department of Pathology, Yale University School of Medicine, New Haven, Connecticut

Edward J. Holupka, PhD
Department of Radiation Oncology, Beth Israel Deaconess Medical Center, Boston, Massachusetts

Irving D. Kaplan, MD
Department of Radiation Oncology, Beth Israel Deaconess Medical Center, Boston, Massachusetts

Ronald Kaleya, MD, FACS
Department of Surgery, Montefiore Medical Center, Albert Einstein College of Medicine, Bronx, New York

John H. Leamon, PhD
Department of Pathology, Yale University School of Medicine, New Haven, Connecticut

Steven A. Leibel, MD
Department of Radiation Oncology, Memorial Sloan-Kettering Cancer Center, New York, New York

C. Clifton Ling, PhD
Department of Medical Physics, Memorial Sloan-Kettering Cancer Center, New York, New York

Lance A. Liotta, MD, PhD
Laboratory of Pathology, National Cancer Institute, National Institutes of Health, Bethesda, Maryland

Paul M. Lizardi, PhD
Department of Pathology, Yale University School of Medicine, New Haven, Connecticut

David G. Maloney, MD, PhD
Fred Hutchinson Cancer Research Center and the University of Washington, Seattle, Washington

Peter W. McLaughlin, MD
Lymphoma Department, M.D. Anderson Cancer Center, The University of Texas, Houston, Texas

Franco Muggia, MD
Kaplan Comprehensive Cancer Center, New York University Medical Center, New York, New York

Eva Musulen, MD
Advanced Diagnostic Technology Unit, Parc Tauli Corporation, Sabadell-Barcelona, Spain

Karolina A. Palucka, MD, PhD
Baylor Institute for Immunology Research, Dallas, Texas

Cloud P. Paweletz, BS
Department of Chemistry, Georgetown University, Washington DC

T. S. Ravikumar, MD
Department of Surgery, Montefiore Medical Center, Albert Einstein College of Medicine, Bronx, New York

Peter T. Scardino, MD
Department of Urology, Memorial Sloan-Kettering Cancer Center, New York, New York

Margaret R. Spitz, MD
Department of Epidemiology, M.D. Anderson Cancer Center, The University of Texas, Houston, Texas

Thomas R. Spitzer, MD
Bone Marrow Transplant Program, Massachusetts General Hospital, Harvard Medical School, Boston, Massachusetts

Craig B. Thompson, MD
Abramson Family Cancer Research Institute, University of Pennsylvania, Philadelphia, Pennsylvania

Guido Tricot, MD, PhD
The Myeloma and Transplantation Research Center/Arkansas Cancer Research Center at the University of Arkansas for Medical Sciences, Little Rock, Arkansas

David C. Ward, PhD
Department of Genetics, Yale University School of Medicine, New Haven, Connecticut

Qingyi Wei, PhD
Department of Epidemiology, M.D. Anderson Cancer Center, The University of Texas, Houston, Texas

Xifeng Wu, PhD
Department of Epidemiology, M.D. Anderson Cancer Center, The University of Texas, Houston, Texas

Michael J. Zelefsky, MD
Department of Radiation Oncology, Memorial Sloan-Kettering Cancer Center, New York, New York

Gene Analysis Using DNA Microarrays

Cloud P. Paweletz

Verena E. Bichsel

Lance A. Liotta

Traditionally, tumors have been classified on the basis of histology and immunohistochemistry. However, staining patterns that are microscopically observed cannot predict biological behavior or clinical outcome.[1] For example, two patients who harbor histologically similar tumors may have two different clinical outcomes or may respond differently to the same therapeutic treatment strategy. Histology alone is insufficient to guide clinical treatment strategies, because the outward manifestation of the neoplastic process is the product of a complex tissue microenvironment in which positive and negative protein interactions are taking place among cancer cells, organ parenchymal cells, stroma, blood vessels, and the extracellular matrix. After somatic genetic progression, defects in the cancer cell genome trigger proteomic derangements that drive survival, growth, invasion, and metastasis. The complicated changing pattern of cancer cell messenger RNA (mRNA) transcripts, a result of its genetic defects combined with the microenvironmental stimuli at the tumor-host interface, may provide clues about the molecular events that are the basis for the clinical behavior of the patient's individual cancer.

A NEW PARADIGM IN TUMOR BIOLOGY?

Instead of studying one gene at a time, investigators are surveying hundreds or thousands of transcripts using complementary DNA (cDNA) microarrays and oligonucleotide arrays. Microarrays are propelling oncology toward a future in which patients are managed based on a molecular classification of their individual tumors. Gene expression patterns contain information about transcriptionally regulated genes that track with or cause the disease. In addition, they hold information about the tumor's cell of origin and differentiation status. Expression profiling will enhance our current tumor classification system by identifying individual genes or gene profiles that track with disease or clinical outcome.[2-4] Concomitantly, this may also allow for insights into pathogenesis, diagnosis, prognosis, and effective therapeutic targets.[5-10]

Complementary DNA microarrays take their cue from well-established hybridization chemistries between immobilized oligonucleotides and fluorescently tagged RNA populations.[11] More precisely, cDNA probes first are chosen and amplified by polymerase chain reaction from a database containing sequences that are relevant to the study. For the purpose of cancer research, the GenBank[12] or UniGene[13] databases have proven extremely useful for the synthesis and amplification of probes that will be arrayed and subsequently analyzed. After cDNA sequences have been synthesized, they are robotically arrayed at distinct, spatially addressable regions on a solid support, such as glass, charged nylon, or nitrocellulose. Many companies offer pre-made cDNA and gene arrays for those who do not have a microarrayer in house with which to print arrays themselves (Table 1.1).

After an appropriate array has been chosen, total RNA from normal and tumor cell populations (i.e., tumor vs normal cell lines, tumor-enriched vs tumor-devoid tissue fractions, or microdissected normal vs tumor cells) are isolated, purified, and fluorescently cy-3- and cy-5-labeled. Subsequently, the array is allowed to hybridize with labeled RNA, is excited at the appropriate wavelengths (cy-5, ~ 649 nm; cy-3, ~ 550 nm), and is analyzed by scanning confocal microscopy. The raw data present as monochromatic images that represent the signal intensity of the appropriate channel (cy-5, ~ 670 nm; cy-3, ~ 560 nm). To visualize mRNA abundance, a false color (cy-5, red; cy-3, green) will be applied to the monochro-

TABLE 1.1 Commercial Sources for Microarrays

Company Name	Product Name	Contact Web Site
Affymetrix, Inc.	GeneChip arrays	http://www.gene-chips.com/
AlphaGene	MICROMAX	http://www.alphagene.com/
DNAmicroarray.com	Made-to-order microarrays	http://www.dnamicroarray.com/
Clontech	Atlas arrays	http://www.clontech.com/
Gene Logic, Inc.	READS	http://www.genelogic.com/
OriGene Technologies, Inc.	SmartArray	http://www.origene.com/
Hyseq, Inc.	HyChip	http://www.hyseq.com

matic images, and the arrays will be overlaid. The measured cy-3/cy-5 light output correlates directly to an increase (> 1, red), decrease (< 1, green) or no change (1, yellow) in gene expression (Fig. 1.1; see color plates, p. 24). The background appears black. Normalization between microarrays usually is based on housekeeping genes such as *GAPDH*, actin, or other genes known not to change. However, standardization for microarray experiments is not confined to single genes alone but rather is dependent on the experiment itself. For example, Alizadeh et al[14] (vide infra) measured relative gene expressions in diffuse large-cell B-cell (DLBCL) lymphoma biopsy samples ($N = 40$) and normalized the relative gene expression of each sample to total RNA of a common control probe that contained an RNA pool of nine lymphoma cell lines. Nonetheless, RNA isolation, printing, labeling, and hybridization to microarrays is not uniform between laboratories, and a wide source of reliable information for microarray preparation, printing, RNA labeling, and hybridization is now available on the World Wide Web (Table 1.2).[15]

The goal of microarray-based experiments in oncology is to create a *gene expression profile* that represents the dynamic makeup of each gene in the genome from tissues, cell lines, disease stages, or treatments. To accomplish this task, a two-dimensional *gene expression matrix,* in which rows represent genes and columns represent samples, must be designed (Fig. 1.2; see color plates, p. 24). The design of this matrix is a complicated process that involves the identification of each mRNA spot and a measurement of its intensity. Once the gene expression matrix has been designed, two approaches are then used to correlate gene expressions

TABLE 1.2 Internet Sources of Information About Microarray Preparation and Analysis

Internet Address	Type of Information
http://www.nhgri.nih.gov/DIR/LCG/15K/HTML/protocol.html	A continually updated site that provides information about RNA quality, RNA extraction, labeling, hybridization, and analysis
http://brownlab.stanford.edu/	An excellent starting point to find all relevant information regarding microarrays
http://www.tigr.org/tdb/microarray	A good site that provides alternative protocols and introduction to microarrays.
http://www.lab-on-a-chip.com/files/corepage.htm/	An excellent source of information pertaining to published papers, news, events, products, discussion forums, and careers utilizing microarrays.
http://www.bsi.vt.edu/ralscher/gridit	A collaborative site between Virginia Tech and North Carolina State University that contains a large amount of information related to microarray-based research. Also provides an opportunity to sign on to three microarray discussion groups

with sample characteristics: the similarities or differences can be measured in either rows or columns. To elucidate the subtle pattern changes of either all rows or all columns, the Euclidean distance for all objects must be measured. Thus, we consider each variable in gene expression matrices as objects in n-dimensional space or as n-dimensional vectors.[16] After the similarity of the gene expression profile has been determined, one can analyze these data in either a supervised or an unsupervised fashion. In unsupervised analysis, we cluster objects that exhibit similar properties into groups by either hierarchic[17] or K-mean clustering[18] algorithms. Hierarchic clustering algorithms start by joining two clusters with the closest Euclidean distances in n-dimensional space and proceed by recalculating the distances between residual clusters and the newly formed cluster. The threshold distance that is defined by the user determines the number of clusters.

The K-mean algorithm, on the other hand, uses the Euclidean vectors of all objects to cluster the data set. The vector space is divided into K parts (defined prior to analysis by the user), after which the algorithm calculates the center in each of these K subsets. Clusters then are designed based on the closeness of each Euclidean vector to the center of the subsets.

Supervised analysis, on the other hand, attempts to create classifiers such as decision trees that assign predefined classes to gene expression profiles.[19] The remainder of this review explains recent advances made using supervised and unsupervised analysis of microarray experiments in pathogenetic analysis of cancers.

TRANSCRIPTIONAL PROFILING OF CANCERS

Golub et al[19] were among the first to attempt to correlate gene expression profiles with classification of tumors. In the course of their studies, these researchers decided to test whether obtained gene expression patterns can be subdivided into "class discovery" and "class prediction" categories. For the purpose of this study, *class discovery* was defined as the search of expression profiles that correspond to previous unrecognized tumor types, whereas *class prediction* attempts to correlate gene expression profiles with already established tumor classifications. Using acute leukemia as a proof-in-principle example, Golub et al[19] succeeded in distinguishing acute myeloid leukemia (AML) from acute lymphoblastic leukemia (ALL) on the basis of gene expression alone in 36 of 38 bone marrow samples (27 ALL and 11 AML). To accomplish this task, 6817 genes were correlated on the basis of gene expression similarity and were analyzed by what Golub termed a *neighboring analysis algorithm*. Briefly, this analysis defines an optimum expression pattern of a particular gene that is uniformly high in the reference sample and low in the test sample and tests whether there exists a cluster of genes that is similar to the optimum expression pattern rather than displaying a random pattern. Using this analysis, the researchers found 1100 genes that are more likely to correlate with ALL and AML patterns rather than random patterns. Of that class, they chose 50 reference genes that correctly predicted tumor classification in these samples (36 of 38). The number of references genes used is somewhat arbitrary, as 10–200 so-called predictor genes yielded 100% accuracy. Independent verification of this procedure was carried out using 34 leukemia samples (24 bone marrow and 10 peripheral blood) in which 29 of 34 were identified correctly with an accuracy of 100%.

An underlying philosophical question that arises by attempting to discover cancer subtypes using cDNA microarrays (i.e., class discovery) is whether expression patterns reflect a "true" state of biology. The researchers reasoned that if a gene cluster were found that represented a novel tumor classification, it could be tested, verified, and redefined by the already established gene predictors used during class prediction. The researchers proceeded first to cluster tumors by a "self-organizing map" algorithm.[20-22] The resulting clusters then were cross-validated by predictor genes that were used previously during class prediction. Using a self-organizing map algorithm, they clustered the initial 38 samples into two classes using the original 6817 genes. On closer investigation, Golub et al[19] found that the two new classes generally followed already established classifications, with cluster 1 containing 24 of 25 ALL cases and cluster 2 containing 10 of 13 AML cases. Subsequently, cross-validation of these new classes using class prediction accurately identified all but one case.

A final conclusion that was drawn by the researchers projected that gene expression profiling may provide insights into the pathogenesis of tumors, such as stage and origin, that previously was not attainable by standard histologic staining.[19] More important, these correlations were performed in an unbiased forum in which no prior biological information was readily available.

Alternatively, tumor classification has been performed using cultured tumor cell lines. Ross et al.[23] used cDNA microarrays containing 9703 cDNA probes to study 60 cell lines that currently are used as part of the preclinical trial study set for evaluation purposes for anticancer drugs at the National Cancer Institute. Using gene expression clustering alone, the authors were able to correlate ostensible cell type and origin to cancer cell lineage. Furthermore, growth rate and drug metabolism seems to correlate to specific features found in these expression patterns. When these expression patterns were compared to normal and tumor breast tissues, the investigators found that although the gene expression patterns varied from cancer tissue to cancer tissue, recognizable features could be found between human cancerous tissue and specific human cancer cell lines.[23]

The first clinical correlation between gene expression patterns and clinical outcome was demonstrated by Alizadeh et al[14] in DLBCLs. The DLBCL is the most common subtype of non-Hodgkin's lymphoma, with 40% of patients having prolonged survival as compared with the remaining 60%. Alizadeh et al[14] found two distinct gene expression patterns indicative of different stages of B-cell differentiation. One type was characteristic of germinal-center B cells, and the other type expressed genes that normally are induced during in vitro activation of peripheral B cells. The two expression profiles correlated with high and low 10-year survival rates of the patients, respectively. This remarkable divergence in clinical behavior suggests that the two kinds of lymphomas should be regarded as distinct diseases. Gene expression profiles represent a big step forward in clinical diagnosis, as traditional methods such as immunohistochemistry fail to detect subtle molecular changes. DLBCL patients may benefit in the near future from improved intervention strategies, as transcriptional analyses may become an integral part in the diagnosis of lymphoma.

Many other researchers, using cDNA or oligonucleotide microarrays, are involved in deciphering genetic events that are taking place during tumorigenesis. Their experiments range from uncovering downstream transcriptional targets to identifying novel tumor suppressor genes to pharmacological screenings. A number of published references should be considered good starting points for readers who are interested in designing their own gene expression experiments using microarrays both in tissue and tumor cell lines.[24-42]

PATHOGENIC ANALYSIS USING cDNA MICROARRAYS

Perou et al[43] were among the first to use cDNA microarray experiments to gain direct molecular insights into tumorigenesis. These researchers proposed that phenotypic diversity has an underlying genetic diversity, and thus one would be able to gain insight into disease characteristics such as grade, clinical course, and treatment by analyzing gene expression profiles. Microarray analysis of 8102 genes of 65 breast tumor samples from 42 patients revealed distinct patterns for each tumor. More precisely, cDNA that was prepared from RNA from each tumor sample was fluorescently cy-5-labeled and compared to a reference (cy-3-labeled) that contained RNA isolated from 11 different cell lines. Twenty of the tumors were sampled before and after doxorubicin chemotherapy. Clustering analysis indicated a high degree of similarity within samples derived from the same patient as compared with those from different patients. By analyzing hierarchical relationships, tumors were classified into those that were estrogen receptor–positive and those that were estrogen receptor–negative.

Following the same scheme, Bittner et al[10] proposed that unrecognizable cancer "taxonomy" may be elucidated by hierarchical clustering of gene expression profiles. In their experiments, 31 melanoma biopsy samples and 7 control samples were hybridized against a microarray that contained 8150 (6971 unique) genes. Using this microarray, Bittner et al[10] demonstrated that mathematically these 31 melanoma samples can be subdivided into two major groups of 12 and 19 species that formed close clusters. On closer investigation, these researchers found that many genes that are differently expressed also are regulated in cultured melanomas that form tubular networks in vitro, a feature that may point to an aggressive phenotype. Melanoma biopsies that clustered outside this vascular-like group showed reduced motility and reduced aggressiveness. A recurrent theme was the lack of any correlation between hierarchical clustering and melanoma morphology. Thus, hierarchical analysis of cancer may be a novel assay for the understanding of tumor aggressiveness and progression.

GENE EXPRESSION ARRAYS USING MICRODISSECTED TISSUE SAMPLES

Although exciting results indicating that gene expression profiles track with disease have been obtained with tumor cell lines or heterogeneous tissue samples, it is widely accepted that molecular analyses will be the most accurate if the analysis is performed on cells that undergo tumorigenesis in actual human tissue.[44,45] Cultured cells, though chosen to reflect a particular tumor, are separated from their in vivo environment, such as soluble growth factors or the extracellular matrix. Surrounding cell populations are not simply innocent bystanders during tumor growth and invasion, but rather play an important supportive role. Cell-to-cell interaction and autocrine and paracrine stimuli between cells ultimately determine whether a cell (1) remains quiescent, (2) proliferates, (3) differentiates, (4) undergoes programmed cell death, (5) adapts to a differentiated state, or (6) migrates. Changes in gene expression governing this homeostasis may therefore determine such important events as tumor growth or invasion. Thus, cultured tumor cell lines cannot accurately reflect the actual status of cells in human tissue. Nonetheless, two possible strategies have been chosen to circumvent the use of cell lines and thereby still allow the use of gene expression profiles for tumor classification.

First, gene expressions of tumors may be analyzed by global gene expression analyses. Global gene expression surveys assume that information of interacting cell populations can be investigated by analyzing gene expression patterns from heterogeneous tissue samples. Total RNA from tissue fragments (i.e., high tumor content vs low tumor content) is isolated, labeled, and probed on an array, and the status of gene expression is quantified. However, imagining that genes from cell subpopulations also are included and thus may contaminate the results is not difficult. Heuristic algorithms,[10,14,42] routinely used to estimate the proportion of original tumor cells by incorporating known genes of specific subpopulations, provide a means that allows the use of heterogeneous tissue fragments.

An alternative strategy is to microdissect cell populations of interest (i.e., normal, tumor, hyperplastic, dysplastic, and endothelial cell populations) and to analyze their gene expression profile with respect to one another (Fig. 1.3; see color plates, p. 24). Thus, one can easily obtain information about genetic events underlying tumor progression without the need for extensive heuristic algorithms. Many techniques exist that aid in tissue microdissection, and these are constantly being developed further to improve ease and speed of use. Earlier methodologies entailed the gross removal of tissue by hand, whereas two predominant techniques currently employ the use of lasers. The first, known as *selective ultraviolet radiation fractionation*, requires the application of an ultraviolet-absorbent ink to cells from which genetic material is warranted to protect against ultraviolet radiation, after which an ultraviolet laser is employed to destroy genetic material of unwanted surrounding tissue.[46]

A second microdissection technique is a positive selection method (i.e., selecting what the user wants rather than destroying surrounding cells), which has recently been used in genomic and proteomic studies of individual cancer cells. This method is termed *laser capture microdissection* (LCM). In LCM, a stained slide is placed under an inverted microscope, where the tissue can be visualized in real time.[47] An ethylene vinyl acetate cap is placed onto the tissue, and the user moves the slide until the area of interest is in the path of the laser. To procure cells of interest, an infrared laser is fired that allows for expansion of the polymer and subsequent embedding of the cells. This procedure can be repeated until all the cells of interest have been captured, after which these cells can be lysed off the cap.

Gene expression experiments performed by global gene expression analysis of tissue fragments and microdissection have their own advantages and disadvantages. The most relevant advantage of global gene expression analysis is that it is not hindered by the amount of input material. However, we may not accurately know the actual proportion of diseased cell populations to surrounding contaminating cell populations. For example, a change in a low-abundance mRNA may not be readily observed as its signal is "overshadowed" by high-abundance mRNA species that is not part of the tumor population. The decisive advantage that microdissection has over global gene expression is that cell-specific transcriptional profiles from patient-matched normal, hyperplastic, carcinoma in situ, and invasive carcinoma cells can be independently investigated and compared to one another. However, the use of microdissected cell populations to probe cDNA microarrays is somewhat hindered, as the amount of total RNA needed usually exceeds the amount of RNA that can practically be obtained by microdissection. This holds true especially if one wants to analyze gene expression profiles from premalignant lesions, such as low-grade dysplasia. Thus, methods are designed to amplify transcript populations from microdissected cell populations linearly, so that these can be used to hybridize cDNA.[48,49]

The first successful integration among LCM, cDNA microarrays, and linear probe amplification of an entire transcript population was demonstrated by Luo et al.[48] Independent microdissections, amplifications using T7 RNA polymerase, and gene expression analyses of small and large dorsal root ganglia were performed, and similar gene expression signal intensities with r^2 values ranging from 0.9688 to 0.9399 were observed. However, a bias may still exist during probe amplification. Thus, if a nonamplification approach is warranted, one can always microdissect between 50,000 and 100,000 cells, synthesize direct-labeled cDNA as the array probe, and analyze the expression profiles from nonamplified cell populations.

Sgroi et al[50] were among the first to analyze distinct LCM-procured tumor cell population and cDNA microarrays without any amplification-based method, using a direct radioactively labeled cDNA probe. In their study, total RNA from approximately 20,000 microdissected breast normal epithelial, invasive, and malignant metastatic cells (to the lymph node) were isolated and radioactively labeled during reverse transcription, and the corresponding single-stranded cDNA probe was hybridized against two different cDNA arrays that contained a total of 8084 genes. To gain insight into genetic events that underlie in vivo breast cancer progression, the expression profile between target cell populations was compared. Hybridization of these arrays revealed that 90 genes were regulated differently by a magnitude of twofold or more (overall expression change ranged from eightfold to fortyfold) when normal cell populations were compared to their corresponding invasive cell populations. When normal cell populations were compared to metastatic cell populations, 112 genes were found to change at least twofold or more. Four genes (of a total of 212) were found to be differentially expressed in both the invasive and metastatic cell populations, and 83 of the genes were expressed sequence tags. Genes that were identified showed a broad range of functional activity. For example, apolipoprotein D, annexin I, tissue factor, and RANTES were all found to be differentially regulated. These molecules have been previously associated with immune cell movement and homing, so it could make sense that they act in cancer progression. The genes identified in this study now constitute previously unknown therapeutic and diagnostic targets. Furthermore, quantitative reverse transcriptase–PCR from the same isolated RNA and immunohistochemistry from the same tissue validated these findings.

In another experiment that used LCM-procured cells and cDNA microarrays, Leethanakul et al[51] probed radioactively labeled and amplified cDNA against a cDNA microarray that contained known human cancer and housekeeping genes. In this study, 5000 cells from representative sets of head and neck carcinomas were microdissected and their gene expression profiles analyzed. The cell sets contained hyperplastic cell populations as well as invasive carcinoma (well and moderately differentiated) of the tongue, poorly differentiated laryngeal carcinoma, and moderately differentiated pharyngeal carcinoma. Corresponding normal cells of each tissue set were microdissected from the same anatomical site. Using this array, the investigators found that genes that are involved in the mitogen-activated protein kinase, *wnt*, and *noth* pathways are up-regulated with increasing severity of tumorigenesis. Furthermore, the researchers found a decrease (two- to twentyfold reduction) in expression of cytokeratins 2E, 2P, 6A-F, 7, 13, 14, 15, 17, 18, and 19.

The advantage of microdissection-based approaches in studying expression profiles as they occur during tumorigenesis has been elaborated by Cole et al.[52] These researchers proposed the use of LCM to develop a three-dimensional model of cancer progression by characterizing genetic changes of all cell populations throughout an entire prostate gland. By analyzing these changes, it should be possible to combine physical and molecular characteristics of cell populations; that is, it may be possible to determine which genes drive the transition from dysplastic lesions to invasive carcinoma.

THE FUTURE

Although substantial progress over existing tumor classifications has been accomplished using gene expression profiling, genetic information alone will not reveal all the information necessary to understand the molecular mechanism governing tumor growth and invasion. The activated (e.g., phosphorylated) state of signal pathway checkpoints in vivo cannot be ascertained from gene expression alone. Nevertheless, the state of such pathways may be a key determinant of diseased cellular physiology. Genes involved in determining chemotherapeutic responsiveness and, hence, reasons for differential clinical outcome have yet to be discovered. Knowledge about upstream events in gene expression, about defects in the protein circuitry of the cell, would unveil the effects of altered gene expression. This knowledge would eventually lead to the discovery of new accurate targets for therapy, development of new therapeutic regimens with the least toxicity and greatest efficacy, and new biological markers that can serve as early detection surrogates. Furthermore, that there is not necessarily any direct correlation between mRNA expression and protein levels in vivo is well-known.[49] Emerging proteomic technologies allow for scanning of cellular proteins in simple, short, reproducible, and quantitative chemical assays. Protein and tissue microarrays now are being designed to allow investigation of large sets of proteins and protein interactions in parallel, similar to gene expression arrays recently used in functional genomics.[53-64]

Tissue arrays have traditionally been used as complementary arrays to cDNA microarrays.[55] Once a potential tumor marker has been identified by gene expression analyses, validation of that marker in the actual tissue is necessary. Traditionally, this was done by immunohistochemical studies conducted in sequence. Punch-based tissue arrays allow for simultaneous investigation of analytes in hundreds of samples by immunohistochemistry and in situ hybridization methodologies. These tissue arrays are based on up to 1000 cylindrical biopsies, each from different patients, that are precisely arrayed into a 45 mm × 20 mm donor block for further in situ analyses. The potential of the approach was first tested with arrays, each containing 645 samples, that were screened for known breast tumor markers. The data obtained confirmed many of the clinicopathologic correlations of gene amplifications that had already been established by whole-tissue analysis.

To characterize cellular metabolism directly at the protein level, Chaurand et al[65] described the use of mass-spectrometric analysis on primary tissue. Tissue sections from several mouse organs were mounted on a conductive polyethylene membrane and digested in situ, and peptide profiles were generated by matrix-assisted laser desorption ionization at defined areas. Distinct peptide and protein patterns were observed for different regions of colon. Database searches matched to known proteins 35 of the 100 peptides detected in the range from 2000 to 30,000 Da. From some of the lower-mass peptides, a primary amino acid sequence could be obtained. These peptide mass profiles, similar to cDNA microarrays, represent the molecular signature of a cell in a defined tissue environment at a defined time. The ability to study proteins in human tissue is crucial for unveiling processes that lead to aberrant cellular behavior and disease.

In our laboratory, we use surface-enhanced laser desorption ionization mass spectrometry to generate protein mass profiles from laser-capture microdissected tissue. Reproducible protein fingerprints were generated for different human epithelial tumors, as well as from different progression states of human prostate tumor.[66] Intriguingly, the speed and ease of matrix-assisted laser desorption ionization and surface-enhanced laser desorption ionization mass spectrometry directly imply the use of mass spectrometry for diagnosis of disease in the clinical laboratory. Future technical improvements will define the power of these methods in identifying the most specific and efficient targets for therapy.

However, investigators already are moving beyond mere protein arrays to more functional arrays that aim to measure biochemical activities. For example, kinase arrays have been designed that attempt to characterize the status of all kinases in a given species; alternatively, all substrates of a particular kinase are being analyzed.[67,68] It is merely a matter of time until these arrays will find their way into the field of tumor biology.

CONCLUSION

Evolving research interests in oncology can be divided into three main phases. The first involves the identification and sequencing of previously unknown genes that underlie tumorigenesis. Thus, novel oncogenes or tumor suppressor genes may be discovered that may provide insights into the pathogenic state of individual tumors. The second phase attempts to correlate gene expression or protein profiles with the genomic or functional status of oncogenic signaling pathways within tissue or individual cell populations. The third phase can be described as *circuitry building*.[69] In the last and most encompassing phase, all the information obtained from the first and second phases is incorporated in a "road map" that underlies tumorigenesis. This phase may provide the most complex but, simultaneously and seemingly contradictorily, simplified and unified overview of tumors and tumor progression.[70] The promise of all this is that heuristic algorithm analyses of all the information obtained from gene expression arrays, proteomic arrays, and functional arrays may provide to individual patients tailor-made treatments with the promise of higher efficacy and lower toxicity.

REFERENCES

1. Holland JF et al. Cancer Medicine (5th ed). New York: Williams & Wilkins, 1999:1–17.
2. Marx J. DNA arrays reveal cancer in its many forms. Science 2000;289:1670–1672.
3. Khan J, Bittner ML, Chen Y et al. DNA microarray technology: the anticipated impact on the study of human disease. BBA-Rev Cancer 1999;1423:M17–23.
4. Afshari CA, Nuwaysir EF, Barrett JC. Application of complementary DNA microarray technology to carcinogen identification, toxicology, and drug safety evaluation. Cancer Res 1999;59:4759–4760.
5. Pease AC, Solas D, Sullivan EJ et al. Light generated oligonucleotide arrays for rapid DNA sequence analysis. Proc Natl Acad Sci USA 1994;91:5022–5026.
6. DeRisi J, Penland L, Brown PO et al. Use of cDNA microarray to analyze gene expression patterns in human cancers. Nat Genet 1996;14:457–460.
7. Khan J, Simon R, Bittner M et al. Gene expression profiling of alveolar rhabdomyosarcoma with cDNA microarrays. Cancer Res 1998;58:5009–5013.
8. Lipshutz RJ, Fodor SP, Gingeras TR et al. High density synthetic oligonucleotide arrays. Nat Genet 1999;21[suppl 1]:20–24.
9. Perou CM, Jeffrey SS, van de Rijn M et al. Distinctive gene expression patterns in human mammary epithelial cells and breast cancers. Proc Natl Acad Sci USA 1999;96:9212–9217.
10. Bittner M, Meltzer P, Chen Y et al. Molecular classification of cutaneous malignant melanoma by gene expression profiling. Nature 2000;406:536–540.
11. Southern E, Mir K, Shchepinov M. Molecular interactions on microarrays. Nat Genet 1999;21[suppl 1]:5–9.
12. Benson DA, Boguski MS, Lipman DJ et al. GenBank. Nucleic Acid Res 1997;25:1–6
13. Schuler GD, Boguski MD, Stewart EA et al. A gene map of the human genome. Science 1996;274:540–546.
14. Alizadeh AA, Eisen MB, Davis RE et al. Distinct types of diffuse large B-cell lymphoma identified by gene expression profiling. Nature 2000;403:503–511.
15. Hegde P, Qi R, Abernathy K et al. A concise guide to cDNA microarray analysis. Biotechniques 2000;29:548–562.
16. Brazma A, Vilo J. Gene expression data analysis. FEBS Lett 2000;480:17–24.
17. Eisen M, Spellman PT, Botstein D et al. Cluster analysis and display of genome-wide expression patterns. Proc Natl Acad Sci USA 1998;95(25):14863–14868.
18. Tavazoie S, Hughes JD, Campbell MJ et al. Systematic determination of genetic network architecture. Nat Genet 1999;22:281–285.
19. Golub TR, Slonim DK, Tamayo P et al. Molecular classification of cancer: class discovery and class prediction by gene expression monitoring. Science 1999;286:531–537.
20. Claverie JM. Computational methods for the identification of differential and coordinated gene expression. Hum Mol Genet 1999;8:1821–1832.
21. Tamayo P, Slonim D, Mesirov J et al. Interpreting patterns of gene expression with self-organizing maps: methods and application to hematopoietic differentiation. Proc Natl Acad Sci USA 1999;96:2907–2912.
22. Toronen P, Kolehmainen M, Wong G et al. Analysis of gene expression data using self-organizing maps. FEBS Lett 1999;451:142–146.
23. Ross DT, Scherf U, Eisen MB et al. Systematic variation in gene expression patterns in human cancer cell lines. Nat Genet 2000;24:227–235.
24. Harkin DP. Uncovering functionally relevant signaling pathways using microarray-based expression profiling. Oncologist 2000;5:501–507.

25. Su YA, Bittner ML, Chen Y et al. Identification of tumor suppressor genes using human melanoma cell lines UACC903, UAC903(+6), and SRS3 by comparison of expression profiles. Mol Carcinog 2000;28:119–127.
26. Wikman FP, Lu ML, Thykjaer T et al. Evaluation of the performance of p53 sequencing microarray chip using 140 previously sequenced bladder tumor samples. Clin Chem 2000;46:1555–1561.
27. Nelson PS, Han D, Rochon Y et al. Comprehensive analyses of prostate gene expression: convergence of expressed sequence taq databases, transcript profiling and proteomics. Electrophoresis 2000;21:1823–1831.
28. Forozan F, Mahlamaki EH, Monni O et al. Comparative genomic hybridization analysis of 38 breast cancer cell lines: a basis for interpreting complementary DNA microarray data. Cancer Res 2000;60:4519–4525.
29. Simeonova PP, Wang S, Toriuma W et al. Arsenic mediates cell proliferation and gene expression in the bladder epithelium: association with activating protein-1 transactivation. Cancer Res 2000; 60:3445–3453.
30. Elek J, Park KH, Narayanan R. Microarray-based expression profiling in prostate tumors. In Vivo 2000;14:173–182.
31. Ono K, Tanaka T, Tsunoda T et al. Identification by cDNA microarray of genes in ovarian carcinogenesis. Cancer Res 2000;60:5007–5011.
32. Heiskanen MA, Bittner ML, Chen Y et al. Detection of gene amplification by genomic hybridization to cDNA microarrays. Cancer Res 2000;60:799–802.
33. Scherf U, Ross DT, Waltham M et al. A gene expression database for the molecular pharmacology of cancer. Nat Genet 2000;24:236–244.
34. Welford SM, Gregg J, Chen E et al. Detection of differentially expressed genes in primary tumor tissue using representational differences analysis coupled with microarray hybridization. Nucleic Acids Res 1998;26:3059–3065.
35. Kudoh K, Ramanna M, Ravatn R et al. Monitoring the expression profile of doxorubicin-induced and doxorubicin-resistant cancer cells by cDNA microarray. Cancer Res 2000;60:4161–4166.
36. Xu J, Stolk JA, Zhang X et al. Identification of differentially expressed genes in human prostate cancer using subtraction and microarray. Cancer Res 2000;60:1677–1682.
37. Alon U, Barkai N, Notterman DA et al. Broad patterns of gene expression revealed by clustering analysis of tumor and normal colon tissues probed by oligonucleotide arrays. Proc Natl Acad Sci USA 1999;96:6745–6750.
38. Heller RA, Schena M, Chai A et al. Discovery and analysis of inflammatory disease related genes using cDNA microarrays. Proc Natl Acad Sci USA 1997;94:2150–2155.
39. Villaret DB, Wang T, Dillon D et al. Identification of genes overexpressed in head and neck squamous cell carcinoma using a combination of complementary DNA subtraction and microarray analysis. Laryngoscopy 2000;110(3, pt 1):374–381.
40. Clark EA, Golub T, Lander E et al. Genomic analysis of metastasis reveals an essential role for RhoC. Nature 2000;406:532–535.
41. St Croix B, Rago C, Velculescu V et al. Genes expressed in human tumor endothelium. Science 2000;289:1197–1202.
42. Wellmann A, Thieblemont C, Pittaluga S et al. Detection of differentially expressed genes in lymphomas using cDNA arrays: identification of clustering as a new diagnostic marker for anaplastic large-cell lymphomas. Blood 2000;96:398–404.
43. Perou CM, Sorlie T, Eisen MB et al. Molecular portraits of human breast tumours. Nature 2000; 406:747–752.
44. Page MJ, Amess B, Townsend R et al. Proteomic definition of normal luminal and myoepithelial

breast cells purified from reduction mammoplasties. Proc Natl Acad Sci USA 2000;96: 12589–12594.
45. Ornstein DK, Gillespie JW, Paweletz CP et al. Proteomic analysis of laser capture microdissected human prostate cancer and *in vitro* prostate cell lines. Electrophoresis 2000;21:2235–2242.
46. Shibata D, Hawes D, Li ZH et al. Specific genetic analysis of microscopic tissue after selective ultraviolet radiation fractionation and the polymerase chain reaction. Am J Pathol 1992;141: 539–543.
47. Emmert-Buck MR, Bonner RF, Smith PD et al. Laser capture microdissection. Science 1996;274: 998–1001.
48. Luo L, Salunga RC, Guo H et al. Gene expression profiles of laser-captured adjacent neuronal subtypes. Nat Med 1999;5:117–122.
49. Ohyama H, Zhang X, Kohno Y et al. Laser captured microdissection-generated target sample for high-density oligonucleotide array hybridization. Biotechniques 2000;29:530–536.
50. Sgroi DC, Teng S, Robinson G et al. In vivo gene expression profile analysis of human breast cancer progression. Cancer Res 1999;59:5656–5661.
51. Leethanakul C, Patel V, Gillespie J et al. Distinct pattern of expression of differentiation and growth-related genes in squamous cell carcinomas of the head and neck revealed by the use of laser capture microdissection and cDNa arrrays. Oncogene 2000;19:3220–3224.
52. Cole KA, Krizman DB, Emmert-Buck MR. The genetics of cancer—a 3D model. Nat Genet 1999; 21[suppl 1]:38–41.
53. Anderson L, Seilhamer J. A comparison of selected mRNA and protein abundances in human liver. Electrophoresis 1997;18:533–537.
54. Fodor SPA, Read JL, Pirrung MC at al. Light directed, spatially addressable parallel chemical synthesis. Science 1991;251:767–773.
55. Kononen J, Bubendorf L, Kallioniemi A at al. Tissue microarrays for high-throughput molecular profiling of tumor specimens. Nat Med 1998;4:844–847.
56. MacBeath G, Koehler AN, Schreiber SL. Printing small molecules as microarrays and detecting protein-ligand interactions en masse. J Am Chem Soc 1999;121:7966–7968.
57. Ge H. UPA: a universal protein array. Nucleic Acid Res 2000;28:e3.
58. Englert CR, Baibakov GV, Emmert-Buck MR. Layered expression scanning: rapid molecular profiling of tumor samples. Cancer Res 2000;60:1526–1530.
59. Lueking A, Horn M, Eickhoff H at al. Protein microarrays for gene expression and antibody screening. Anal Biochem 1999;270:103–111.
60. Arenkov P, Kukhtin A, Gemmell A. Protein microarrays: use of immunoassays and enzymatic reactions. Anal Biochem 2000;278:123–131.
61. Ekins RP, Chu FW. Multianalyte microspot immunoassay—microanalytical compact-disk of the future. Clin Chem 1991;37:1955–1967.
62. Rowe AC, Tender LM, Feldstein MJ et al. Array biosensor for simultaneous identification of bacterial, viral, and protein analytes. Anal Chem 1999;71:3846–3852.
63. Jones WV, Kenseth JR, Porter MD at al. Microminiaturized immunoassays using atomic force microscopy and compositionally patterned antigen arrays. Anal Chem 1998;70:1233–1241.
64. Haab BB, Dunham MJ, Brown PO. Protein microarrays for highly parallel detection and quantitation of specific proteins and antibodies in complex solutions. Genome Biol 2000;1:1–22.
65. Chaurand P, Pearsall RS, Stoeckli M et al. Identification of tumor specific biomarkers in colon cancer by MALDI mass spectrometry. FASEB 2000;14:A328–A328.
66. Paweletz CP, Gillespie JW, Ornstein DK et al. Rapid protein display profiling of cancer progression directly from human tissue using a protein biochip. Drug Dev Res 2000;49:34–42.

67. MacBeath G, Schreiber SL. Printing proteins as microarrays for high-throughput function determination. Science 2000;289:1760–1763.
68. Zhu H, Klemic JF, Chang S et al. Analyte of yeast protein kinases using protein chips. Nat Genet 2000;26:283–289.
69. Berns A. Turning on tumors to study cancer progression. Nat Med 1999;5:989–990.
70. Hanahan D, Weinberg RA. The hallmarks of cancer. Cell 2000;100:57–70.

Chapter 2

Progress in the Molecular Diagnosis of Cancer

Eva Musulen

José C. Costa

In the last two decades, unparalleled progress has been made in our understanding of cancer. We have acquired fundamental insights that enable us to approach every aspect of cancer, from etiology to the cell cycle to drug resistance, in totally different and novel ways. The development of technology, more specifically biotechnology and bioinformatics, opens new avenues by which to treat complex problems and is augmenting our capabilities at a vertiginous speed. The simple fact that we have had to add *in silico* to *in vivo* and *in vitro* as an expression for describing hypothesis-driven data mining provides a measure of the depth of change brought about by computational biology in the postgenomic period.

Of the disciplines involved in the study of cancer as a disease and in the care of individual cancer patients, pathology is particularly concerned with diagnostic tests. For the last two centuries, diagnostic pathologists have used histopathology as the cardinal diagnostic tool, and we rely on pathologic examination to establish the nature of a tumor. In most instances the histotypic classification of a neoplasm is one of the most important determinants of therapy and prognosis. Determining a precise date for the crystallization of the field known as *molecular diagnostics of cancer* is difficult but, since the mid-1980s, an increasing number of publications have reported on the diagnosis of cancer by molecular means. Not surprisingly, molecular oncology—the study of the causes and mechanism of cancer at the molecular level—found the principles it uncovered being rapidly translated to the science of diagnostics.

The first technologic advance that affected molecular diagnostics was the polymerase chain reaction (PCR). After its appearance, pathologic diagnosis, an endeavor essentially based on morphology, shifted to an integrative activity, merging the progress in molecular oncology and advanced tissue analysis with conventional morphology. More recently, advances in high-throughput technologies make it plausible to reduce to practice the molecular fingerprinting of tumors. We now have a new way to diagnose and classify malignancy. These comprehensive approaches at the molecular level hold great promise, because they reveal not only the basic mechanisms underlying the biological behavior of tumors but also potential therapeutic targets. Correlative knowledge becomes knowledge based on the causal mechanisms.

In this chapter, we review some of the salient technologies that are changing the field of molecular diagnostics of cancer. We also look at their current uses and predict some future applications.

SAMPLING OF HUMAN TISSUES FOR MOLECULAR ANALYSES: PROCURING TISSUE THROUGH MICRODISSECTION

The surgical pathologist must "think molecularly" to ensure that tissue is handled in a way that will not jeopardize morphologic evaluation and at the same time will allow for the use of molecular technologies. In practice, it is usually possible to divide the material for conventional processing without compromising the procurement of frozen tissue or cells for comprehensive analysis. In an effort to render histopathologic processing of tissue compatible with advanced diagnostics, a number of fixatives have been tested and, in some laboratories, ethanol-based fixatives have replaced 4% formaldehyde solution.

When macroscopic division of tissue is not possible, microdissection of tissue sections or cell preparations can procure the necessary material for analysis. Microdissection can be performed manually or by the use of micromanipulation devices and can be enabled through microscopes and laser technology. Laser capture microdissection[1] and laser microbeam systems[2] are designed to identify and physically isolate microscopic regions in a tissue section. After capture, the targeted region can be processed for nucleic acid extraction or proteomic analysis.[3] Microdissection can be navigated by capturing tissue from immunostained sections so that cells or regions of the tumor can be selected on the basis of a phenotypic marker that identifies a specific subpopulation of cells. This methodology, when executed on frozen sections, allows for the analysis of gene expression using array technology.[4] A major contribution of microdissection is the avoidance of contamination of tumor samples by stromal elements. Conversely, the host stromal reaction can be analyzed at the molecular level, and the characteristics of immune cells surrounding the edge of the tumor can be determined by purifying these cells from the rest of the tissue. Microdissection is crucial in the evaluation of preneoplastic lesions such as dysplasia and carcinoma in situ. Because gross identification of these alterations is difficult, one must rely on microscopical definition to capture a representative cell population that can be studied with comprehensive approaches. It has been suggested that exhaustive histologic navigation of the microprocurement of tissue will produce the most informative sets of gene expression data.[5] Microdissection also allows for detailed analysis of tumor microheterogeneity. Subclones emerging in tumors can be genetically defined and their geographic extension mapped with accuracy (Fig. 2.1; see color plates, p. 24). It is possible to foresee the day when analysis of tumor heterogeneity will determine the presence of a subpopulation of resistant cells, and therapy will be modulated accordingly.

Unbiased amplification technologies that globally amplify nucleic acids are essential for the analysis of microdissected specimens or the study of low numbers of cells obtained by fine-needle aspiration or brushing of mucosae. Whole-genome amplification and random primed PCR reactions have been used successfully to obtain material representative of the genome or of the transcriptome.[6] With the advent of these techniques, it can be anticipated that microdissection will become routinely used in diagnostics. For instance, current trends in the diagnosis and management of breast cancer yield smaller tumors and, in many instances, dividing the biopsy specimen is difficult. The malignant lesions (e.g., invasive carcinoma) are so small that tumor cells can be procured only through microscope-guided dissection. An added advantage of microdissection is that DNA amplification products can be sequenced directly, as they are likely to be free of contamination by normal tissue. It seems very likely that specialized diagnostic chips (e.g., lymphochips) will be directly coupled to the amplificand products derived from samples procured by microdissection and that diagnosis, classification, and selection of therapies will be achieved efficiently and prognosis improved.

TISSUE MICROARRAYS: SPEEDING UP THE VALIDATION OF DISCOVERIES

Tissue microarray is a new high-throughput method that permits the study of a large number of tumor samples in a unique test or assay.[7] Typically, 1000 disc-shaped histologic sections of tissue, 0.6 mm in diameter, are arrayed on a slide (Fig. 2.2; see color plates, p. 24). This is achieved by cutting histologic sections from a master array block that will yield, on average, 200–300 sections. The master array block is constructed by housing core biopsies obtained from conventional tissue blocks in the receptacle silos of the recipient master array block. This ingenious technology has two advantages: First, obtaining a biopsy of the donor block preserves the diagnostic value of the original specimen. Second, the tissue in the original block is greatly amplified, as three cores will yield 600 discs that can be analyzed. Any morphologic treatment applied to paraffin-embedded tissue can be used in tissue microarrays, including immunohistochemistry, fluorescent in situ hybridization (FISH), in situ hybridization with DNA and RNA probes, and terminal deoxy transferase nick end-labeling. The ability to subject 1000 tissue samples to simultaneous analysis under the same conditions facilitates reproducibility and saves reagent costs. When properly annotated cases are used to construct a tissue microarray, an invaluable reagent is generated. The cohort of cases arrayed may be ideally suited to generate data on the prognostic value of a novel biomarker or to determine its prevalence among different tumor types, provided that the array contains the most common 200 histologic tumor types. Even when the characteristics of tumors are highly heterogeneous, it has been suggested that three samples of a donor block will yield representative data.[8] The cumulative experience of the published studies to date strongly suggests that tissue microarrays will expedite the discovery and validation of tumor markers. Inasmuch as they accelerate the validation of new diagnostic reagents and speed up their characterization, tissue microarrays have a significant impact on the generation of individual diagnostic tests. For example, tissue microarrays are an efficient way to test and validate the value of new antibodies recognizing posttranslational modifications of proteins.[9-13]

STRUCTURAL GENETIC ALTERATIONS FOUND IN TUMOR DNA

Malignant tumors are caused by genetic disturbances of the somatic cells. Hence, not surprisingly, a major focus of cancer research in the recent past has been uncovering genetic defects in tumors. A variety of techniques have been applied to the study of the structural genomic alterations found in tumor cells or tumor tissue (Table 2.1). Among the more traditional techniques, cytogenetics and FISH are routinely applied to diagnostic questions. Whereas cytogenetics, including spectral karyotypic analysis,[14] requires the culture of tumor cells to generate metaphases, FISH has the advantage of probing cells in all phases of the cell cycle and can be carried out either in cytologic preparations or in tissue sections. It has been used successfully in pathology for the study of gene translocations, deletions, and amplifications. The results obtained by FISH in the case of Her2neu amplification in breast cancer correlate well with the levels of expression of the Her2neu protein estimated by immunohistochemistry.[15]

The introduction of microarray technology, based on the capacity of complementary DNA strands to hybridize when one of them is immobilized by tethering to a solid support, has revolutionized the study of genomics. The miniaturization, fidelity of the hybridization, and resolution of the detection systems have made possible the high-throughput analysis of thousands of genetic alterations in a single experiment.[16,17] Two approaches have been taken to the manufacture of DNA arrays: One uses robots to spot complementary DNA (cDNA) clones on a surface such as nylon or, more commonly, glass. The alternative method synthesizes oligonucleotides in situ using complex masks and photolithographic techniques. These two approaches differ in the length of the DNA: Spotting uses relatively large nucleic acid components, longer than 100 nucleotides, and the arrays so constructed often are designed for gene expression analysis. The shorter

TABLE 2.1 Diagnostic Methods by Which to Analyze Structural DNA Alterations

Approach	Nature of Alteration	Level of Alteration	Alteration Detected	High Throughput
DNA content	Structural and numeric	Genome	Ploidy, clonality	No
Flow cytometry	Numeric	Genome		No
Cytogenetics (G binding)	Structural and numeric	Chromosomes	Translocation, deletion, inversion, amplification	No
Spectral karyotyping (SKY)	Structural and numeric	Chromosomes, subchromosomal	Translocation, deletion, inversion, amplification	No
Comparative genomic hybridization (CGH)	Numeric	Chromosomes, subchromosomal	Deletion, amplification	No
Array CGH	Numeric	Genes	Deletion, amplification	Yes
Fluorescent in situ hybridization (FISH)	Structural and numeric	Genes	Translocation, deletion, amplification, ring chromosome	No
Southern blot	Structural and numeric	Genes	Clonality, mutation, translocation	No
LOH	Structural	Genes	Losses	No
AP-PCR	Structural	Genes	MIS	Yes
Array sequencing	Structural	Nucleotides	Point mutation, deletion	Yes

AP-PCR, arbitrary primed–polymerase chain reaction; LOH, loss of heterozygosity.

nucleic acids synthesized in situ are well suited for sequencing but also are efficient in RNA expression experiments. A recently devised variety of arrays uses short sequences of oligonucleotides, each specifying a different mutated sequence of a gene, to analyze genomic alterations. Using this method, Wen et al[18] detected alterations in the p53 gene in a series of ovarian tumors and compared the results with those obtained by conventional DNA sequence analysis. This oligoarray approach yielded a 92% sensitivity and a 100% specificity with a 94% accuracy rate, whereas the conventional DNA sequence analysis showed an 82% sensitivity and a 100% specificity with an 87% assurance rate.[18] Thus, the high-throughput approach matched the efficiency of the slower and more labor-intensive methodology.

DNA microarrays are a powerful tool for detecting point mutations within a gene, but they have not been adequately efficient to detect the deletions, insertions, or frameshift mutations that occur in the context of a short repeated sequence or in relation to inactivated tumor suppressor genes. The introduction of new polymerases in the PCR step and of ligases to enable PCR–ligase detection reactions (PCR/LDR) and the use of generic "zip-code" arrays to identify the product of the PCR/LDR add significantly to DNA microarray technology. An advantage of the zip-code arrays is that array construction is generic (i.e., one array can be used to study many genes) and that they can be adapted to the simultaneous detection of different point mutations in a single gene (Fig. 2.3; see color plates, p. 24). In multiplex mode, zip arrays are capable of detecting a mutated allele present as a minor constituent of a mixture of alleles (see Fig. 2.3). The same strategy can be used to create a universal DNA microarray capable of detecting with a high sensitivity insertions and deletions in repeat sequences and in a background of normal DNA.[19] Favis et al[20,21] have detected mutations in *K-ras*, *BRCA1*, *BRCA2*, and *p53* by applying that method successfully in a large population of tumors. A limitation of oligonucleotide microarrays has been decreased sensitivity owing to the presence of short repetitive sequences that are susceptible to mutation through DNA polymerase slippage. Although still unresolved, evidence suggests that this barrier can be surmounted.[22]

DNA arrays of bacterial artificial chromosomes (BACs) or yeast artificial chromosomes can be used as a substrate for comparative genomic hybridization experiments. This is a powerful approach because recurring structural alterations such as amplification of deletions are detected throughout the genome. Arrays of oligonucleotides can also be used for comparative genomic hybridization (array comparative genomic hybridization) and constitute a powerful way to look for structural alterations at the gene or subgene level.[23]

FUNCTIONAL ALTERATIONS: RNA EXPRESSION STUDIES

Gaining a comprehensive picture of molecular alterations underlying the malignant behavior of tumors requires the characterization of changes in the expression of the entire set of genes active in a given cell type. Ultimately, the phenotypic diversity of tumor cells is caused by variation in the patterns of gene expression. Definition of the myriad changes in expression caused by the more limited set of structural alterations found in tumors is likely to change the classification of cancer and may identify therapeutic targets for chemical intervention. In addition, defining discrete subsets of gene expression patterns within a morphologically defined tumor category may provide the key to prognosticating the behavior of the tumor and predicting its response to existing therapeutic regimens.

A number of technical advances in the last 10 years, including differential display, nucleic acid subtraction, serial analysis of gene expression, and expression microarrays, have made possible the comprehensive study of gene expression patterns in different cell and tumor types. A powerful technology is based on the use of arrayed cDNA libraries or oligonucleotides that hybridize to a mixture of differentially labeled test and reference RNAs.[24–26] This approach enables quantitative gene expression analysis with high sensitivity and specificity and yields large data sets that can be processed using different bioinformatic tools. Expression arrays can determine the gene expression patterns present in one sample by using a standard reference set of messenger RNAs or can compare two different samples (e.g., tumor vs normal). The test sample is amplified and labeled with a green fluorescent dye, and the reference is amplified and labeled with a red fluorochrome; the two labeled products are mixed and hybridized in the same array (Fig. 2.4; see color plates, p. 24). The comparison of the fluorescence of the two signals is relative to the abundance of the gene expressed in each specific sample. Because thousands of genes can be analyzed in a single array experiment, one can easily envision how this technology can radically transform tissue analysis.

One of the consequences of the application of cDNA microarrays has been the further characterization of some of the anonymous expressed sequence tags (ESTs). Changes in the expression levels of these unidentified genes in known samples can contribute greatly to our understanding of their function. The ESTs deposited in public databases represent 50%–90% of all human genes. The data are growing and recently, through the Cancer Genome Anatomy Project, these sequences have been deposited in the dbEST (http://www.ncbi.nlm.nih.gov/dbEST/index.html), a division of GenBank, in which an automated process called *UniGene* compares ESTs and assembles overlapping sequences into clusters in a manner similar to shotgun sequencing projects (http://www.ncbi.nlm.nih.gov/UniGene/index.html).

The application of high-density synthetic oligonucleotide arrays follows the same principles that are applied to cDNA arrays. Because of the smaller size of the oligonucleotides, more than 40,000 genes can be interrogated on a surface measuring 1.28 × 1.28 cm, and experimental versions of this approach are capable of displaying 1 million probes per array. It seems reasonable to predict that in the near future, the level of expression of the entire genome may be examined in a single experiment.[27] New methods that enhance fluorescence, such as rolling-circle amplification, are likely to improve the sensitivity and discriminating power of microarray hybridization (see also Chapter 4, this volume).[28]

PROTEINS: FROM MONOCLONAL ANTIBODIES TO PROTEOMICS

Immunohistochemical (IHC) methods, now largely integrated in the routine of diagnostic laboratories, are based on the recognition of cellular antigens, often using monoclonal antibodies enhanced by a variety of strategies designed to amplify the detection of bound antibody molecules. Although limited to the simultaneous demonstration of two antigens in a single histologic section, IHC has brought great advances to the diagnosis and classification of tumors through the recognition of specific cellular differentiation proteins. Not usually regarded as molecular tools by most users, antibodies are nevertheless capable of probing molecular structure in great detail. For example, antibodies against the C- and N-terminal regions of the nucleophosmin (*NPM*) gene recognize chimeric fusion proteins distinct from the nucleophosmin–anaplastic lymphoma kinase (*NPM/ALK*) gene in a subgroup of anaplastic large-cell lymphomas.[29] Antibodies also can probe functionally significant posttranslational modifications of protein molecules. Antibodies to the phosphorylated cytoplasmic domain of the Her2neu receptor are likely to reflect the amount of functional receptor better than do antibodies that do not discriminate between the active (phosphorylated) and inactive forms of the receptor.[30] The somewhat limited capacity to study tissues by using batteries of monoclonal antibodies applied to consecutive sections is likely to be replaced by high-throughput proteomics. *Proteomics* is the comprehensive analysis of the proteins present in a cell or tissue type and thus represents gene expression analysis at the protein level. Following the complete sequencing of the human genome, attention is focusing on gaining information on the complete set of proteins expressed in a particular cell type or in a particular functional state of a cell. Posttranscriptional mechanisms that control the rate of protein synthesis and the half-life of proteins make measurement of protein expression central to the analysis of biological processes and the understanding of disease.

Traditionally, the comprehensive technique applied to protein analysis has been two-dimensional gel electrophoresis followed by tryptic digestion of the spots of interest and sequencing by biophysical methods. This approach contributes to the study of disease pathogenesis,[31] but systematic technical studies carried out on yeast protein preparations indicate that the present standard approaches can detect and identify only abundant proteins. More refined methods will be needed to detect and quantify accurately regulatory proteins that are, as a rule, expressed in low abundance. Recently, methods other than two-dimensional gel electrophoresis have been proposed as front ends for mass spectrometry (MS) and matrix-assisted laser desorption ionization–time of flight (MALDI-TOF) instruments. Specially coated surfaces can be prepared to bind subsets of proteins that then are analyzed by MALDI-TOF. The proteins of interest can be captured on a chip array directly from the biological source. After washing, the proteins retained on the chip are characterized by MALDI/MS. Protein profiles obtained from different cell types can be compared and may serve as specific signatures for a given functional state. Antibodies can be arranged on the surface of a silicon chip as probes to recognize antigens of native and posttranslationally modified proteins. Libraries of antibodies can be generated by phage display and spotted on glass substrate and the bound proteins recognized by sandwich approaches.[32,33] Signal amplification strategies such as immuno-rolling-circle amplification are likely to play a role in making protein chips a reality.[34]

SELECTED APPLICATIONS OF MOLECULAR MARKERS: DIAGNOSTIC MOLECULAR PATHOLOGY

This section provides some examples of the ways in which recently acquired knowledge and the most novel technologies are being applied to the diagnosis of cancer. The progressive discovery of a series of fusion genes created by the translocations characteristic of specific types of neoplasm has provided diagnosticians with specific tumor markers. Whether detected by cytogenetics or IHC, the demonstration of specific genetic lesions has begun to remodel tumor nosology, as illustrated in the following examples: Ewing sarcoma and peripheral neuroectodermal tumors are members of the same entity as a reflection of a spectrum of neural differentiation.[35] The "ALKomas" are now recognized as a separate entity within the heterogeneous group of anaplastic large-cell lymphomas, based on the presence of the fusion gene NPM-ALK.[36] Congenital fibrosarcoma and mesoblastic nephroma represent different sites of the same tumor caused by the *ETV6-NTRK3* gene fusion product.[37] Classification of liposarcomas by the presence of translocation t(12;16)(q13:p11) has permitted the grouping of round cell and myxoid variants as types distinct from pleomorphic and well-differentiated variants.[38]

Proof of the concept that global expression analysis of tumors is a promising tool for the classification of tumors has been obtained for leukemia, lymphoma, and breast carcinoma.[39–41] Golub et al[39] and others[40,41] provide evidence that class discovery and class prediction, two different tasks, can be accomplished by algorithms applied to comprehensive expression analysis data sets. A discovery procedure automatically identified the criteria to discriminate between acute myeloid leukemia and acute lymphoblastic leukemia. These results were the first to show the feasibility of cancer classification based on gene expression patterns. Perhaps the most remarkable aspect is that the algorithms analyzing the gene expression data generated the correct solution independent of biological knowledge. The practical utility of this approach has been elegantly demonstrated for diffuse large-cell lymphomas. Attempts to define subgroups on the basis of morphology and IHC have failed, as have attempts to predict the response to therapy in a population of patients in which fewer than half are cured. The

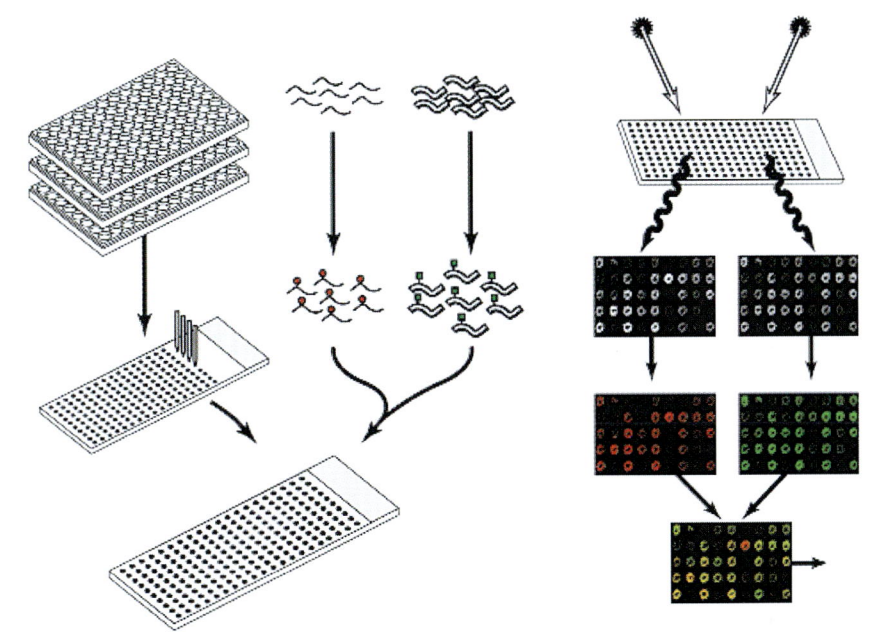

FIGURE 1.1 cDNA microarray printing and analysis. cDNA probes are amplified by polymerase chain reaction and, subsequently, are robotically immobilized at distinct, spatially addressable regions on a solid support. Parallel RNA from normal and tumor cell populations is isolated, purified, and fluorescently cy-3- and cy-5-labeled. The array then is allowed to hybridize with labeled RNA and is analyzed by exciting the array at the appropriate wavelengths. The raw data present as monochromatic images that represent the signal intensity of the appropriate channel. To visualize messenger RNA abundance, a false color (cy-5, red; cy-3, green) will be applied to the monochromatic images, and the arrays will be overlaid to visualize changes in gene expressions. (Adapted from reference 11.)

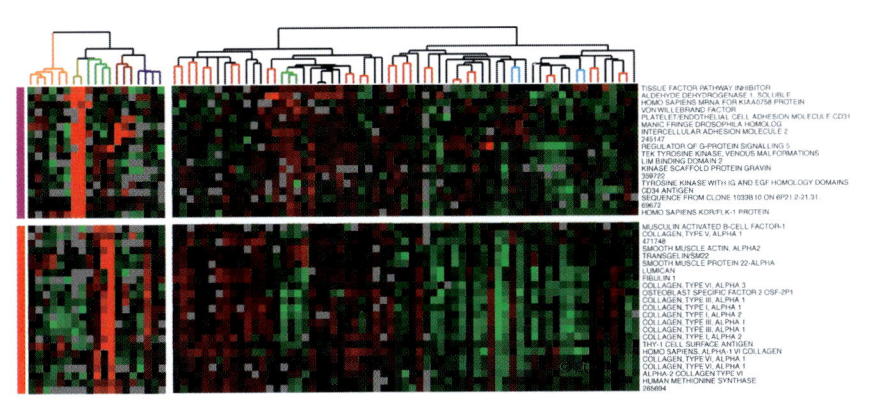

FIGURE 1.2 Example of a gene expression matrix. Forty-two individual samples were hybridized on an array that contained 8102 human genes. The image presented in this figure shows a small section of the gene expression matrix. In this case, each row represents a different gene, whereas each column represents an independent sample. RNA abundance is presented by a color code: Red squares indicate abundance levels that are above the median, whereas green squares indicate an abundance below the median. (Adapted from reference 43.)

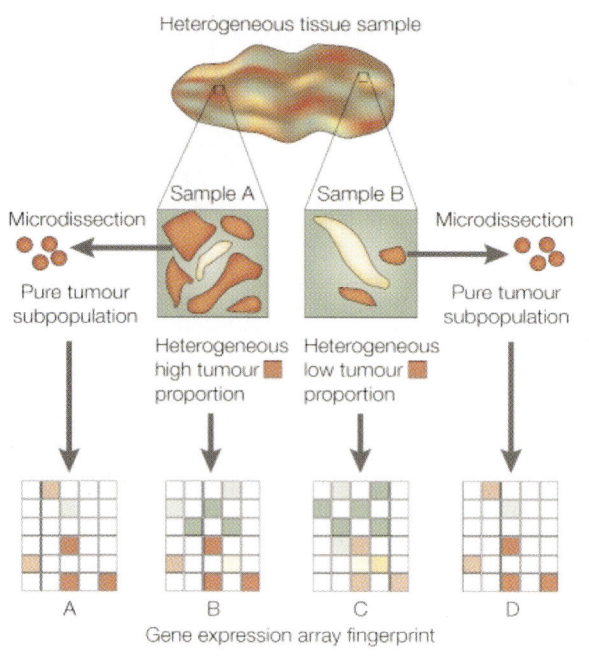

FIGURE 1.3
Global gene analysis vs. microdissection-based gene analysis. If gene profiles are performed on crude specimens (samples A and B; arrays B and C), the different proportion of genes derived from the respective tissue subpopulations will be reflected. First microdissecting the subpopulation of interest will enrich the cell population of interest, which in turn yields a profile specific for the chosen population (arrays A and D). (Adapted from reference 71.)

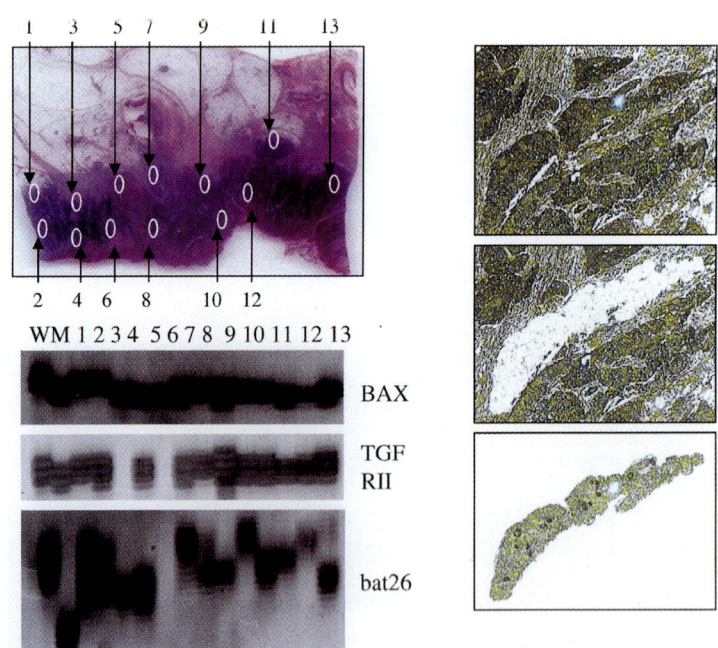

FIGURE 2.1 Analysis of tumor heterogeneity by microdissection. Areas of a tumor section can be targeted (*left upper panel*) and groups of approximately 200 cells can be captured (*right panel*) and analyzed for genetic heterogeneity using microsatellite sequences (as shown in the *left lower panels*).

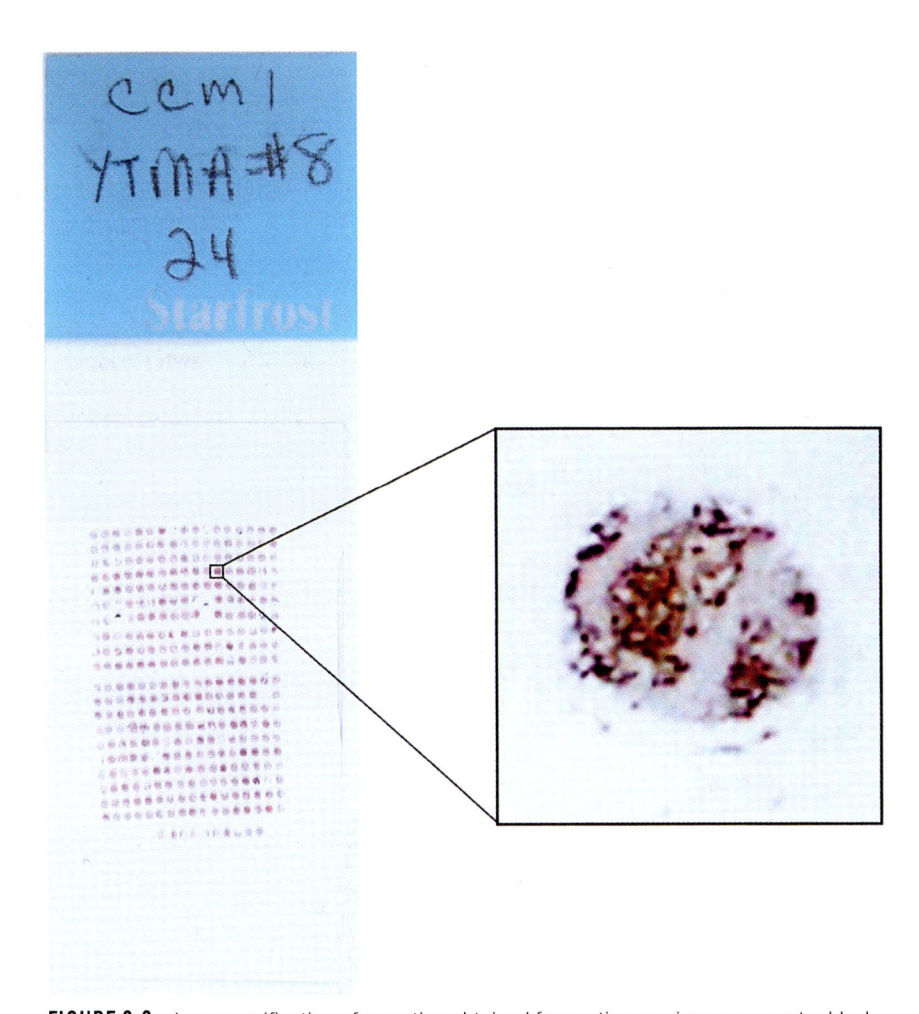

FIGURE 2.2 Low magnification of a section obtained from a tissue microarray master block. Each tissue disc corresponds to an individual case. The cohort assembled on the array can be examined by immunohistochemistry, as shown in the magnified disc (cytokeratin stain ×20).

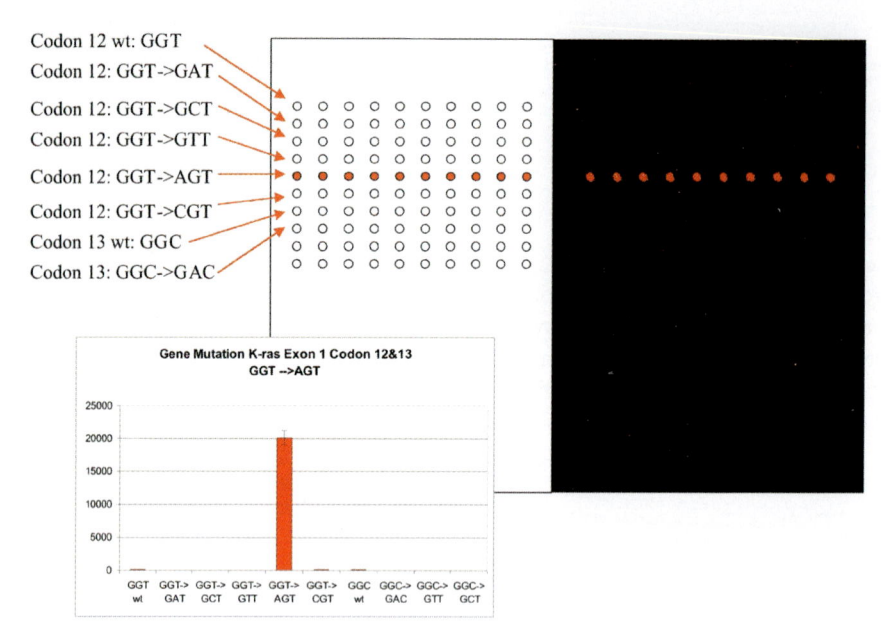

FIGURE 2.3 A genetic zip-code array designed to detect common mutations in the *K-ras* gene. The specific zip-code addresses arrayed on a glass slide as indicated on the *upper left panel*. Hybridization of the polymerase chain reaction/ligase reaction product reveals a single mutation (*upper right panel*) with little or no signal at the addresses specific for other mutations (*left lower panel*).

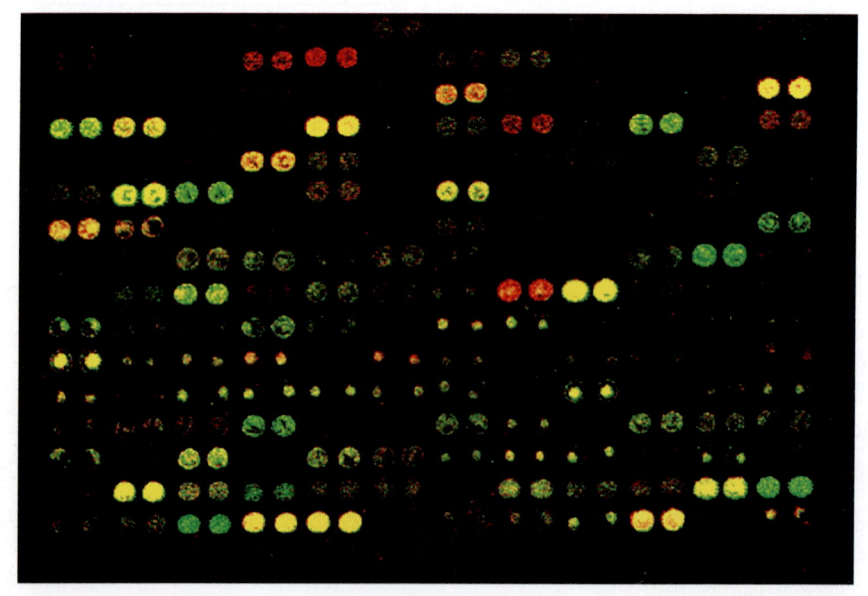

FIGURE 2.4 Expression microarray comparing the gene expression patterns in two related breast cancer cell lines. Red signal indicates overexpression; yellow, equally expressed in both cell lines; and green, loss of expression.

experiments carried out by the Stanford and National Institutes of Health groups use a specially constructed "lymphochip."

To construct this specialized chip, 12,069 of the 17,856 clones in the array were chosen from a germinal center B library. The results demonstrate that diffuse large-cell B-cell lymphoma is composed of two subgroups that can be distinguished from each other by the expression pattern of hundreds of genes and suggest that the two groups correspond to two separate stages of physiologic B-cell differentiation and activation. Most remarkably, the taxonomy created by gene expression analysis defines two prognostically relevant groups that are not identified by the International Prognostic Indicator.[40] Gene expression patterns have also proven apt to the profiling of breast tumors, a complex tumor type with notoriously wide variation in biological behavior.[41] By analyzing two sequential samples in 20 patients, Perou et al[41] have been able to define an "intrinsic" set of genes that define the individuality of each tumor. This set also defined a higher-order relationship between different tumors and indicated the existence of four previously unrecognized distinct tumor types. Bittner et al[42] have applied the same general strategy to melanoma and identified a distinctive subtype of tumor. Clinical application of comprehensive expression analysis will require attention to issues such as reproducibility of results. The use of at least three replicates in experiments analyzing a single specimen has been recommended.[43]

The identification of mutations in primary tumor tissue is facilitated by the use of microarrays designed to investigate hot regions of a gene. Although not infallible, this type of assay will make possible the study of large series of lesions as compared to manual sequencing.[44] The possibility of combining amplification of multiple probes, in a multiplex reaction, with the detection of products by PCR/LDR and generic zip-code arrays constitutes another promising avenue for the genotyping of tumors. The generic zip-code array is a good tool for identifying point mutations in samples containing a low proportion of mutated cells, and so this high-throughput technology might eventually play a role in screening populations at high risk for developing a specific type of tumor. For example, in a population at high risk for colorectal cancer, the detection in the stool of mutations in the *ras* and *p53* genes can be an alternative to colonoscopy. The detection of gene mutations with high sensitivity using single-strand conformation polymorphism analysis has proven useful in the study of samples obtained by fine-needle aspiration. The detection of *K-ras* gene mutations in cytologic samples from the pancreaticobiliary tract is an effective adjunct in the diagnosis of pancreatic cancer. It is most valuable when the morphology is inconclusive and results in a test with a 55% sensitivity, 97% specificity, and 96% positive predictive value for the presence of carcinoma.[45] The design of high-throughput zip-code type arrays will greatly enhance this diagnostic approach. When a point mutation constitutes a quasi-specific tumor marker, the ability to find the needle in the haystack is central to the detection of minimal residual disease. Given the very rapid progress in many technologies, it appears safe to predict that molecular staging and grading will become the standard of practice in the near future. Indeed, evidence indicates that the introduction of molecular diagnostics for the small round cell tumors of children has significantly improved patient management and prognosis.[46]

CONCLUSION

The practice of advanced molecular diagnostics will depend on informatics. Analysis of the large data sets generated by microarray experiments requires computational resources that have, in part, been developed as a response to the need to interpret the data generated by biologists and physicians using the new discovery tools.[47,48] Whereas in the past the function of a gene was explored from the vantage point of a hypothesis, today it is possible to let the very large data sets reveal systemic relationships that can be uncovered and seen only through the proper bioinformatic lenses. Considerable challenges remain in the theoretic domain of computational biology as well as in the domain of the clinical application of high-throughput techniques. Even in the realm of research, no consensus has been reached regarding the ways to compare results obtained by different technologies or to communicate and publish results and use public database systems. These problems will be even more daunting when the diagnostic technologies reviewed are applied in the clinic.

The prospect of coupling specific molecular therapies to molecular tumor profiles undoubtedly will fuel clinical investigation and, eventually, will lead to the reduction of the practice of diagnostics to that based on high-throughput comprehensive technologies. New informatic tools will be needed to manage the vast amount of molecular information concerning the tissue biopsy of a patient and perhaps his or her genotype and to integrate it in a staging and grading system. It is hoped that these integrated data sets will result in a specific patient-tailored treatment recommendation and in an improved prognosis and prediction of the patient's response to therapy.

REFERENCES

1. Emmert-Buck MR, Bonner RF, Smith PD et al. Laser capture microdissection. Science 1996;274: 998–1001.
2. Bohm M, Wieland I, Schutze K, Rubben H. Microbeam MOMeNT: non-contact laser microdissection of membrane-mounted native tissue. Am J Pathol 1997;151:63–67.
3. Ohyama H, Zhang X, Kohno Y et al. Laser capture microdissection generated target sample for high density oligonucleotide array hybridization. Biotechniques 2000;29:530–536.
4. Fend F, Emmert-Buck MR, Chuaqui R et al. Immuno-LCM: laser capture microdissection of immunostained frozen sections for mRNA analysis. Am J Pathol 1999;154:61–66.
5. Cole KA, Krizman DB, Emmert-Buck MR. The genetics of cancer—a 3D model. Nat Genet 1999; 21[Suppl 1]:38–41.

6. Trenkle T, Welsh J, Jung B, Mathieu-Daude F, McClelland M. Non-stoichiometric reduced complexity probes for cDNA arrays. Nucleic Acids Res 1998;26:3883–3891.
7. Kononen J, Bubendorf L, Kallioniemi A et al. Tissue microarrays for high-throughput molecular profiling of tumor specimens. Nat Med 1998;4:844–847.
8. Camp RL, Charette LA, Rimm DL. Validation of tissue microarray technology in breast cancer. Lab Invest 2000;80:1943–1949.
9. Bubendorf L, Kononen J, Koivisto P et al. Survey of gene amplifications during prostate cancer progression by high-throughput fluorescence in situ hybridization on tissue microarrays. Cancer Res 1999;59:803–806.
10. Moch H, Schraml P, Bubendorf L et al. High-throughput tissue microarray analysis to evaluate genes uncovered by cDNA microarray screening in renal cell carcinoma. Am J Pathol 1999;154:981–986.
11. Bubendorf L, Kolmer M, Kononen J et al. Hormone therapy failure in human prostate cancer: analysis by complementary DNA and tissue microarrays. J Natl Cancer Inst 1999;91:1758–1764.
12. Richter J, Wagner U, Kononen J et al. High-throughput tissue microarray analysis of cyclin E gene amplification and overexpression in urinary bladder cancer. Am J Pathol 2000;157:787–794.
13. Schraml P, Konomen J, Budendorf L et al. Tissue microarrays for gene amplification surveys in many different tumor types. Clin Cancer Res 1999;5:1966–1975.
14. Speicher MR, Gwyn Ballard S, Ward DC. Karyotyping human chromosomes by combinatorial multi-fluor FISH. Nat Genet 1996;12;368–375.
15. Couturier J, Vincent-Salomon A, Nicolas A et al. Strong correlation between results of fluorescent in situ hybridization and immunohistochemistry for the assessment of the ERBB2 (HER-2/neu) gene status in breast cancer. Mod Pathol 2000;13:1238–1243.
16. Gray JW, Collins C. Genome changes and gene expression in human solid tumors. Carcinogenesis 2000;21;443–452.
17. Epstein CB, Butow RA. Microarray technology-enhanced versatility, persistent challenge. Curr Opin Biotechnol 2000;11:36–41.
18. Wen WH, Bernstein L, Lescallett J et al. Comparison of TP53 mutations identified by oligonucleotide microarray and conventional DNA sequence analysis. Cancer Res 2000;60:2716–2722.
19. Gerry NP, Witowski NE, Day J et al. Universal DNA microarray method for multiplex detection of low abundance point mutations. J Mol Biol 1999;292:251–262.
20. Favis R, Day JP, Gerry NP et al. Universal DNA array detection of small insertions and deletions in BRCA1 and BRCA2. Nat Biotechnol 2000;18:561–564.
21. Favis R, Barany F. Mutation detection in K-ras, BRCA1, BRCA2, and p53 using PCR/LDR and a universal DNA microarray. Ann N Y Acad Sci 2000;906:39–43.
22. Hacia JG, Edgemon K, Fang N et al. Oligonucleotide microarray based detection of repetitive sequence changes. Hum Mutat 2000;16:354–363.
23. Pollack JR, Perou CM, Alizadeh AA et al. Genome-wide analysis of DNA copy-number changes using cDNA microarrays. Nat Genet 1999;23:41–46.
24. Khan J, Saal LH, Bittner ML et al. Expression profiling in cancer using cDNA microarrays. Electrophoresis 1999;20:223–229.
25. Duggan DJ, Bittner M, Chen Y et al. Expression profile using cDNA microarrays. Nat Genet 1999;21[suppl 1]:10–14.
26. Brown PO, Botstein D. Exploring the new world of the genome with DNA microarrays. Nat Genet 1999;21[suppl 1]:33–37.
27. Lipshutz RJ, Fodor SPA, Gingeras TR, Lockhart DJ. High density synthetic oligonucleotide arrays. Nat Genet 1999;21[suppl 1]:20–24.

28. Lizardi PM, Huang X, Zhu Z et al. Mutation detection and single-molecule counting using isothermal rolling-circle amplification. Nat Genet 1998;19:225–232.
29. Falini B, Puldorf K, Pucciarini A et al. Lymphomas expressing ALK fusion protein(s) other than NPM-ALK. Blood 1999;10:3509–3515.
30. Thor AD, Liu S, Edgerton S et al. Activation (tyrosine phosphorylation) of ErbB-2 (HER-2/neu): a study of incidence and correlation with outcome in breast cancer. J Clin Oncol 2000;18:3230–3239.
31. Chambers G, Lawrie L, Cash P, Murray GI. Proteomics: a new approach to the study of disease. J Pathol 2000;192:280–288.
32. Borrebaeck CAK. Antibodies in diagnostics—from immunoassays to protein chips. Immunol Today 2000;21:379–382.
33. MacBeath G, Schreiber SL. Printing proteins as microarrays for high-throughput function determination. Science 2000;289:1760–1763.
34. Schweitzer B, Wiltshire S, Lambert J et al. Immunoassays with rolling circle amplification: a versatile platform for ultrasensitive antigen detection. Proc Natl Acad Sci USA 2000;97:10113–10119.
35. De Alava E, Gerald WL. Molecular biology of the Ewing's sarcoma/primitive neuroectodermal tumor family. J Clin Oncol 2000;18:204–213.
36. Drexler HG, Gignac SM, von Wasielewski R et al. Pathobiology of NPM-ALK and variant fusion genes in anaplastic large cell lymphoma and other lymphomas. Leukemia 2000;14:1533–1559.
37. Knezevich SR, Garnett MJ, Pysher TJ et al. ETV6-NTRK3 gene fusions and trisomy 11 establish a histogenetic link between mesoblastic nephroma and congenital fibrosarcoma. Cancer Res 1998;58:5046–5048.
38. Tallini G, Akerman M, Del Cin P et al. Combined morphological and karyotypic study of 28 myxoid liposarcomas. Implications for a revised morphological typing (a report from the CHAMP Group). Am J Surg Pathol 1996;20:1047–1055.
39. Golub TR, Slonim DK, Tamayo P et al. Molecular classification of cancer: class discovery and class prediction by gene expression monitoring. Science 1999;286:531–537.
40. Alizadeh A, Eisen M, Davis R et al. Distinct types of diffuse large B-cell lymphoma identified by gene expression profiling. Nature 2000;403:503–511.
41. Perou CM, et al. Molecular portraits of human breast tumours. Nature 2000;406:747–752.
42. Bittner M, Meltzer P, Chen Y et al. Molecular classification of cutaneous malignant melanoma by gene expression profiling. Nature 2000;406:536–540.
43. Lee MLT, Kuo FC, Whitmore GA, Sklar J. Importance of replication in microarray gene expression studies: statistical methods and evidence from repetitive cDNA hybridizations. Proc Natl Acad Sci USA 2000;97:9834–9839.
44. Ahrendt SA, Halachmi S, Chow JT et al. Rapid p53 sequence analysis in primary lung cancer using an oligonucleotide probe array. Proc Natl Acad Sci USA 1999;96:7382–7387.
45. Dillon DA, Johnson CC, Topazian MD et al. The utility of Ki-ras mutation analysis in the cytologic diagnosis of pancreatobiliary neoplasms. Cancer J 2000;6:294–301.
46. Krushner BH, LaQuaglia MP, Cheung NKV et al. Clinically critical impact of molecular genetic studies in pediatric solid tumors. Med Pediatr Oncol 1999;33:530–535.
47. Boguski MS. Biosequence exegesis. Science 1999;286:453–455.
48. Brazma A, Vilo J. Minireview: gene expression data analysis. FEBS Lett 2000;480:17–24.

Dendritic Cells and Cancer Immunization

Karolina A. Palucka

Jacques Banchereau

Vaccines may constitute the greatest achievement of modern medicine. They have eradicated smallpox and spared countless people from tetanus, measles, and hepatitis. Consequently, the great hope is that they also could contribute to our fight against cancer and that we could create effective cancer vaccines. Vaccines are composed of antigens and adjuvants (i.e., activators of the immune system). Adjuvants play a critical role in determining the quantity and quality of the response to the antigen, and the identification of appropriate adjuvants represents a universal problem in vaccine development. Owing to their unique ability to induce and sustain immune responses, dendritic cells often are called *nature's adjuvants* and, as such, represent an essential component of any vaccination strategy. In fact, a majority of current immunization strategies in cancer—be they peptides, naked DNA, viral vectors, or cytokine-transfected tumor cells—have a common denominator: targeting of dendritic cells. Thus, we might as well focus our attention on developing immunization strategies using dendritic cells as vehicles rather than targeting them randomly. However, as our knowledge of dendritic cell biology increased, investigators became aware of their complexity (e.g., different subsets with different functions). This outcome actually might explain why certain vaccines could not be built using empirical strategies, and it brings about the necessity for their rational manipulation to achieve protective or therapeutic immunity. We discuss dendritic cell biology in the context of immunization against cancer and address the parameters that must be considered to ensure the optimal outcome of dendritic cell–based vaccination protocols.

DENDRITIC CELLS

Discovery and Function

For nearly 20 years after their discovery, dendritic cells had to be isolated from tissues to be studied and, as they represent a minor cell population in all tissues, progress was rather slow.[1] In 1992, culture systems that were identified permitted in vitro generation of large numbers of mouse[2] and human dendritic cells.[3] These milestones allowed considerable progresses in understanding dendritic cell biology.[4-6] Currently, human dendritic cells are generated in vitro (1) from bone marrow progenitors cultured in granulocyte-macrophage colony-stimulating factor (GM-CSF) and tumor necrosis factor and (2) from blood monocytes cultured with GM-CSF and interleukin-4 (IL-4) or IL-13.[5]

Just as lymphocytes are composed of different subsets with specific effector functions (B cells, natural killer cells, and T cells), dendritic cells are composed of distinct subsets with specific regulatory functions. The picture is complicated further as four stages of dendritic cell development have been delineated: (1) bone marrow progenitors; (2) circulating precursor dendritic cells; (3) tissue-residing immature dendritic cells, the main property of which is to capture antigens; and (4) mature dendritic cells, present within secondary lymphoid organs, the main property of which is antigen presentation (Fig. 3.1).[1,4,5] Besides replenishing the pool of tissue-residing immature dendritic cell, circulating dendritic cell precursors play a critical role in the immediate reaction to pathogens and in the shaping of immune response. Indeed, monocytes, the most abundant precursors of myeloid dendritic cells in blood, long have been recognized as initial effectors of lipopolysaccharide-related inflammatory responses. Another circulating precursor population, CD11c−IL-3Rα+ plasmacytoid dendritic cells, recently were shown to be a major source of interferon-α (IFN-α) in response to virus.[7,8] The emerging picture is that of the plasticity of the dendritic cell system revealed by (1) specialization of dendritic cell precursors to respond to different pathogens, virus, or bacteria; and (2) the dual function of these cells at two distinct stages of differentiation, as exemplified by ability of precursor dendritic cell to secrete large amounts of proinflammatory or antiviral cytokines and ability of mature dendritic cell to activate and modulate T-cell responses (discussed later).

Distinct Functions at Different Maturation Stages

Immature dendritic cells capture antigens by several pathways: (1) macropinocytosis; (2) receptor-mediated endocytosis via C-type lectins or Fcγ receptors; (3) phagocytosis of particulate live and nonlive antigens;[4,5] and (4) internalization of heat shock proteins.[9] Captured antigens are directed to endosomal compartments for major histocompatibility complex (MHC) class II loading and subsequent presentation to CD4 T cells.[10,11] In most cells, MHC class I molecules

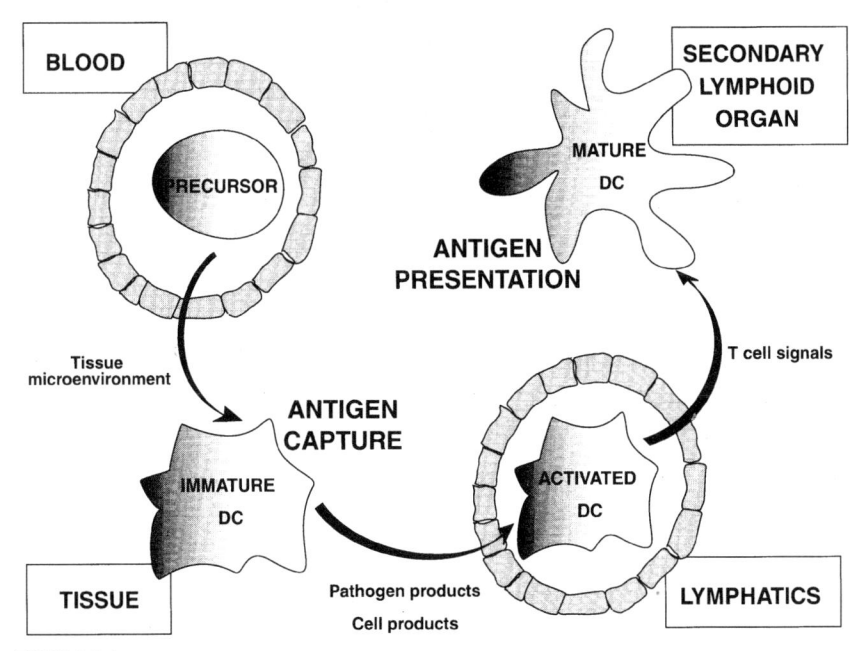

FIGURE 3.1 Dendritic cells (DCs) originate from hematopoietic progenitors. Circulating precursors give rise to immature tissue-residing antigen-capturing DCs. After antigen capture and activation, DCs migrate to lymphoid organs. Mature antigen-presenting DCs display peptide–major histocompatibility complexes and costimulatory molecules, allowing selection, expansion, and differentiation of antigen-specific lymphocytes.

associate only with peptides derived from endogenous proteins but not with peptides from exogenous proteins taken up by the cell. Here again, dendritic cells are unique, as they have evolved a property of loading class I molecules with peptides derived from exogenous antigens. This mechanism, called *cross-presentation* or *cross-priming*, now has been shown to be relevant for presentation of antigens from immune complexes or dying cells.[12–15]

Mature dendritic cells migrate to secondary lymphoid organs, where they present peptide–MHCs to naïve T cells, thereby eliciting primary immune response. The initial contact between dendritic cells and resting T cells seems to be mediated by a transient, high-affinity interaction between specific ICAM-3 grabbing nonintegration (SIGN) molecule on dendritic cells, and intercellular adhesion molecule-3 on T cells[16] and is followed by involvement of other adhesion molecules and their corresponding ligands, (intercellular adhesion molecule-1/leukocyte function–associated antigen-1, leukocyte function–associated antigen-3/CD2). After T-cell receptor engagement, an intimate contact, often called *the immunologic synapse*, evolves where multiple interactions between costimulatory molecules on dendritic cells and their ligands on T cells result in final dendritic cell maturation and T-cell activation.[17] The induced antigen-specific CD4 T cells then orchestrate other effectors of the immune system, including CD8 T cells, B cells, and natural killer cells. However, dendritic cells can present antigens directly to CD8 T cells and can induce proliferation of naïve B cells and their differentiation into plasma cells.[5] Thus, dendritic cells induce a diverse immune response involving multiple effectors of both cellular and humoral immunity.

Subsets

In mice, the concept of dendritic cell subsets came with the description of a dendritic cell subset in the thymus that developed from a population of thymic lymphoid progenitor cells in vivo.[18] As of today, at least three distinct pathways of dendritic cell development are being considered in mice: myeloid dendritic cells, Langerhans cells (LCs), and lymphoid dendritic cells.[19]

In humans, the existence of distinct dendritic cell subsets (Fig. 3.2) came from several directions based on the analyses of (1) skin dendritic cells,[20] (2) dendritic

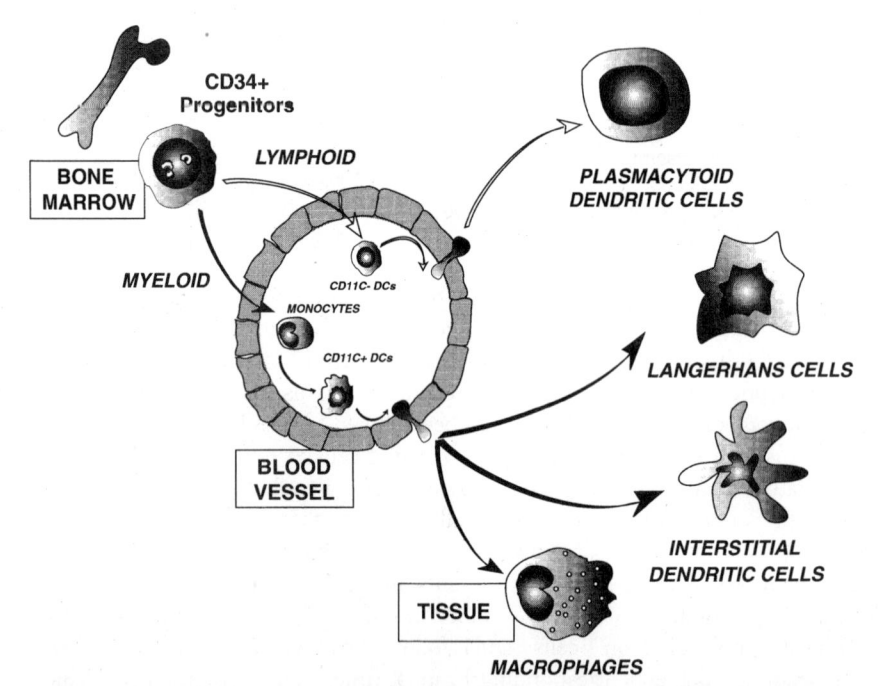

FIGURE 3.2 Dendritic cell (DC) progenitors give rise to myeloid (monocytes and CD11c+ DCs) and lymphoid (CD11c− plasmacytoid DCs) precursors. On interaction with inflamed endothelium, monocytes differentiate into CD11c+ blood DCs, which give rise to Langerhans cells, interstitial DCs, and macrophages. Differentiation of plasmacytoid DCs from CD34+ progenitors[85] can be blocked by Id2 and Id3 overexpression, suggesting their lymphoid origin.[86]

cells generated in vitro by culture of CD34+ hematopoietic progenitors,[21] and (3) blood dendritic cell precursors.[22] Human skin contains two subsets with distinct localization: LCs within the epidermis, characterized by the expression of CD1a and Birbeck granules, and interstitial (dermal) dendritic cells, lacking Birbeck granules but expressing coagulation factor XIIIa. These two subsets also emerge in cultures of CD34+ hematopoietic progenitors driven by GM-CSF and tumor necrosis factor[21] and, most interestingly, these subsets have both common and unique functions.[23] In particular, interstitial dendritic cells, but not LCs, are able to induce the differentiation of naïve B cells into immunoglobulin-secreting plasma cells. Though no unique function has yet been attributed formally to LCs, there are hints that they may be particularly efficient activators of cytotoxic CD8 T cells.

Three subsets of dendritic cell precursors circulate in the blood: CD14+ monocytes, lineage-negative CD11c+ precursor dendritic cell, and CD11c⁻IL-3Ra+ plasmacytoid dendritic cells (see Fig. 3.2).[5,24] Both monocytes and CD11c+ subset can give rise to interstitial dendritic cells, LC, and macrophages.[23,25,26] Plasmacytoid dendritic cells have unique properties, such as the expression of lymphoid antigens,[27] the ability to produce large amounts of type I IFN (as discussed),[7] and the ability to polarize a fraction of the T cells toward IL-4 and IL-5 production (type 2 cells); hence the nomenclature DC2.[28]

Type 1 and Type 2 T Cells Whereas IFN-γ- and IL-2-producing Th1 cells lead to protective antitumor immunity, Th2 cells producing IL-4 and IL-10 may be associated with nonprotective responses.[29] Therefore, understanding of how distinct dendritic cell subsets regulate T-cell polarization is paramount for development of dendritic cell–based cancer vaccines. In mice, the lymphoid dendritic cells induce naïve T cells to produce IFN-γ, thus promoting type 1 responses (Th1) in a process involving IL-12.[30] Myeloid dendritic cells do not produce IL-12 and induce T cells to release IL-4, thus favoring type 2 responses (Th2).[31,32] In humans, the picture is less clear. CD40-ligand-activated monocyte-derived dendritic cells prime Th1 responses via an IL-12-dependent mechanism, whereas IL-3+CD40-ligand-activated plasmacytoid dendritic cells have been shown to secrete negligible amounts of IL-12 and prime Th2 responses.[28] However, the polarizing effects of dendritic cell subsets may be susceptible to microenvironmental signals that could instruct a given dendritic cell subset to elicit different Th responses. Indeed, monocyte-derived dendritic cells can induce T cells to make IL-4, rather than IFN-γ, when (1) the dendritic cells are used at low numbers[33]; (2) the dendritic cells are exposed to such factors as prostaglandin E2, corticosteroids, or IL-10; or (3) on prolonged activation in vitro.[6,34–36] Furthermore, when stimulated by virus, plasmacytoid dendritic cells secrete IFN-α, which drives Th1 responses in humans,[37] and mature into dendritic cells that can induce T cells to produce IFN-γ and IL-10.[8] Thus, both the type of dendritic cell subset and microenvironmental signals are important for Th polarization.

Regulatory T Cells Though Th1 and Th2 cells have been considered as the two extremes of T-cell polarization,[38] other subsets of CD4 T cells with regulatory function have been identified: transforming growth factor-β-producing Th3 cells[39,40] and IL-10-producing Tr1 cells.[41] Regulatory T cells specific for tumor antigens have been found in melanoma.[42,43] Furthermore, repetitive in vitro stimulation with Ag-loaded antigen-presenting cells, immature dendritic cells in particular,[44] can lead to the emergence of regulatory T cells, producing large amounts of IL-4 and IL-10, the supernatant of which can block the activation of fresh T cells. IL-10 also may convert dendritic cell function to the induction of antigen-specific anergy, thus leading to the state of tolerance against tumor tissue.[45,46]

Dendritic Cells and Tumor Immunity

The immune system evolved to protect us from harmful pathogens. This formidable task relies on a concerted action of both antigen-nonspecific innate immunity and antigen-specific adaptive immunity.[47] Those two systems are linked by dendritic cells. The innate system includes phagocytic cells, natural killer cells, complement, and IFNs and is characterized by the ability to recognize pathogen or tissue injury (or both) rapidly and by the ability to signal the presence of "danger" to cells of the adaptive immune system. In turn, the adaptive immunity is characterized by the ability to rearrange genes of the immunoglobulin family, permitting creation of a large diversity of antigen-specific clones, and by immunologic memory. The inflammatory reaction occurring on pathogen invasion—the danger signal[48]—leads to dendritic cell activation, migration, and maturation, culminating in the induction of immunity and pathogen elimination. In this context, tumors are "silent." As they do not provide a danger signal, dendritic cells have no reason to migrate to the lymphoid organs and to initiate an immune response. Furthermore, much like normal tissues, tumors themselves do not provide costimulation and, finally, most of the tumor-associated antigens (TAAs) are derived from self-antigens, expressed for instance during tissue differentiation.[49,50] Hence, the immune system is rendered tolerant to such antigens.

Thus, inducing effective antitumor immunity—as yet an elusive goal—has to be seen as inducing autoimmunity.[51,52] Indeed, although rare, tumor-related autoimmune responses exist and manifest themselves as paraneoplastic neurologic disorders. Discovery of onconeural antigens[53] and the identification of onconeural antibodies led to the proposal that paraneoplastic cerebellar degeneration, associated with breast and ovarian cancer, is an autoimmune disorder mediated by the humoral arm of the immune system. Furthermore, the presence of cdr-2-specific CD8+ cytotoxic T lymphocytes (CTLs) circulating in the blood of these patients has been demonstrated.[54]

Dendritic Cells as Tumor Vaccine

In animal models, dendritic cells loaded with TAA are able to induce protective-rejection antitumor responses.[55-61] A number of ongoing and reported clinical trials have use TAA-loaded dendritic cells as a vaccine in human cancer.[62,63] Some clinical responses have been observed in preliminary trials, including (1) a pioneer study based on injection of blood-derived dendritic cells loaded with lymphoma idiotype[64]; (2) administration of peptide-pulsed antigen-presenting cells generated by culturing monocytes with GM-CSF[65]; (3) vaccination with monocyte-derived dendritic cells loaded with melanoma peptides[66,67]; and (4) vaccination of prostate cancer patients using monocyte-derived dendritic cells pulsed with prostate-specific membrane antigen peptide[68] or blood dendritic cells loaded with recombinant protein consisting of tumor antigen (prostatic acid phosphatase) and GM-CSF.[69] In particular, intranodal injection of immature monocyte-derived dendritic cells pulsed with synthetic melanoma peptides or tumor lysate–induced delayed-type hypersensitivity toward vaccine antigens in 11 patients.[66] Most recent study demonstrates that vaccination with melanoma peptide–loaded mature monocyte-derived dendritic cells leads to substantial immune responses in blood.[67] Our preliminary results demonstrate that vaccinating stage IV melanoma patients with dendritic cells derived from CD34+ hematopoietic progenitors and pulsed with multiple antigens, including keyhole-limpet hemocyanin (KLH) protein, flu-matrix peptide, and melanoma peptides, leads to significant primary and recall immune responses in blood.[70]

PARAMETERS OF DENDRITIC CELL VACCINES

Trials reported to date prove the safety and tolerability of administration of TAA-loaded dendritic cells in cancer patients and substantiate limited clinical responses. Furthermore, dendritic cells loaded with influenza-matrix peptide and KLH have been shown to be safe and immunogenic in healthy volunteers.[71,72] In view of these encouraging results, several parameters, illustrated in Figure 3.3, have to be established. They include: (1) the subset of dendritic cell and the method of generation (ex vivo culture or in vivo mobilization); (2) the dendritic cell dose, route, and frequency of injection; (3) the optimal dendritic cell activation-maturation status; (4) the source and the preparation of both TAA and dendritic cell loading strategy; (5) the combination of dendritic cell vaccination with other therapies (e.g., such biological response modifiers as IL-2 or IFN-α); (6) the evaluation of vaccine efficacy, particularly at these early stages of dendritic cell vaccine development; (7) the determination of vaccine potency (e.g., feasibility of using TAA-specific T-cell lines to determine TAA presentation by loaded dendritic cells in large-scale trials); and finally (8) the duration of vaccination. Two crucial parameters that must be analyzed, preferably in randomized trials, include the nature of the TAA and the optimal methods for dendritic cell loading and the endpoints and determination of vaccine efficacy.

TAA Delivery to Dendritic Cells

Several antigen delivery systems have been employed so far (Table 3.1)[62,72,73]: peptides of known sequences,[57,58] undefined acid-eluted peptides from autologous

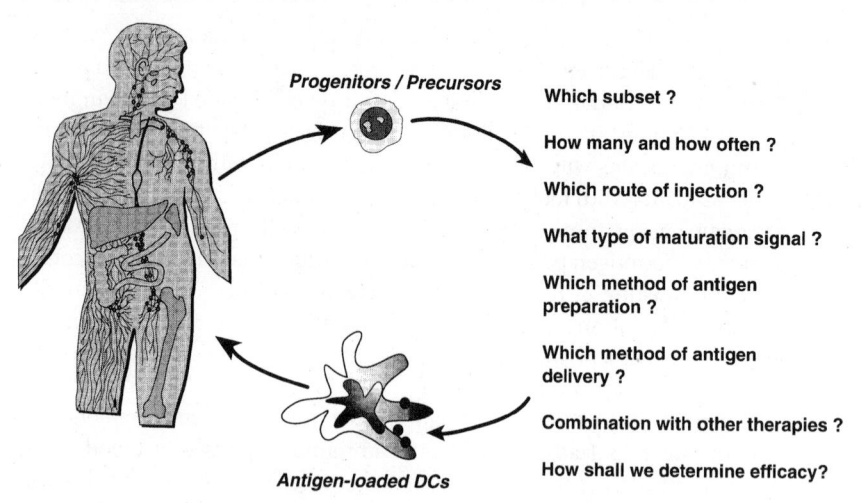

FIGURE 3.3 Ultimate parameters of cancer vaccine are the rate of tumor elimination and the long-term disease-free survival. Early trials show that dendritic cell (DC) administration is safe and leads, under certain conditions, to immune responses and to limited clinical responses. We now need to resolve the remaining questions.

tumor,[74] tumor lysates,[75] viral vectors,[76] tumor cell–derived RNA,[55] fusion of dendritic cells with tumor cells,[77] and tumor peptide pulsed dendritic cell–derived exosomes (subcellular structures containing high levels of MHC molecules and peptides).[78] The approach used most commonly is based on loading of empty MHC class I molecules with exogenous peptides. This is, however, limited by peptide restriction to a given HLA type, induction of CTL responses only, and limitation of the induced responses to defined TAA.[79] In contrast to the peptide-based approach, unfractionated tumor material (killed tumor cells, tumor RNA) may provide both MHC class I and class II epitopes and does not require the identification of TAA.[80] Furthermore, antigen presentation by MHC class I and class II leads to the diversification of immune responses and engages other effectors (as discussed). Recent studies demonstrate that dendritic cells can capture killed tumor cells and can elicit MHC class I–restricted CTL responses against tumor antigens.[12,14,15,54] Such an approach could provide a very attractive strategy for dendritic cell–based vaccination protocols whereby tumor-derived epitopes could be presented without the need for molecular characterization of TAA per se. Tumor death may lead also to the unraveling of subdominant or cryptic epitopes that, when processed and presented by dendritic cells, either may reach the proper activation threshold for memory T-cells or may lead to priming of naïve T cells. In this context, the use of allogeneic tumor cell lines, rather than autologous tumor, eventually will permit the identification of novel-shared TAAs. Tumor-derived antigens may be delivered also to dendritic cells by fusing dendritic cells and tumor cells. An intriguing example is found in a recently published study in metastatic renal cancer, in which, in 4 of 17 patients, vaccination with allogeneic dendritic cell–autologous tumor hybrids led to resolution of all metastatic tumor lesions.[81]

Other strategies include transfer of genetic material either per se (e.g., tumor RNA) or expressed in viral vectors.[73] Indeed, dendritic cells pulsed with tumor-derived RNA elicit tumor-specific CTL responses, thus offering an interesting alternative to ensure responses against unique, patient-specific TAA.[82,83] Several viral vectors encoding model antigens as well as tumor antigens were used in vivo in mice and the results, in terms of tumor rejection, are promising.[76]

Our own studies suggest the importance of using multiple tumor antigens and control antigens.[70] Indeed, of 18 HLA-A*0201+ patients who had metastatic melanoma and were injected subcutaneously with autologous dendritic cells derived from CD34+ progenitors and pulsed with peptides derived from four melanoma antigens (MelanA/MART-1; tyrosinase; MAGE-3; and gp100), influenza matrix peptide, and KLH, two who failed to respond to control antigens did not respond to tumor antigens and experienced rapid tumor progression. Thus, evaluating response to control antigens will not only provide information as to vaccine potency but will help to identify patients who are unlikely to profit from a given vaccine. Furthermore, of 17 patients with evaluable disease, 6 of 7 with immunity to two or fewer melanoma antigens had progressive disease 10 weeks after study entry, in contrast to tumor progression in only 1 of 10 patients with immunity to more than two melanoma antigens. These observations suggest the importance of loading dendritic cells with multiple TAA.

Vaccine Efficacy

Possibly the most difficult problem of immunotherapy protocols is determination of efficacy. Though the ultimate efficacy should be measured by the rate of tumor regression or duration of disease-free survival—or at least time to disease progression—these endpoints require sufficiently long follow-up. Indeed, tumor regression mediated by the immune system may take a long time to manifest itself. Thus, several years of follow-up likely will be necessary to conclude whether a given immunotherapy protocol is improving the clinical outcome. Hence, the search for so-called surrogate markers that would permit early measurements and be predictive of clinical outcome. Until now, in vitro measurements of tumor- or vaccine-specific immune responses have not proven to be helpful surrogate markers.[84] Responses measured in the most easily accessible organ, such as blood, have not shown correlation with the clinical outcome. However, the results of our study suggest that measurement of responses in the blood may constitute a relevant and predictive marker.[70] Indeed, patients with immune response to two or fewer melanoma antigens, measured by IFN-γ enzyme-linked immunospot (ELISPOT) in peripheral blood mononuclear cells, were those who experienced

TABLE 3.1 Various Antigen Delivery Systems

Method	Strengths	Limitations
Peptides	Well-defined antigens that allow precise analysis of elicited tumor immunity	HLA restriction; responses limited to only a few T-cell clones and to defined TAA
Proteins	Well-defined antigens; presentation of MHC class II epitopes and induction of CD4 T-cell responses; patient-specific responses (e.g., idiotype)	Responses limited to known TAA; not yet established whether loading DCs with proteins permits presentation of MHC class I epitopes
Tumor cell preparations: tumor lysate, killed tumor cells, exosomes	Presentation of multiple epitopes, potentially both MHC class I and class II, including both known and unknown antigens; identification of novel TAA	
	Autologous tumor: tailored vaccine, patient-specific epitopes (e.g., point mutations)	*Autologous tumor:* not always available; limited number of shared epitopes; T-cell repertoire may be deleted; true tumor rejection antigens?
	Allogeneic tumor: practically unlimited supply of TAA; pharmacologic-grade antigenic preparations; responses against shared TAA known or unknown; availability of epitopes expressed at various stages of tumor differentiation; large-scale applicability	*Allogeneic tumor:* allosensitization; predominant response against alloantigen at the expense of TAA-specific response

(continued)

TABLE 3.1 Continued

Method	Strengths	Limitations
Live vectors: viral, bacterial	Targeting of DCs in vivo; vector-induced DC maturation	Predominant response against vector and suppression of response to tumor antigens; elimination of TAA-bearing DCs on subsequent immunization; presentation of MHC class II epitopes as yet not optimal
Other vectors: liposomes, pseudoviral particles, toxins	Feasibility of uniform vaccine and large-scale preparations; targeting DCs in vivo	Stability of vehicles; necessity for adjuvants; limited experience with regard to MHC class II presentation
Nucleic acids: DNA, RNA	Practically unlimited supply of TAA; possibility of retrieving TAA from archival pathology material; expression of several TAA both known and unknown; possibility for combined expression of patient-specific (autologous tumor) and shared (allogeneic tumor) TAA; large-scale applicability; possibility to target the antigen to lysosomal compartments	Limited amount of TAA expressed when using DNA; RNA relatively labile; method for RNA amplification may influence immunogenicity

DC, dendritic cell; HLA, human leukocyte antigen; MHC, major histocompatibility complex; TAA, tumor-associated antigens.

early disease progression. The possible explanation for such correlation is that we have used four melanoma antigens, thus avoiding "antigenic escape" of the tumor. Indeed, that the tumor would lose all four antigens is rare. Though preliminary, our observations suggest that evaluation of vaccine-induced immune responses in blood could be a predictive factor for efficacy, thus allowing early conclusions for unsuccessful approaches.

Other Parameters

The remaining issues to be discussed with regard to dendritic cell vaccines include two simple questions: when and how long? It is unlikely that the immune system, even if activated to its best performance, can clear all metastatic tumors in an advanced disease. Therefore, as soon as the safety and tolerability are proven, the trials should move into earlier disease stages and, optimally, to adjuvant setting (e.g., after surgical removal of a major tumor mass), thus in truly residual disease. Only by testing vaccines in the early disease stages will we really be able to conclude as to their clinical efficacy measured by duration of the time to progression or disease-free survival (or both).

Finally, how long shall we continue immunizing patients in whom vaccine induces immune responses and disease stabilization? Matzinger[48] suggested as long as it takes to clear the tumor. Though in full agreement, we would suggest that dendritic cell vaccination, when efficient, should be a lifetime treatment, first therapeutic to clear the tumor and subsequently prophylactic to prevent relapse.

CONCLUSION

Given the fact that the immune system has taken millions of years to evolve efficient pathogen countermeasures, the progress in our efforts to use the immune system to combat cancer is encouraging, even if slow. All three levels of intervention in cancer immunotherapy involve dendritic cells (Fig. 3.4). Everything that we learn from these immunotherapy approaches will permit us in the future to develop an "intelligent missile," a generic cancer vaccine equipped with tumor antigens, chaperons, and dendritic cell activation molecules and with specific ligands that would permit targeting of desired dendritic cell subset. This will keep us busy for a while.

ACKNOWLEDGMENTS

This work was supported by grants from Baylor Health Care Systems Foundation, the Falk Foundation, the Cancer Research Institute, and the National Institutes of Health (CA78846, PO-1 CA84512). We could cite only a fraction of an enormous

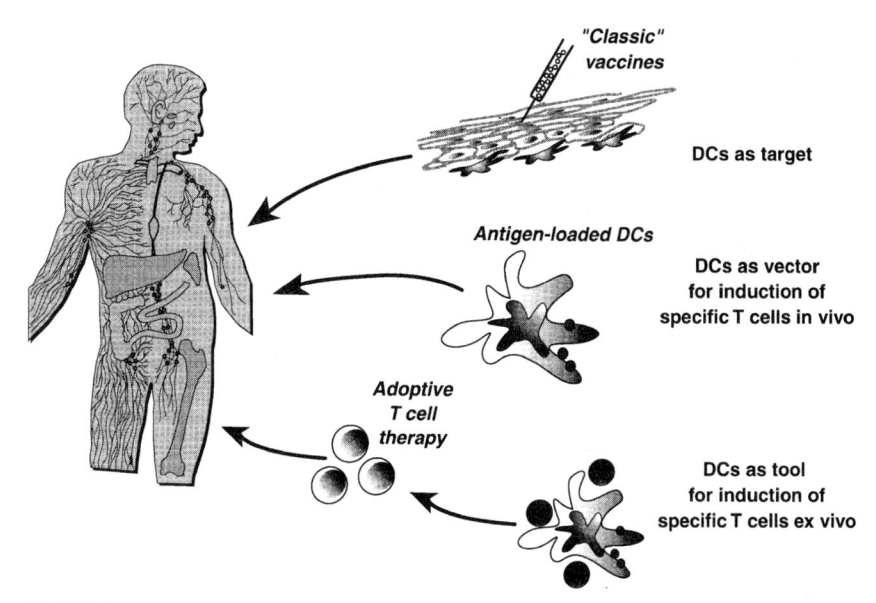

FIGURE 3.4 Three levels of dendritic cell–based immune intervention in cancer: "classic" vaccines that target dendritic cells (DCs) randomly, tumor antigen–bearing DCs as vaccines, and tumor antigen–specific T cells expanded ex vivo by antigen-loaded DCs.

number of studies (more than 10,000 citations in PubMed as of December 2000), all of which contributed to our progress.

REFERENCES

1. Steinman RM. The dendritic cell system and its role in immunogenicity. Annu Rev Immunol 1991;9:271–296.
2. Inaba K, Inaba M, Romani N et al. Generation of large numbers of dendritic cells from mouse bone marrow cultures supplemented with granulocyte/macrophage colony-stimulating factor. J Exp Med 1992;176:1693–1702.
3. Caux C, Dezutter-Dambuyant C, Schmitt D, Banchereau J. GM-CSF and TNF-alpha cooperate in the generation of dendritic Langerhans cells. Nature 1992;360:258–261.
4. Banchereau J, Steinman RM. Dendritic cells and the control of immunity. Nature 1998;392:245–252.
5. Banchereau J, Briere F, Caux C et al. Immunobiology of dendritic cells. Ann Rev Immunol 2000;18:767–812.
6. Lanzavecchia A, Sallusto F. Dynamics of T lymphocyte responses: Intermediates, effectors, and memory cells. Science 2000;290:92–97.
7. Siegal FP, Kadowaki N, Shodell M et al. The nature of the principal type 1 interferon-producing cells in human blood. Science 1999;284:1835–1837.
8. Kadowaki N, Antonenko S, Lau JY, Liu YJ. Natural interferon alpha/beta-producing cells link innate and adaptive immunity. J Exp Med 2000;192:219–226.

9. Srivastava PK, Menoret A, Basu S et al. Heat shock proteins come of age: Primitive functions acquire new roles in an adaptive world. Immunity 1998;8:657–665.
10. Cella M, Engering A, Pinet V et al. Inflammatory stimuli induce accumulation of MHC class II complexes on dendritic cells. Nature 1997;388:782–787.
11. Inaba K, Turley S, Yamaide F et al. Efficient presentation of phagocytosed cellular fragments on the major histocompatibility complex class II products of dendritic cells. J Exp Med 1998;188(11): 2163–2173.
12. Albert ML, Sauter B, Bhardwaj N. Dendritic cells acquire antigen from apoptotic cells and induce class I-restricted CTLs. Nature 1998;392:86–89.
13. Rodriguez A, Regnault A, Kleijmeer M et al. Selective transport of internalized antigens to the cytosol for MHC class I presentation in dendritic cells. Nat Cell Biol 1999;1:362–368.
14. Nouri-Shirazi M, Banchereau J, Bell D et al. Dendritic cells capture killed tumor cells and present their antigens to elicit tumor-specific immune responses. J Immunol 2000;165:3797–3803.
15. Berard F, Blanco P, Davoust J et al. Cross-priming of naive CD8 T cells against melanoma antigens using dendritic cells loaded with killed allogeneic melanoma cells. J Exp Med 2000;192: 1535–1544.
16. Geijtenbeek TB, Torensma R, van Vliet SJ et al. Identification of DC-SIGN, a novel dendritic cell-specific ICAM-3 receptor that supports primary immune responses. Cell 2000;100:575–585.
17. Lanzavecchia A, Sallusto F. From synapses to immunological memory: The role of sustained T cell stimulation. Curr Opin Immunol 2000;12:92–98.
18. Ardavin C, Wu L, Li CL, Shortman K. Thymic dendritic cells and T cells develop simultaneously in the thymus from a common precursor population. Nature 1993;362:761–763.
19. Shortman K. Dendritic cells: Multiple subtypes, multiple origins, multiple functions. Immunol Cell Biol 2000;78:161–165.
20. Cerio R, Griffiths CE, Cooper KD et al. Characterization of factor XIIIa positive dermal dendritic cells in normal and inflamed skin. Br J Dermatol 1989;121:421–431.
21. Caux C, Vandervliet B, Massacrier C et al. CD34+ hematopoietic progenitors from human cord blood differentiate along two independent dendritic cell pathways in response to GM-CSF + TNF alpha. J Exp Med 1996;184:695–706.
22. O'Doherty U, Peng M, Gezelter S et al. Human blood contains two subsets of dendritic cells, one immunologically mature and the other immature. Immunology 1994;82:487–493.
23. Caux C, Massacrier C, Vanbervliet B et al. CD34+ hematopoietic progenitors from human cord blood differentiate along two independent dendritic cell pathways in response to granulocyte-macrophage colony-stimulating factor plus tumor necrosis factor alpha: II. Functional analysis. Blood 1997;90:1458–1470.
24. Pulendran B, Banchereau J, Burkeholder S et al. K. FLT3 ligand and G-CSF mobilize distinct human DC subsets in vivo. J Immunol 2000;165:566–572.
25. Palucka KA, Taquet N, Sanchez-Chapui F, Gluckman JC. Dendritic cells as the terminal stage of monocyte differentiation. J Immunol 1998;160:4587–4595.
26. Ito T, Inaba M, Inaba K et al. CD1a+/CD11c+ subset of human blood dendritic cells is a direct precursor of Langerhans cells. J Immunol 1999;163:1409–1419.
27. Grouard G, Rissoan MC, Filgueira L et al. The enigmatic plasmacytoid T cells develop into dendritic cells with interleukin (IL)-3 and CD40-ligand. J Exp Med 1997;185:1101–1111.
28. Rissoan MC, Soumelis V, Kadowaki N et al. Reciprocal control of T helper cell and dendritic cell differentiation. Science 1999;283:1183–1186.
29. Hu HM, Urba WJ, Fox BA. Gene-modified tumor vaccine with therapeutic potential shifts tumor-specific T cell response from a type 2 to a type 1 cytokine profile. J Immunol 1998;161:3033–3041.

30. Pulendran B, Lingappa J, Kennedy MK et al. Developmental pathways of dendritic cells in vivo: Distinct function, phenotype, and localization of dendritic cell subsets in FLT3 ligand-treated mice. J Immunol 1997;159:2222–2231.
31. Pulendran B, Smith JL, Caspary G et al. Distinct dendritic cell subsets differentially regulate the class of immune response in vivo. Proc Natl Acad Sci USA 1999;96:1036–1041.
32. Maldonado-Lopez R, De Smedt T, Michel P et al. CD8alpha+ and CD8alpha- subclasses of dendritic cells direct the development of distinct T helper cells in vivo. J Exp Med 1999;189:587–592.
33. Tanaka H, Demeure CE, Rubio M et al. Human monocyte-derived dendritic cells induce naive T cell differentiation into T helper cell type 2 (Th2) or Th1/Th2 effectors. Role of stimulator/responder ratio. J Exp Med 2000;192:405–412.
34. Kalinski P, Schuitemaker JH, Hilkens CM et al. Final maturation of dendritic cells is associated with impaired responsiveness to IFN-gamma and to bacterial IL-12 inducers: Decreased ability of mature dendritic cells to produce IL-12 during the interaction with Th cells. J Immunol 1999;162:3231–3236.
35. Vieira PL, de Jong EC, Wierenga EA et al. Development of Th1-inducing capacity in myeloid dendritic cells requires environmental instruction. J Immunol 2000;164:4507–4512.
36. Langenkamp A, Messi M, Lanzavecchia A, Sallusto F. Kinetics of dendritic cell activation: Impact on priming of TH1, TH2 and nonpolarized T cells. Nat Immun 2000;1:311–316.
37. Parronchi P, Mohapatra S, Sampognaro S et al. Effects of interferon-alpha on cytokine profile, T cell receptor repertoire and peptide reactivity of human allergen-specific T cells. Eur J Immunol 1996;26:697–703.
38. Mosmann TR, Coffman RL. TH1 and TH2 cells: Different patterns of lymphokine secretion lead to different functional properties. Annu Rev Immunol 1989;7:145–173.
39. Fukaura H, Kent SC, Pietrusewicz MJ et al. Induction of circulating myelin basic protein and proteolipid protein-specific transforming growth factor-beta$_1$–secreting Th3 T cells by oral administration of myelin in multiple sclerosis patients. J Clin Invest 1996;98:70–77.
40. Kitan A, Chua K, Nakamura K, Strober W. Activated self-MHC-reactive T cells have the cytokine phenotype of Th3/T regulatory cell 1 T cells. J Immunol 2000;165:691–702.
41. Groux H, O'Garra A, Bigler M et al. A CD4+ T-cell subset inhibits antigen-specific T-cell responses and prevents colitis. Nature 1997;389:737–742.
42. Mukherji B, Guha A, Chakraborty NG et al. Clonal analysis of cytotoxic and regulatory T cell responses against human melanoma. J Exp Med 1989;169:1961–1976.
43. Chakraborty NG, Li L, Sporn JR et al. Emergence of regulatory CD4+ T cell response to repetitive stimulation with antigen-presenting cells in vitro: Implications in designing antigen-presenting cell-based tumor vaccines. J Immunol 1999;162:5576–5583.
44. Jonuleit H, Schmitt E, Schuler G et al. Induction of interleukin 10–producing, nonproliferating CD4(+) T cells with regulatory properties by repetitive stimulation with allogeneic immature human dendritic cells. J Exp Med 2000;192:1213–1222.
45. Enk AH, Jonuleit H, Saloga J, Knop J. Dendritic cells as mediators of tumor-induced tolerance in metastatic melanoma. Int J Cancer 1997;73:309–316.
46. Steinbrink K, Jonuleit H, Muller G et al. Interleukin-10-treated human dendritic cells induce a melanoma-antigen-specific anergy in CD8(+) T cells resulting in a failure to lyse tumor cells. Blood 1999;93:1634–1642.
47. Fearon DT, Locksley RM. The instructive role of innate immunity in the acquired immune response. Science 1996;272(5258):50–53.
48. Matzinger P. An innate sense of danger. Semin Immunol 1998;10:399–415.

49. Sogn JA. Tumor immunology: The glass is half full. Immunity 1998;9:757–763.
50. Allison J. Cancer. Curr Opin Immunol 2000;12:569–570.
51. Bowne WB, Srinivasan R, Wolchok JD et al. Coupling and uncoupling of tumor immunity and autoimmunity. J Exp Med 1999;190:1717–1722.
52. Pardoll DM. Inducing autoimmune disease to treat cancer. Proc Natl Acad Sci USA 1999;96:5340–5342.
53. Darnell RB. Onconeural antigens and the paraneoplastic neurologic disorders: At the intersection of cancer, immunity, and the brain. Proc Natl Acad Sci USA 1996;93:4529–4536.
54. Albert ML, Darnell JC, Bender A et al. Tumor-specific killer cells in paraneoplastic cerebellar degeneration. Nat Med 1998;4:1321–1324.
55. Boczkowski D, Nair SK, Snyder D, Gilboa E. Dendritic cells pulsed with RNA are potent antigen-presenting cells in vitro and in vivo. J Exp Med 1996;184:465–472.
56. Flamand V, Sornasse T, Thielemans K et al. Murine dendritic cells pulsed in vitro with tumor antigen induce tumor resistance in vivo. Eur J Immunol 1994;24:605–610.
57. Mayordomo JI, Zorina T, Storkus WJ et al. Bone marrow–derived dendritic cells pulsed with synthetic tumour peptides elicit protective and therapeutic antitumour immunity. Nat Med 1995;1:1297–1302.
58. Porgador A, Gilboa E. Bone marrow–generated dendritic cells pulsed with a class I-restricted peptide are potent inducers of cytotoxic T lymphocytes. J Exp Med 1995;182:255–260.
59. Song W, Kong HL, Carpenter H et al. Dendritic cells genetically modified with an adenovirus vector encoding the cDNA for a model antigen induce protective and therapeutic antitumor immunity. J Exp Med 1997;186:1247–1256.
60. Specht JM, Wang G, Do MT et al. Dendritic cells retrovirally transduced with a model antigen gene are therapeutically effective against established pulmonary metastases. J Exp Med 1997;186:1213–1221.
61. Toes RE, Blom RJ, van der Voort E et al. Protective antitumor immunity induced by immunization with completely allogeneic tumor cells. Cancer Res 1996;56(16):3782–3787.
62. Timmerman JM, Levy R. Dendritic cell vaccines for cancer immunotherapy. Annu Rev Med 1999;50:507–529.
63. Fong L, Engelman E. Dendritic cells in cancer immunotherapy. Ann Rev Immunol 2000;18:245–273.
64. Hsu FJ, Benike C, Fagnoni F et al. Vaccination of patients with B-cell lymphoma using autologous antigen-pulsed dendritic cells. Nat Med 1996;2:52–58.
65. Mukherji B, Chakraborty NG, Yamasaki S et al. Induction of antigen-specific cytolytic T cells in situ in human melanoma by immunization with synthetic peptide-pulsed autologous antigen presenting cells. Proc Natl Acad Sci USA 1995;92:8078–8082.
66. Nestle FO, Alijagic S, Gilliet M et al. Vaccination of melanoma patients with peptide- or tumor lysate–pulsed dendritic cells. Nat Med 1998;4:328–332.
67. Thurner B, Haendle I, Roder C et al. Vaccination with mage-3A1 peptide-pulsed mature, monocyte-derived dendritic cells expands specific cytotoxic T cells and induces regression of some metastases in advanced stage IV melanoma. J Exp Med 1999;190:1669–1678.
68. Salgaller ML, Tjoa BA, Lodge PA et al. Dendritic cell–based immunotherapy of prostate cancer. Crit Rev Immunol 1998;18:109–119.
69. Small EJ, Fratesi P, Reese DM et al. Immunotherapy of hormone-refractory prostate cancer with antigen-loaded dendritic cells. J Clin Oncol 2000;18:3894–3903.
70. Banchereau J, Palucka K, Dhodapkar M et al. Immunological and clinical responses to CD34+ hematopoietic progenitors–derived DC in patients with stage IV melanoma. 2000 (submitted).

71. Dhodapkar MV, Steinman RM, Sapp M et al. Rapid generation of broad T-cell immunity in humans after a single injection of mature dendritic cells. J Clin Invest 1999;104:173–180.
72. Dhodapkar MV, Krasovsky J, Steinman RM, Bhardwaj N. Mature dendritic cells boost functionally superior CD8(+) T-cell in humans without foreign helper epitopes. J Clin Invest 2000;105:9–14.
73. Gilboa E. The makings of a tumor rejection antigen. Immunity 1999;11:263–270.
74. Zitvogel L, Mayordomo JI, Tjandrawan T et al. Therapy of murine tumors with tumor peptide–pulsed dendritic cells: Dependence on T cells, B7 costimulation, and T helper cell 1–associated cytokines. J Exp Med 1996;183:87–97.
75. Fields RC, Shimizu K, Mule JJ. Murine dendritic cells pulsed with whole tumor lysates mediate potent antitumor immune responses in vitro and in vivo. Proc Natl Acad Sci USA 1998;95: 9482–9487.
76. Kirk CJ, Mule JJ. Gene-modified dendritic cells for use in tumor vaccines. Hum Gene Ther 2000; 11:797–806.
77. Gong J, Chen D, Kashiwaba M et al. Reversal of tolerance to human MUC1 antigen in MUC1 transgenic mice immunized with fusions of dendritic and carcinoma cells. Proc Natl Acad Sci USA 1998;95:6279–6283.
78. Zitvogel L, Regnault A, Lozier A et al. Eradication of established murine tumors using a novel cell-free vaccine: Dendritic cell–derived exosomes. Nat Med 1998;4:594–600.
79. Rosenberg SA. Cancer vaccines based on the identification of genes encoding cancer regression antigens. Immunol Today 1997;18:175–182.
80. Mule JJ. Dendritic cells: At the clinical crossroads. J Clin Invest 2000;105:707–708.
81. Kugler A, Stuhler G, Walden P et al. Regression of human metastatic renal cell carcinoma after vaccination with tumor cell–dendritic cell hybrids. Nat Med 2000;6:332–336.
82. Nair SK, Hull S, Coleman D et al. Induction of carcinoembryonic antigen (CEA)-specific cytotoxic T-lymphocyte responses in vitro using autologous dendritic cells loaded with CEA peptide or CEA RNA in patients with metastatic malignancies expressing CEA. Int J Cancer 1999;82:121–124.
83. Nair SK, Heiser A, Boczkowski D et al. Induction of cytotoxic T cell responses and tumor immunity against unrelated tumors using telomerase reverse transcriptase RNA transfected dendritic cells. Nat Med 2000;6:1011–1017.
84. Srivastava P. Immunotherapy of human cancer: Lessons from mice. Nat Immun 2000;1:363–366.
85. Blom B, Ho S, Antonenko S, Liu YJ. Generation of IFN alpha producing pre-DC2 from human CD34+ hematopoietic stem cells. J Exp Med 2000;192:1785–1796.
86. Spits H, Couwenberg F, Bakker AQ et al. Id2 and Id3 inhibit development of CD34+ stem cells into pre-DC2 but not into pre-DC1: evidence for a lymphoid origin of pre-DC2. J Exp Med 2000; 192:1775–1784.

Rolling Circle Amplification Technology: Potential Applications in Cancer Research and Clinical Oncology

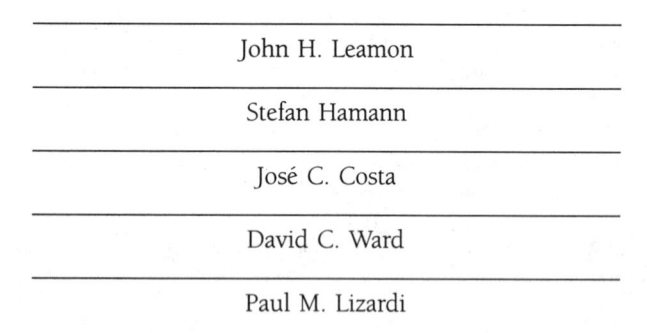

John H. Leamon

Stefan Hamann

José C. Costa

David C. Ward

Paul M. Lizardi

Advances in technologies for the detection of molecular alterations in tissues and cells are having an impact on cancer prevention and treatment at many levels. In basic cancer research, advances in molecular detection have helped to achieve a more detailed understanding of the natural history of the disease. In diagnostics and prevention, advances in detection technology have led to improvements in cancer grading and staging, and in the early assessment of cancer risk. In cancer treatment, improved detection technologies will facilitate the monitoring of chemotherapy, as well as the identification of residual metastatic disease. Some of the most remarkable advances in detection technology over the last fifteen years have occurred in the field of DNA amplification. The polymerase chain reaction (PCR) has rapidly become a key tool for the diagnosis of minimal residual disease in hematologic tumors, as well as in the staging of solid tumors.[1-3] PCR-driven amplification enables the detection of minute amounts of tumor-derived DNA in serum and other body fluids, and the assessment of mutational status for oncogenes and tumor suppressor genes. Reverse transcription PCR (RT-PCR) permits the detection of a variety of altered RNA molecules that play a role in cancer, even if such RNA molecules are present in a solitary tumor cell, among thousands of normal cells.

There are a number of important problems in oncology that have resisted analysis due to the technical difficulties of detecting rare molecular targets. One such problem is the identification of somatically mutated cells, where a point mutation alters an important tumor suppressor or oncogene. While point mutations may be detectable by PCR using extracted DNA from tissue, localization of mutated alleles in cytological preparations is not possible using conventional fluorescent in situ hybridization (FISH) technology. Another critical problem is the detection of altered proteins. A number of potentially relevant protein alterations in cancer involve minute numbers of molecules, often not detectable by existing methods. Thus, a capability for the detection of single-protein molecules would open up new research and clinical applications in oncology. This is of particular relevance for the study of pre-neoplastic lesions. Dysplasias composed of small numbers of cells have not been studied in detail because of technical limitations.

While PCR excels in amplifying DNA molecules in solution, it is not as well suited for surface-based detection assays. With the advent of microarray-based technologies, there has been increasing interest in surface-anchored DNA amplification. A novel technology called rolling circle amplification (RCA)[4] permits the localization of individual molecular recognition events on surfaces. This technology relies on isothermal DNA amplification reactions, which can be adapted to a variety of assay formats in which the amplification products can be generated with either linear or geometric kinetics. In this chapter, we describe the design of a variety of existing RCA-based assays with multiple potential applications in tumor genetic analysis and in cancer immunodiagnostics. We also discuss the advantages as well as the current limitations of RCA-based methods, and speculate on potential future applications in oncology.

LINEAR RCA TECHNIQUES

RCA technology is based on the ability of circular molecules of single-stranded DNA to be copied by any DNA polymerase with strand-displacement activity.

When an oligonucleotide primer, complementary to a circular DNA molecule, binds and is extended by DNA polymerase, the growing strand will elongate along the circumference of the template until it completes a circle by reaching the 5'-end of the primer (Fig. 4.1A). At that point, the strand displacement activity of the DNA polymerase causes the 5'-end of the primer to unwind, freeing the circular DNA to serve as template for continued extension of the 3'-end of the newly-synthesized strand (Fig. 4.1B). As long as there are sufficient deoxynucleotide triphosphates available, the replication reaction will continue, generating a long, single-stranded DNA molecule that contains multiple repeats of the complementary strand of the original circular DNA.

RCA-based assays employ a variety of designs, depending on the nature of the molecular targets, and the preference for surface-based or solution-based detection.[4] The simplest RCA assays are based on linear signal amplification, and employ a single oligonucleotide primer, together with a circular DNA molecule designed to hybridize to the primer. The circular DNA molecule is of arbitrary sequence and typically contains from 60 to 100 bases of DNA, while the primer usually is 20 to 30 bases in length. A specific detector molecule is constructed,

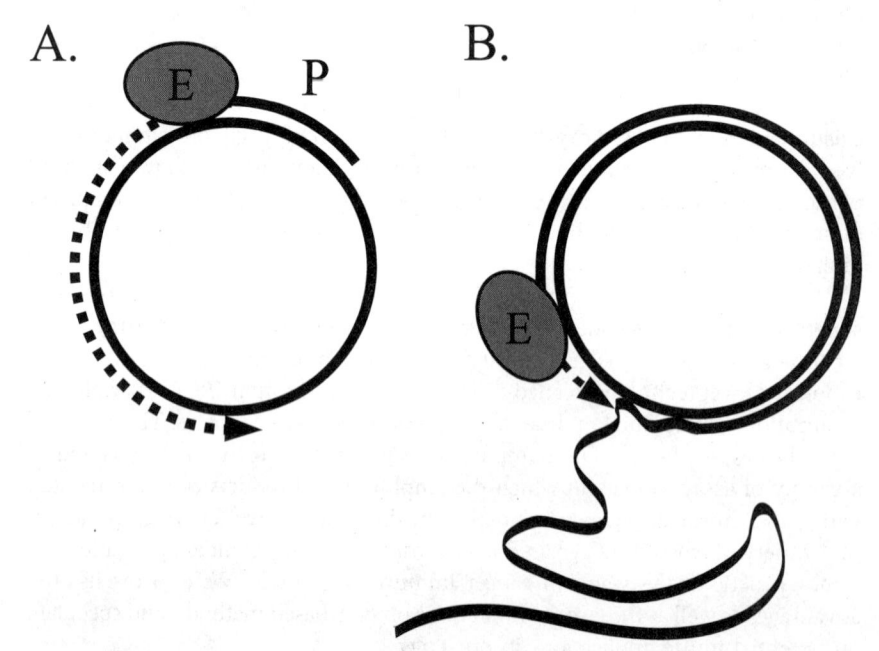

FIGURE 4.1 Principle of rolling circle amplification. (A) A short oligonucleotide serves as a primer (P) for elongation along the circular DNA template. (B) As soon as the enzyme (gray oval with letter E) reaches the 5'-end of the primer, the strand displacement activity unwinds the newly generated strand. A long DNA molecule is thereby generated that contains multiple repeats of the complementary strand of the original circular DNA.

containing an RCA primer tethered either to a DNA probe or to an antibody. When a DNA detector molecule is employed, a single oligonucleotide can be easily generated by chemical synthesis, comprising a specific probe portion and a primer portion, usually connected by an aliphatic carbon spacer. Alternatively, an antibody detector molecule competent for RCA is constructed by covalent synthesis of an adduct between an immunoglobulin and a primer. Antibody-primer adducts typically contain between one and three primer molecules, covalently bound to a single immunoglobulin.[5] Figure 4.2 shows a diagrammatic representation of an immuno-RCA assay. The antibody-primer adduct is contacted with a sample, which may be a histological preparation, or the surface of a microspot. After the antibody-primer adduct binds to the specific cancer antigen of interest, the excess unbound adduct is washed away, and an RCA reaction buffer is added which contains circular DNA, DNA polymerase, and nucleotides. The ensuing rolling circle replication reaction generates a long DNA concatamer that remains attached to the antibody. The amplified DNA can be detected in a variety of ways, including direct incorporation of hapten- or fluorescently-labeled nucleotides, or by hybridization of fluorescently- or enzymatically-labeled complementary oligonucleotide probes that bind to the concatenated DNA repeats generated by RCA.

The assay, shown in Figure 4.2, is easily modified to permit the detection of a DNA target sequence by simply substituting the antibody molecule with a specific DNA probe. All the other reagents used in the assay remain unchanged,

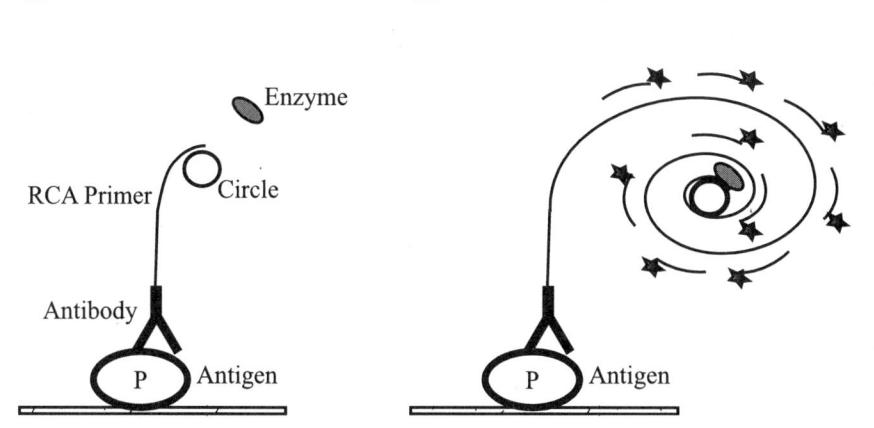

FIGURE 4.2 Schematic representation of immuno-RCA. (A) An antibody-primer conjugate binds to the appropriate antigen. (B) The primer initiates DNA synthesis on the circular template and generates many copies of the circle, which remain tethered to the antibody. The RCA product is subsequently detected by hybridization of fluorescently labeled complementary oligonucleotides (decorators). P denotes a protein antigen.

including the oligonucleotide primer, the circular DNA, and the fluorescent or enzymatic labels. The target DNA sequence must be known in advance, and preferably should be a sequence present in tumor cells and absent in normal cells. One may utilize two different probe designs, one intended for the visualization of small target sequences, and the other for the discrimination of point mutations in genomic DNA. These are illustrated schematically in Figure 4.3A and 4.3B, respectively. When allele discrimination is not required, a single oligonucleotide probe can be used. This probe has one portion, generally 30–50 nucleotides (nt) long, complementary to the target sequence and a second portion, 24–28 nt long, that functions as a primer to initiate rolling circle replication of the circular DNA template required for the RCA reaction. In order to stabilize the association of the RCA products on target DNA molecules and to increase detection efficiency, this probe-primer oligonucleotide is constructed with two 3'-ends, a routine chemical procedure in oligonucleotide synthesis. The polarity reversal permits the 3'-end of the target complementary sequence to be extended at the same time as the primer sequence, resulting in longer, more stable probe-target hybrids. In contrast, allele discrimination assays utilize three oligonucleotides for each locus analyzed. An anchor probe (P1), 30–40 nt long, is synthesized such that its 5'-end is immediately adjacent to the nucleotide in the target to be interrogated as to its wild-type (wt) or mutant (mu) status. The two allele discriminating oligonucleotides (P2 oligos) have inverted (3'-3') polarity with a target complementary sequence, 15–20 bases long, that differs only at the 3'-terminal nucleotide. The primer portions of the two P2 oligonucleotides are attached to the target portions via a spacer and the primers contain sequences complementary to two different circular DNAs. Following hybridization of a mixture of P1 and P2 probes to target DNA, the samples are subjected to a DNA ligation reaction. Since ligation of the P1 oligo to a perfect match P2 is much preferred to a mismatch ligation event, perfect match P1-P2 ligators predominate. Hybrids made with P2 oligonucleotides alone are less stable than those of P1-P2 ligation products and are disrupted under the wash condition employed. In both assay formats, subsequent incubation of a circular DNA (or a mixture of circular templates complementary to primer sequences specific for the wt or the mu allele) with a strand-displacing DNA polymerase results in the production of RCA products. As shown in the diagram, the preferred method for labeling of RCA products is the use of fluorescent oligonucleotide tags that encode the same sequence as the circular DNA, and thus bind specifically to the amplified DNA generated by a unique circular template.

A key feature of RCA assays is the capability for multicolor labeling, and for imaging of amplified DNA molecules originating from a single detection event. An RCA assay may utilize n different primer sequences, corresponding to n specific circular DNAs, where n is a number between 1 and 10. The different primers and circles are incubated together, and they are able to recognize each other specifically by base pairing. For each specific primer and circle, an encoding tag

A. Detection of small sequences

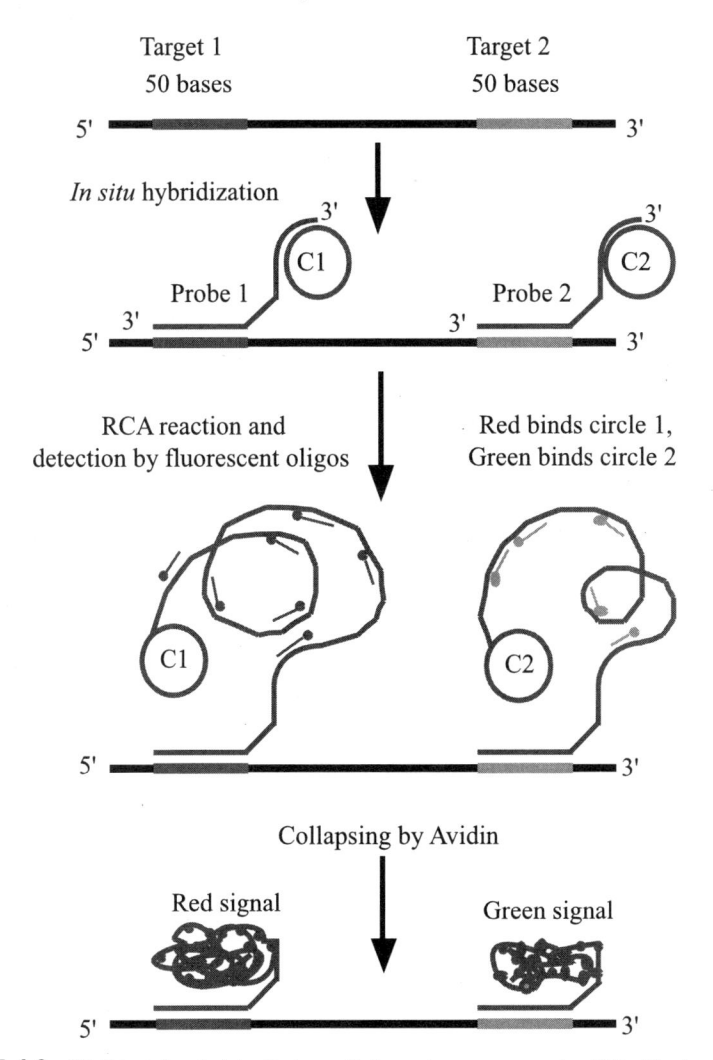

FIGURE 4.3 (A) Principle of detecting small genomic sequences by RCA. Bipolar (3'-3') oligonucleotide probes (Probe 1 and Probe 2) are hybridized to their target sequences and subsequently elongated by RCA. Incorporation of Biotin-dUTP into the DNA permits product-collapsing by Avidin in order to achieve a condensed signal.

B. Mutation Discrimination by RCA

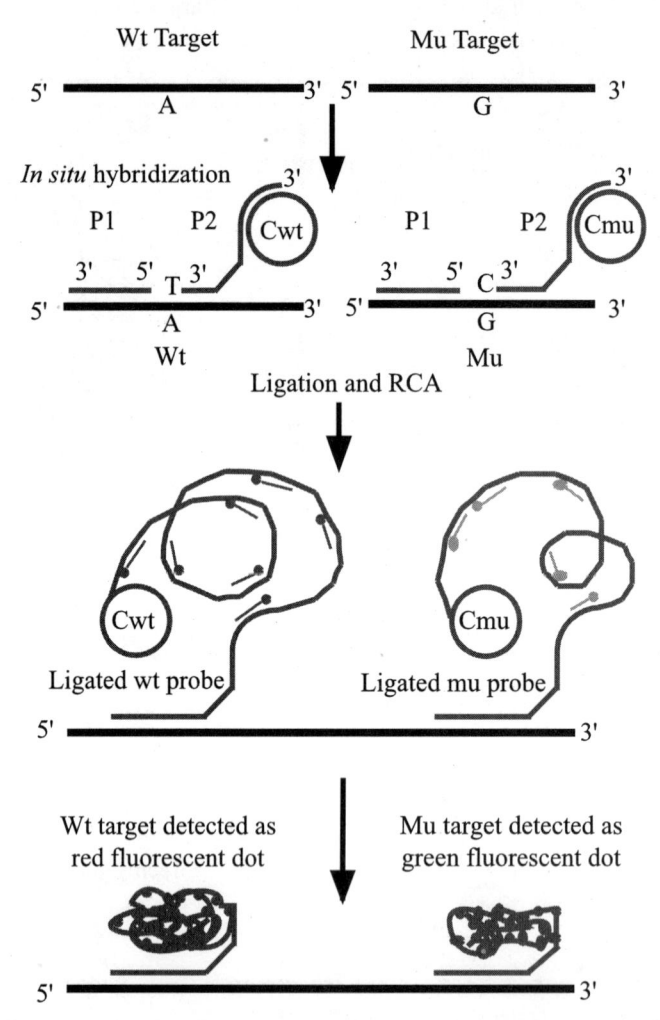

FIGURE 4.3 *Continued* (B) Mutation discrimination utilizing RCA. An anchor probe (P1) is hybridized to the genomic target. The allele-discriminating (3'-3') P2 oligonucleotides are ligated to the anchor probes when perfectly matched to their targets, and serve as primers for RCA after excess unligated P2 probes are washed away.

is also designed, to color-label a unique RCA product by hybridization. As long as RCA detection events are not too numerous, such that they do not overlap on a solid surface, each DNA molecule can be labeled individually, and in different colors, by a process of condensation of amplified circles and hybridization of encoding tags (CACHET). This DNA sequence-driven process in which the circle-specific encoding tags "decorate" each RCA product with its corresponding unique color is illustrated in Figure 4.4. After labeling with encoded decorator tags, the individual signals are readily imaged and counted using an epifluorescence microscope with object-counting software. We will discuss examples of RCA-CACHET applications in which multicolor imaging and single molecule counting may be used to great advantage.

HYPERBRANCHED RCA REACTIONS

A more complex form of RCA involves the use of two different primers, to achieve much greater output of amplified DNA. As in standard RCA, one of the two primers is used to initiate rolling circle replication on a circular template. The second primer present in the reaction is designed to bind specifically to the repeated DNA generated by the first primer (Figure 4.5). This second primer (which must not be complementary to the first primer) will bind to each complementary sequence in the single-stranded DNA, initiating sequential primer extension reactions. As each extending primer runs into the product of a downstream primer, strand displacement ensues, generating single-stranded concatenated repeats of the sequence of the original circular DNA. The displaced strands will in

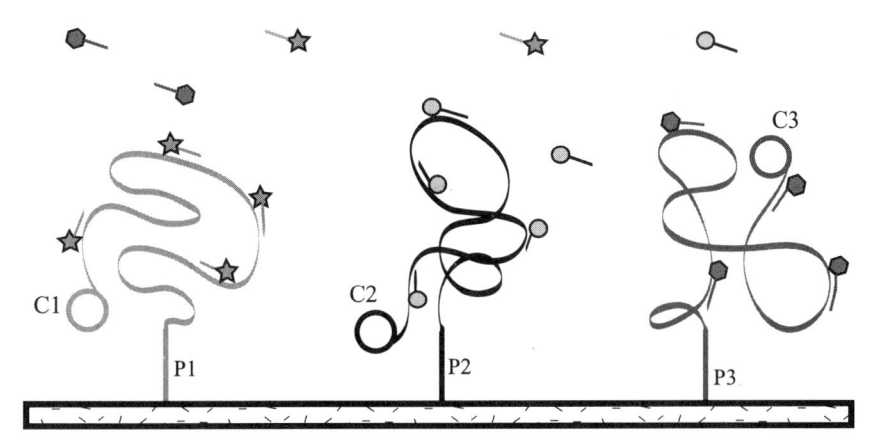

FIGURE 4.4 Principle of multi-color RCA-CACHET. Three different surface-bound primers (P1, P2, and P3) and three corresponding circles (C1-C3) are utilized to generate three different rolling circle products. Since each amplified DNA contains unique sequences, RCA-products can be discriminated by multi-color decoration with differentially labeled oligonucleotides, which bind specifically to their complementary DNA sequences.

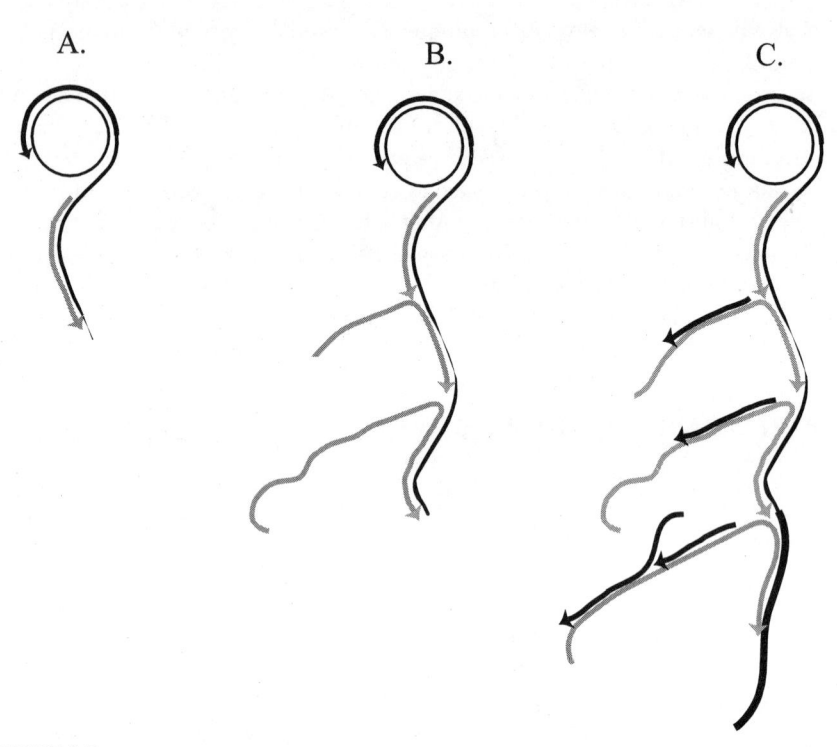

FIGURE 4.5 Schematic representation of hyperbranched rolling circle amplification (HRCA). (A) Primer 1 binds to a circularized oligonucleotide and initiates enzymatic synthesis of the primary single stranded RCA product, shown by the thick black line. This nascent strand contains priming sites for Primer 2, which bind to the RCA product and initiate secondary strand synthesis in the opposite direction (gray arrows). (B) Elongation of the primary strand creates additional sites for Primer 2 and multiple secondary strands are synthesized on a single primary strand. When the elongating 3'-end of one secondary strand encounters the 5'-end of a downstream strand, the downstream strand is detached from the primary strand by enzymatic strand displacement activity. (C) Detached regions of secondary strands contain priming sites for Primer 1 (black arrows) which promote synthesis of complementary strands. Although not shown, strand displacement activity will displace regions of these strands as well, exposing priming sites for Primer 2.

turn contain multiple binding sites for the first RCA primer. Thus, alternate-strand copying and strand displacement processes generate a continuously expanding pattern of DNA branches, many of which remain connected to the original circle. Strand displacement also generates a discrete set of free DNA fragments comprising double-stranded pieces of the unit length of a circle, and multiples thereof. This expanding cascade of strand displacement events is called *DNA hyperbranching*; thus, the complex rolling circle amplification reaction driven by two primers is called *hyperbranched-RCA* (HRCA).

GENETIC AND TRANSCRIPTIONAL ANALYSIS USING RCA

RCA and HRCA have been used with success for a number of applications in genetic analysis and transcription analysis. Some of these applications involve cytological preparations, while others use DNA microarrays or solution assays.

In Situ Detection of Specific Gene Loci Using Short DNA Probes

Short oligonucleotide probes are very difficult to detect using standard FISH methods. Recently, an enzymatic reaction known as tyramide signal amplification[6] has been used with success to amplify the FISH signals from small DNA probes. However, the tyramide signal amplification method is currently limited to the detection of two gene loci, because enzymatic amplification reactions are not easily multiplexed. Zhong et al[7] have demonstrated that three different gene loci may be detected simultaneously in cytological preparations using probes of 50 bases tethered to three specific RCA primers. Different probes, specific for different loci in the cystic fibrosis transmembrane regulator (*CFTR*) gene were used to generate RCA-CACHET signals of different colors, enabling simultaneous detection of the thee gene loci in interphase nuclei. This method can be extended in the future to the detection of gene loss, gene amplification (as occurs in the Her2Neu locus in breast cancer), or DNA translocation events. For example, chronic myelogenous leukemia (CML) is a hematological malignant disorder characterized by the Philadelphia chromosome (Ph) and *Bcr-Abl* gene translocation.[8] It should be possible to design a 30-base DNA probe for previously sequenced break points spanning the *Bcr-Abl* translocation, tethered to a primer competent for RCA, such that the probe will bind only if the translocation sequence is present, but will bind unstably and be washed away if it is not.

In Situ Detection of Point Mutations in Genomic DNA Using Bipartite Probes

The ability of RCA probes to visualize point mutations in interphase cells and DNA fibers has been demonstrated[7] using the P1/P2 probe-ligation scheme illustrated in Figure 4.3B. An anchor probe, P1, and two allele-discriminating probes designed to detect mutations at the G542X locus of the *CFTR* gene were used. Cell lines that were known to be wt, homozygous mu, or heterozygous at this locus were hypotonically swollen and fixed by methanol-acetic acid treatment. DNA ligation reactions and hybridization with a mixture of P1 and P2 probes were carried out simultaneously, and the slides were then subjected to the RCA-CACHET detection procedure. Fluorescent signals were observed, corresponding to each of the mutant and wild type alleles. In each cell line, 100% of the nuclei exhibiting two signals gave the expected genotype. On average, RCA signals were generated from both *CFTR* genes in ~21% of the cells, and from a single copy of the gene in 30%–40% of the cells. The cell lines used in these experiments were not synchronized, so each cell population was expected to have cells in the G_1, S, or G_2 phase of the cell cycle. G_2 cells could be identified readily because 4 RCA signals were generated per locus in each nucleus, as a pair of closely juxtaposed (gemini) signals. Mutations could also be detected in genes other than *CFTR*. Allele-discriminating P1/P2 probe sets were prepared for the A13073C locus in the *p53* gene, the 5382Cins locus in the *BRCA-1* gene, and the C3383A locus in the patched (Gorlin Syndrome) gene. Methanol-fixed preparations were probed by RCA-CACHET in separate experiments to detect each of the loci in interphase nuclei. As with the *CFTR* gene, 100% of the nuclei exhibiting RCA signal from both genes correctly identified the expected genotype. The efficiency of detecting both gene copies in the nucleus of individual cells varied significantly from experiment to experiment. Despite this caveat, the data clearly indicate that genetic mutations can be visualized in a cellular context on a cell-by-cell basis.

Detection of point mutations has also been reported on stretched DNA fibers prepared from normal lymphocytes and a transformed lymphoblast cell line homozygous for the G542X mutation.[7] In these experiments, which employed probes specific for three loci, two of which mapped close to the G542X mutation, the signals generated by RCA were observed as co-linear spots localized as expected on the basis of gene order and genetic map distance. Thus, RCA may be used to map genetic mutations or single nucleotide polymorphisms (SNPs) in DNA from individual DNA strands, which may be useful for haplotyping studies in cancer.

The mutation detection method based on ligation of P1 and P2 probes, followed by RCA, has been tried on metaphase chromosome spreads, so far without success. It seems that the highly condensed state of DNA in chromatin makes the metaphase chromosome inaccessible to the RCA reaction components. Likewise, the detection of point mutations in formalin-fixed histological sections using RCA has not yet been reported. The application of the mutation detection method to formaldehyde-fixed tissue will likely require considerable efforts in protocol optimization.

Somatic Mutation Analysis on DNA Microarrays Using Ligation Detection Reaction Combined with RCA Signal Enhancement

The analysis of the frequency and distribution of somatic mutations in tissues and biological fluids could in principle serve as a biomarker for cancer risk. Unfortunately, high-throughput genetic analysis has so far been possible only for germline mutations and SNPs, which typically represent at least 50% of the DNA in a sample. On the other hand, the detection of somatic mutations requires discrimination of one mutant strand in a context of 100 or more wild type strands, a demanding goal that typically requires time consuming electrophoretic or HPLC separations. The ligation detection reaction (LDR) is a mutation detection method based in the joining of two DNA probe molecules, where one of the probes has an allele-specific oligonucleotide that can be ligated only if it is correctly base-paired to its target. Recently, the LDR has been coupled to generic DNA microarrays that contain oligonucleotides of arbitrary sequence.[9] The arbitrary oligonucleotides have sequences that serve as zip codes to guide individual ligated LDR probes to specific addresses on the microarray surface. The generic zip codes permit the design of LDR assays where different mutations may be targeted, without the need to change the chemical composition of the microarray. LDR can be made extremely specific by increasing the ligation temperature; however, the increase in specificity comes at the expense of reduced ligation efficiency and weaker fluorescence signals. Alternatively, enhanced ligation selectivity can be achieved using mutant ligases that have significantly greater specificity than the wild-type enzyme.[10]

A recent improvement on LDR has been the use of probe molecules that incorporate an RCA primer as part of their design. The allele-specific probe, which contains the complement of the zip oligonucleotide, remains unchanged, while the second probe is made longer, to be able to serve as primer for RCA. After ligation, the LDR oligonucleotides are contacted with the microarray of zip oligos, which immobilize ligated probes and their associated primers. Circular oligonucleotides are then added, and an RCA reaction is performed to generate fluorescent signals that are indicative of successful ligation. The increased signal intensity provided by RCA permits the LDR experiments to be performed at higher ligation temperatures, resulting in markedly improved allele-discrimination. Ladner et al[11] have demonstrated a very sensitive assay for the detection of somatic mutations in DNA from colon using a highly multiplexed LDR-RCA probe design coupled to generic zip microarrays.

RNA Expression Profiling on DNA Microarrays with RCA Signal Enhancement

Recent advances in robotics and microfabrication have permitted the construction of DNA microarrays on the surface of standard microscope slides. These microarrays contain thousands of individual DNA spots—each spot comprising a specific DNA probe—capable of binding a unique gene product. The probes are typically derived from the 3′-end of specific mRNAs of known sequence. In a DNA microarray experiment, the glass slide is contacted with fluorescently tagged cDNA representations of total RNA pools from test and reference cells or tissue, which bind specifically to each probe on the surface, thereby allowing one to determine the relative amount of each transcript present in the pool. Since a measurement of relative mRNA abundance is based on a direct comparison between a "test" cell and a "reference" cell, its value is independent of the amount of DNA probe immobilized on the microarray surface. The analysis of mRNA expression profiles using microarrays of human DNA clones offers unprecedented opportunities for understanding the molecular alterations that underlie cancer.[12–15] There are precedents in the literature supporting the feasibility of performing ab initio tumor classification using comprehensive analysis of gene expression in a limited number of tumor samples. Published studies on lymphoma classification, based on analysis of mRNA expression profiles obtained from DNA microarray experiments, have revealed the emergence previously undetected subclasses of disease.[16] Using DNA microarrays, Alizadeh and colleagues[16] conducted a systematic characterization of gene expression in B-cell malignancies. They showed that there is diversity in gene expression among the tumors of diffuse large B-cell lymphoma (DLBCL) patients, apparently reflecting the variation in tumor proliferation rate, host response, and differentiation state of the tumor. They identified two molecularly distinct forms of DLBCL that have gene expression patterns indicative of different stages of B-cell differentiation and activation. Considerable heterogeneity was found within each of the two subgroups; it is not clear to what extent this heterogeneity reflects differences in the patients' genetic makeup, as opposed to additional tumor subclasses.

Rolling circle amplification has recently been adapted to DNA microarray experimental protocols with the goal of improving both the sensitivity and the precision of gene expression measurements. Such improvements are of considerable importance for cancer research applications where the amount of biological material is limited to a very small number of cells. Figure 4.6 demonstrates this microarray protocol, which combines linear amplification of mRNA with on-slide amplification by RCA and introduces an innovative method for analysis of very weak fluorescent signals generated by low-abundance mRNAs. cDNA is generated from total RNA using standard methods and is amplified using a linear transcriptional amplification method originally developed by Eberwine.[17] The amplified RNA is then copied by random priming by reverse transcriptase, using a special primer with 8 randomized bases at the 3'-end and a unique 5' DNA tail sequence. The random-primed cDNA is hybridized on the microarray, and then two types of tether-RCA primers are added, which are complementary to the tail sequence of each type of random primer. The two different tether-RCA primers and their cognate DNA circles are designed to enable a two-color labeling scheme. RCA is performed on the microarray surface, and the surface-anchored, amplified DNA is labeled using the CACHET method. For the subset of microarray spots corresponding to low copy number mRNAs, it is possible to resolve RCA-amplified hybridization signals as tiny discrete objects by imaging at high resolution (0.5 microns or better). Thus, when signals are weak, RCA signals can be detected and counted individually, to provide a direct measure of the number of hybridization events on the microarray surface. We have implemented in our laboratory at Yale a two-stage microarray imaging strategy using first a conventional laser scanner, and then a microscope-based scanner. In the first scanning stage, we record the entire microarray image using aggregate fluorescence intensity. We then export the image into a software package that reads the TIFF file and finds

20X Fluorescence Microscopy Imaging

Cy3 RCA Signal　　　　CY 5 RCA Signal

Standard Cy3/Cy5 Microarray Scan

Cy3 RCA Signal　　　　Cy5 RCA Signal

60X Fluorescence Microscopy Imaging

Discrete Hybridization Events

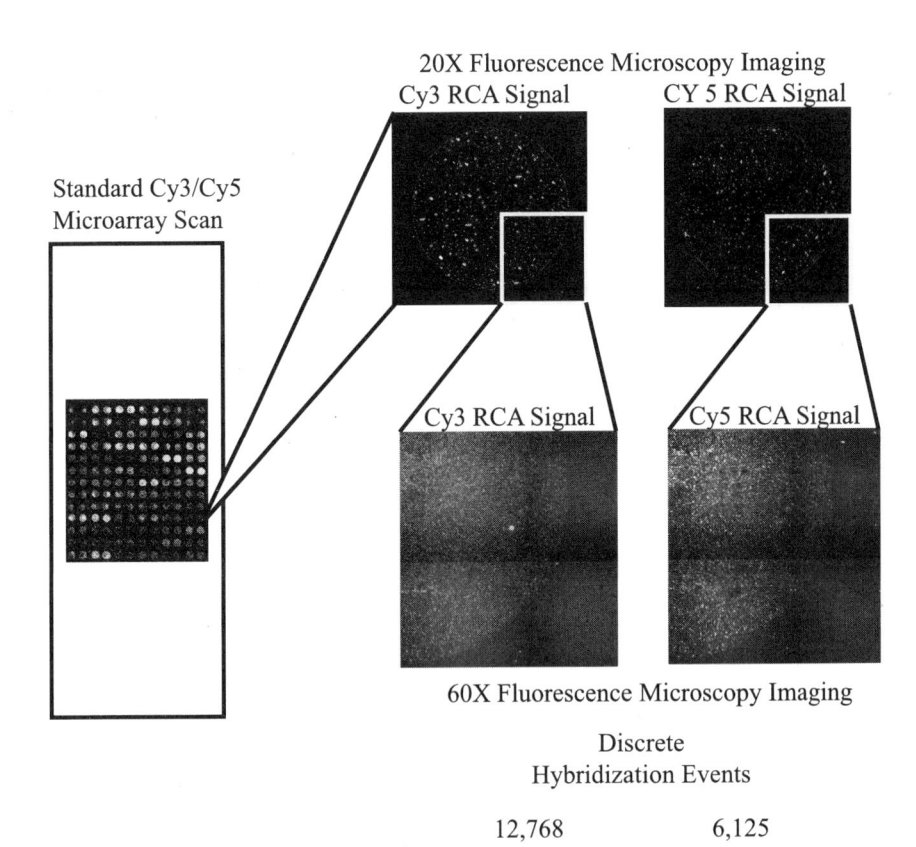

12,768　　　　6,125

FIGURE 4.6 Illustration of single molecule counting used in conjunction with standard aggregate fluorescence microarray imaging. A microarray containing hybridizations of varying fluorescent intensity is initially scanned with a commercially available laser-scanning unit. For hybridizations of high fluorescent intensity, aggregate fluorescence ratios of Cy3 to Cy5 are sufficient to determine relative abundance. Signals with fluorescent intensities too weak to provide reliable data are revisited with an automated fluorescent microscope. Individual hybridization events for each wavelength are detected and enumerated, and a relative ratio is accurately determined from the object counts.

all the spots, assigning x and y coordinates to all gene positions in the microarray. Software thresholding identifies the weak signals and marks them for a second round of imaging. The slide is then placed in a microscope, and the subset of low-intensity spots are re-visited and imaged at 60× (oil) magnification (Fig. 4.6). The single-molecule RCA objects are separated from background noise by image processing software, and the total number of hybridized molecules is determined by automated object counting. This method, called digital hybridization quantitation (DHQ) generates reliable RNA expression data for weak signals that would otherwise have a large coefficient of variation. Recent experimental work shows that RCA-enhanced microarray analysis using DHQ permits high-quality expression analysis in tissue samples containing as few as 1000 cells, without the use of PCR amplification. With more efficient linear pre-amplification of mRNA, and additional refinement of the DHQ method, we envision being able to perform reliable mRNA expression analysis in samples of 100 cells or fewer.

Analysis of Gene Copy Number by Array-CGH with RCA Signal Enhancement

Variation in gene dosage contributes to many diseases. Cancer is a salient example: copy number changes can increase the number and significance of oncogenes, or reduce the number and protective effect of tumor-suppressor genes. Detection of copy number changes, therefore, has emerged as a useful tool for identifying critical genes in cancer progression and assessing an individual's genetic risk of the disease.[18] Comparative genomic hybridization (CGH) is a method that measures the gene dosage of each gene in the genome, and thus permits the identification of gain or loss of gene copies, as occurs in loss of heterozygosity or gene amplification, respectively. Standard CGH[19] is based on hybridization of labeled DNA on metaphase chromosomes and is performed as follows: (1) DNA is prepared from two tissue samples, i.e. normal and tumor, and labeled separately with each of two fluorescent dyes suitable for detection by FISH. (2) The two labeled DNA preparations are mixed in equimolar amounts, and hybridized on normal metaphase spreads. (3) Imaging of the labeled chromosomes is performed for each of the two dyes, and the ratio of the fluorescence intensities is measured across the length of each chromosome. Most regions along the chromosome exhibit a constant ratio of fluorescent intensity, reflecting the invariant gene dosage across that region of the genome. However, any regions in which the cancer DNA has an abnormal gene dosage, caused by loss or gain of DNA sequences, will be distinguished by an altered ratio of fluorescence on the corresponding locus of the normal chromosome. This change in fluorescence ratio reflects precisely the change in gene dosage between the two labeled DNA preparations. CGH has been used successfully to identify chromosomal changes associated with many cancers, including breast[20] and prostate.[21,22] Despite these advances, the research applications of standard CGH have been limited by its relatively low resolution, identifying only chromosomal changes greater than 10 megabases in length,[19] and the complex nature of the chromosome-based image analysis required to obtain quantitative data.

It has been demonstrated recently that CGH can be performed by substituting metaphase chromosomes with DNA microarrays.[18,23] In array-CGH (A-CGH), gene loss or gain can be assessed by the ratio of the fluorescent probes at each microarray spot, provided that the microarray contains a sufficient number of cloned DNA segments to sample all the gene regions of interest. A-CGH utilizes labeling techniques and DNA chips similar to those used in mRNA expression profiling. Briefly, genomic DNA is isolated from two populations of cultured cell or tissue samples; one is the control, or reference population, the other the experimental, or tester, population. The DNA from each population is labeled with a unique fluorophore and hybridized to a microarray comprising thousands of DNA clones, which may be derived from P1 artificial chromosomes (PAC), bacterial artificial chromosomes (BAC), cosmids, or PCR-amplified gene segments of interest. The amount of material hybridized to any one of the immobilized clones determines the fluorescent signal at that location, and the copy number of that particular gene is calculated as the normalized ratio of the total fluorescence of the tester population compared to that of the reference population. The resolution of A-CGH is defined by the map distances of the DNA clones on the array. The improved resolution of A-CGH over standard CGH has permitted the detection of 75 Kb deletions or insertions.[18,23,24]

Although A-CGH methodology and data acquisition are similar to other biochip based techniques, analysis of A-CGH data is more demanding than mRNA expression profiling. The mammalian genome is at least ten times more complex than the expressed sequence set, yet from this diverse mixture, A-CGH must be able to discriminate single copy gene dosage changes relative to the diploid state. Hence, A-CGH requires reliable analysis of subtle fluorescent ratio differences. The theoretical maximum ratio difference for low copy number loss of heterozygosity changes is 0.5.[25] However, in actual experiments with tissue, observed ratio differences are significantly smaller due to the presence of mixed genomes in heterogeneous cell populations and the influence of background fluorescence arising from the hybridization process.[25] Analysis is further complicated by the low level of fluorescent signal produced by standard A-CGH hybridization. While mRNA derived from a single gene may exist in many copies per cell, CGH is limited to a maximum of two copies of genomic DNA per diploid cell. Thus, although A-CGH analysis must reliably score subtle ratio differences, the actual signals most often generated by an A-CGH experiment are of low intensity and characterized by occasional fluorophore bias[26] as well as high standard deviation within replicates.[27]

The sensitivity and reliability of the A-CGH system could be improved by increasing the amount of fluorescently labeled material applied to the array. If the sample size is not limiting, this can be accomplished by increasing the total amount of tissue DNA analyzed. However, this is obviously not a viable option for small samples, such as those provided through biopsy or the precisely selected, low abundance samples resulting from laser capture microdissection (LCM).[28] While A-CGH typically requires the use of 300,000 cells for each experiment, we have recently demonstrated that by using RCA signal enhancement and the DHQ single molecule counting method described above, it becomes possible to reduce the number of cells in the experimental sample by a factor of 6 (50,000 cells). In A-CGH using RCA and the DHQ method, the ratio measurement is less influenced by fluorescence background, which can be distinguished for RCA signals by image analysis. One obtains ratio measurements that are more precise than the standard method, which relies on measurements of aggregate fluorescence intensity. In the future, it may be possible to combine the RCA-enhanced A-CGH method with existing techniques for whole genome amplification, which generate approximately 100 copies of the entire genome,[23,28-31] thereby reducing the sample requirements for array CGH to as few as 500 cells. Thus, A-CGH, coupled with RCA signal enhancement, could be a powerful approach for assessing loss of heterozygosity in relatively small biopsies, including fine needle aspirates of the breast or other tissues.

Analysis of Cancer Mutations Using Padlock Probes and HRCA

Thomas and coworkers[32] have described methods for detection of point mutations using HRCA. They used so-called "padlock" probes, which consist of a long oligonucleotide with probe sequences at both ends. The two probe sequences are designed to bind to a DNA target with opposing polarity and precise apposition of the ends, enabling ligation of the termini, with consequent formation of a circular DNA molecule. The circular molecule thus becomes topologically intertwined with its target after ligation, and cannot be separated from it, hence the term *padlock*. Two otherwise identical padlock probes can be made with different nucleotides at their 3'-end such that the ligation and circularization reaction will only take place if there is a perfect match with a mutated allele in the target DNA. Using allele-discriminating padlock probes, Thomas et al were able to detect mutated alleles in *p53* DNA targets, as well as in c-*KIRAS2* DNA targets. After the allele-discriminating ligation step, the circularized probes were detected by amplification by HRCA using two suitable primers. One of the primers was designed as an energy-transfer primer, which generates a fluorescent signal only when incorporated into the amplified product. Using this HRCA-based fluorescent assay, they were able to detect mutated alleles in the presence of a 500-fold excess of wild type DNA.

Analysis of Single Nucleotide Polymorphisms Using HRCA

Genotyping and haplotyping of human DNA has emerged as an important component in the developing field of pharmacogenomics. Single nucleotide variations in different individuals, point mutations, or SNPs can play a significant role in both disease susceptibility and response to therapeutic drugs. It has been estimated that the 3×10^9 bp human genome contains one SNP every 300–400 nucleotides on average, and the construction of a high density SNP map has been a major undertaking in both academic and commercial sectors, including the Wellcome Trust SNP Consortium, a two-year, multi-million dollar initiative. For high-throughput genotyping of DNA, an assay must be simple, scalable, and easily automated. Molecular Staging Inc. (New Haven, CT) has developed a high-throughput HRCA assay that determines genotype directly from genomic DNA.

Point mutations and SNPs are detected by padlock probe ligation as described above. The ligation step has been optimized to score the correct sequence with a 100,000-fold signal to noise ratio, yielding an assay with high accuracy (Faruqi et al, manuscript in preparation). This exquisitely sensitive assay allows genotyping of as few as several hundred gene copies present in a few nanograms of genomic DNA sample. The circularized padlock probes are detected after amplification by HRCA using molecular beacon type primers (Amplifluor™, Intergen Company, Purchase, NY). Molecular beacon oligonucleotides have a hairpin stem that brings the 3'- and 5'-ends of the oligonucleotide together as a duplex structure. In this configuration, a fluorophore, attached to the 3' terminal nucleotide, is juxtaposed to a quencher species, attached to the 5'-terminal nucleotide, such that fluorophore emission is suppressed. Upon hybridization to the RCA product, the fluorophore and quencher are physically separated, and fluorescence occurs. Amersham Pharmacia Biotech, in collaboration with Molecular Staging, has developed this method for high-throughput genotyping of large numbers of individuals and genetic loci. The assay system, called SNiPer, integrates SNP scoring with robotic liquid handling and automated microtiter plate manipulation.[33]

PROTEIN ANALYSIS USING IMMUNO-RCA

RCA methods are directly applicable to the analysis of protein antigens in any of the conventional assay formats, such as enzyme-linked immunosorbent assay (ELISA), microbead, microarray, flow cytometry, immunohistochemistry, and immunofluorescence. Any specific antibody can be coupled (preferably covalently) to an RCA oligonucleotide capable of priming an RCA reaction. The primer can be attached either to the primary antibody or, preferably, to a secondary antibody used for signal production. Indirect detection using a secondary antibody has the advantage of providing a more universal approach for immunoassays, requiring a single immunoglobulin-primer adduct. For example, a goat anti-mouse IgG coupled covalently to an RCA primer can be used for the detection of virtually all mouse monoclonal antibodies raised against any epitope or hapten of interest. Similarly, an anti-biotin antibody coupled covalently to an RCA primer can be used to assess the presence of any biotinylated biomolecule, including antibodies, lectins, other proteins, nucleic acids, or haptens. The fact that a large variety of primer-circle pairs suitable for RCA have already been constructed and validated makes multicolor assays highly feasible. Outlined below are several examples of immuno-RCA applications.

Immunohistochemistry and Immunofluorescence Analysis

Immuno-RCA is very well suited for the detection of specific antigens by immunohistochemistry or immunofluorescence using methods that largely resemble conventional assays. In a typical experiment, antibody-primer adducts are contacted with the surface of standard histological sections on microscope slides, followed by washing to remove unbound material. An RCA reaction is then performed for 45 minutes at 37°C, and the amplified DNA is detected by addition of either (1) an enzyme such as HRP or alkaline phosphatase, coupled to an oligonucleotide that is complementary to the repeated DNA generated by RCA, or (2) a fluorescent dye coupled to an oligonucleotide. Enzyme-based signal generation yields extremely high sensitivity, since it combines the amplification of DNA provided by RCA with additional enzymatic amplification. On the other hand, fluorescence detection offers a higher potential for multiplexing, since most modern epifluorescence microscopes are equipped for the simultaneous detection of four or more fluorescent dyes. Immunohistochemical assays coupled to RCA have been used with success for the detection of CD20, PSA, and CD23 (Gusev et al, Am J Pathol, submitted).

PSA Detection Using Immuno-RCA

Prostate specific antigen (PSA) is routinely used for the screening of men for prostate cancer and for persistence or recurrence of disease after therapy.[34] Although elevation of PSA levels in peripheral blood in advanced disease can usually be monitored by standard immunodiagnostic procedures such as ELISA, which has a sensitivity limit of approximately 100 pg/mL, this level of sensitivity may be insufficient for detecting residual disease after radical prostatectomy.[35] A recent publication[5] documents a model immuno-RCA assay designed to detect PSA using a glass slide microspot format. Goat anti-PSA polyclonal Ab was immobilized on thiol-silane-coated microscope slides that had been activated with a heterobifunctional crosslinker. Purified human PSA in various concentrations was added, and the slide was incubated at 37°C, then washed to remove unbound protein. A mouse monoclonal anti-PSA Ab was used to form the second part of the immuno-sandwich complex. This complex was detected with a polyclonal rabbit anti-mouse IgG Ab that had been conjugated to an oligonucleotide containing a sequence for priming an RCA reaction. The assay was shown to detect as little as 0.1 pg/mL PSA (300 zeptomoles), which is two to three orders of magnitude more sensitive than standard immunoassays for PSA.

Prostate-associated membrane antigen (PSMA) is a prostate-restricted membrane glycoprotein that is expressed in normal prostatic epithelial cells, and elevated in poorly-differentiated, metastatic, and hormone-refractory carcinomas. PSMA has been proposed as a candidate biomarker for prostate cancer risk, although recent studies have cast doubt on its specificity.[36] There is considerable interest in developing tests in which PSA and PSMA are measured simultaneously; however, PSMA is present at very low levels in serum and so far has required the use of a western blot technique for reliable detection. The high sensitivity of the immuno-RCA based assay for PSA suggests that it may be possible to develop a test where both PSA and PSMA are measured simultaneously. Recent public announcements by Cytogen corporation (Princeton, NJ) indicate that an RCA-based commercial kit for simultaneous detection of PSA and PSMA is under development.

FUTURE PROSPECTS

Potential Applications of RCA in Flow Cytometry

Flow cytometry and fluorescence-based cell sorting are powerful and widely used methods for the analysis of transformed cells in the circulation. These methods are particularly valuable for diagnosis and for detection of minimal residual disease in hematologic cancers. An opportunity exists to apply the power of immuno-RCA to achieve immunofluorescence labeling of very low copy number proteins, located on the surface or in the interior of the cell, which are not presently detectable by flow cytometry. For example, certain proteins with important roles in cancer, such as the BRCA-2 transcription factor, are present in relatively small numbers inside the cell, and cannot be detected readily using standard surface-labeling flow cytometry. Certain candidate cancer biomarkers are most informative when detected in their phosphorylated form. Because the phosphorylated fraction often represents only 1%–3% of the protein mass, detection by immunofluorescence using specific anti-phosphoprotein antibodies is often not possible due to insufficient sensitivity. Immuno-RCA based methods have the potential to enable the detection of rare transcription factors or phosphorylated forms of proteins, despite their low abundance in cells or their intracellular location. Other potential applications in flow cytometry involve the use of RCA as a method to detect cells on the basis of the presence of cancer-specific DNA sequence markers, as exemplified by the Bcr-Abl translocation locus.

Analysis of Circulating Tumor Cells

As our ability to identify molecular alterations in tumors improves, it will be possible to detect circulating tumor cells with an increasingly broad panel of biomarkers earmarked specifically for each patient's tumor. One might envision that circulating tumor cells could be isolated from blood using magnetic particles coated with antibodies for tumor-specific antigens.[37] This recently developed method is based on the use of paramagnetic particles coated with a monoclonal antibody against an epithelial surface marker. Once captured and released, the tumor cells could be assayed for point mutations known to be present in the original tumor, using in situ mutation detection by ligation-mediated RCA. Alternatively, a panel of multiple tumor antigens could be detected in situ on cytological preparations of captured cells, using a high-sensitivity, multicolor immuno-RCA assay.

Detection of Somatic Mutations on Histological Preparations

In situ detection of mutations in histological preparations remains an attractive but elusive goal in oncology. Presently it is possible to detect such mutations by microdissection of areas containing very small numbers of cells, followed by PCR and single strand conformational polymorphism (SSCP) or DNA sequencing analysis. It would be an important advance to detect mutations directly in tissue, on a cell-by-cell basis. For example, a capability for in situ detection of point mutations at hot spots in the k-*ras* gene would permit the observation of patches of colon tissue where clonal expansion of mutated cell populations has taken place. The direct observation of clonal expansion events in tissue would help to understand the complex dynamics that precede overt colorectal cancer. As mentioned earlier, use of RCA for detection of point mutations on formaldehyde-fixed tissue has not yet given satisfactory results. So far, most ongoing RCA work has focused on mutation detection using genomic DNA targets. A promising avenue for future research is the use of mRNA as a target for the detection of point mutations. Although ligation reactions on RNA targets are less efficient than on DNA targets, RNA molecules are more abundant than genomic DNA targets, and conditions that increase the efficiency DNA probe ligation on an RNA guide sequence have been reported recently.[38] Using optimized ligation conditions, it should be possible to detect mutations in RNA targets using the same P1/P2 RCA probe system that has enabled discrimination of point mutations for DNA targets using cytological preparations.

A capability for detection of mutations on a cell-by-cell basis will be useful in the study of micrometastases and minimal residual disease, where mutated loci will have been predetermined in the primary lesion, providing the necessary information for the design of lesion-specific RCA probes. The technology will also enable the study of pre-neoplastic lesions now defined exclusively on a morphological basis, in cases where frequent mutations are known to arise at hot spots, for which a battery of specific RCA probes may be designed. Through the study of somatically mutated cells on a cell-by-cell basis, the knowledge of epithelial or other cell populations at risk will be significantly enhanced.

Studying Cancer Microheterogeneity In Tissue

The problem of tissue heterogeneity has been recognized as a barrier to more complete understanding of the early stages of cancer. However, it is now possible to obtain homogeneous tissue samples for analysis using LCM.[39] As mentioned earlier, RCA-enhanced expression analysis using DNA microarrays enables mRNA profiling experiments to be performed using samples of approximately 500 cells, such as those that may be obtained by LCM. The LCM sample may consist of selected epithelial cells of a breast duct, individual crypts from the colon, or any well-defined anatomical element of tissue. The mRNA expression profiles, which comprise numerical values of relative expression levels for each gene in a list of several thousand, may then be analyzed using hierarchical clustering, or other algorithms that help the investigator to discern differences between stages or different modalities of disease. By performing large-scale sampling in tissues at risk for cancer, patterns may begin to emerge that are indicative of the early changes in the natural history of the disease.

Antibody Microarrays for the Simultaneous Detection of Hundreds of Tumor Antigens

Our ability to perform reliable measurements of circulating tumor antigens in serum has been limited by the technology available for reliable detection. The availability of ultra-sensitive assays based on immuno-RCA creates an opportunity for evaluating previously unrecognized circulating antigens that may serve as prognostic markers. A very promising format for the detection of multiple serum markers is the use of antibody microarrays. Methods have been described for the immobilization of hundreds of different antibodies on the surface of glass slides, using a standard microarray format.[40,41] As large batteries of antibodies become available for detection of important cancer biomarkers, one can envision the use of microarrays with hundreds of antibodies. Serum samples would be deposited on these microarrays, allowing antigens to bind specifically to each of the different immobilized antibodies. Detection could then be performed using an immuno-RCA sandwich assay. Sandwich assays performed on antibody microarrays should offer specificity equivalent to an ELISA, because the immobilized antibody serves to capture the antigen via a surface epitope, while a second specific antibody provides an additional molecular recognition event at a different epitope on the same antigen molecule. Assuming that the second (solution) antibody layer consists of a panel of mouse monoclonal antibodies, the detection system is completed by using a rabbit anti-mouse antibody (which will bind to all of the mouse monoclonals) tethered to an RCA primer. The ample linear dynamic range of immuno-RCA (five orders of magnitude) will facilitate the accurate quantification of cancer antigens present at widely different abundance levels. The practical feasibility of microarray-format assays employing RCA has already been demonstrated by a recent publication where a panel of multiple allergens was spotted on glass slides, and patient sera were tested for the presence of specific anti-allergen IgEs using an immuno-RCA detection system.[42]

Potential Utility of RCA and HRCA Based Methods for Biomarker Studies in Specific Cancers

An important feature of HRCA currently under development is the capability for real-time detection of multiplexed reactions. As is the case for PCR, real-time monitoring of HRCA reactions provides a capability of quantitative assays, where the kinetics of each reaction is recorded and related to the amount of starting

DNA target. As with PCR, such assays will permit quantitation over at least six orders of magnitude, and will be completed in a relatively brief time period. Such applications are likely to become commonplace as HRCA-specific instrumentation for real-time fluorescence detection becomes available.

Blood and bone marrow are easily accessible materials for tests on the status of hematologic tumors. Thus, DNA amplification by PCR has proven a powerful tool for the analysis of cancer markers with well defined sequence alterations, such as chromosomal translocations. Tests based on PCR or RT-PCR have the capability to detect a single cell harboring a translocation event in the context of a million normal cells. Assays for the presence of minimal residual disease have been employed after induction chemotherapy,[43,44] bone marrow transplantation,[45,46] and in the evaluation of either bone marrow or peripheral blood progenitor cell (PBPC) preparations for contamination by residual tumor cells. There is evidence that that low levels of residual disease detectable by PCR may be clinically significant with respect to risk of relapse. Most of the tests based on PCR assays could be performed using HRCA as a detection method. Like PCR, HRCA has the ability to amplify DNA present at a level of a few molecules per test sample. However, HRCA will require additional development efforts before its levels of sensitivity and reliability are competitive with PCR. An important potential advantage of HRCA is reduced cost, since the reaction does not require the use of expensive thermocycling equipment.

RT-PCR has also been used to evaluate the prognosis of melanoma patients who are clinically disease-free but likely to develop recurrent metastatic disease. The detection of circulating melanoma cells in blood is used as a surrogate marker of subclinical residual disease. Multimarker melanoma reverse transcriptase-PCR (RT-PCR) assay may incorporate primers for the detection of tyrosinase, MAGE-3, TRP-1, TRP-2 and several other candidate melanoma marker transcripts.[47] It is possible to design similar reverse transcriptase detection assays based on HRCA, instead of PCR. Like PCR, HRCA may be multiplexed, enabling detection of several target sequences in a single test tube assay.

Based on the literature, there are several molecular markers which might be used for the prognosis of breast cancer. Among possible molecular prognostic markers are: *BRCA-1, BRCA-2, p53,* and *erbB* oncogenes, loss of heterozygosity, microsatellite instability, transforming growth factor-α, and the multiple drug resistance (*MDR*) gene.[48] Fluid extruded from the nipple has been proposed as a surrogate sample, in lieu of a biopsy, that may facilitate assessment of cancer risk.[49] Microspot assays based on immuno-RCA would permit the simultaneous detection of dozens of breast prognostic protein markers in fluid from a small volume of nipple extrusion. As mentioned earlier, antibody microarrays will provide a format for evaluating hundreds of markers in a single assay. This approach will become more attractive as the number of prognostic biomarkers for cancer increases. Thus, a single universal microarray-based assay with hundreds of antibodies for specific cancer biomarkers could be implemented using a highly sensitive immuno-RCA sandwich detection system. Such a system could be used for assessment of biomarkers in several cancers, including breast, prostate, hepatic and gastrointestinal neoplasms.

REFERENCES

1. Seiden M, Sklar J. PCR- and RT-PCR-based methods of tumor detection: potential applications and clinical implications. In: DeVita VT Jr, Hellman S, Rosenberg SA, eds. Important Advances in Oncology. New York: Lippincott-Raven, 1996.
2. Pelkey T, Frierson H, Bruns D. Molecular and immunological detection of circulating tumor cells and micrometastases from solid tumors. Clin Chem 1996;42:1369–1381.
3. Ghossein RA, Rosai J. Polymerase chain reaction in the detection of micrometastases and circulating tumor cells. Cancer 1996;78:10–16.
4. Lizardi PM, Huang X, Zhu Z et al. Mutation detection and single-molecule counting using rolling-circle amplification. Nat Genet 1998;19:225–232.
5. Schweitzer B, Wiltshire S, Lambert J et al. Immunoassays with rolling circle amplification: a versatile platform for ultrasensitive antigen detection. Proc Natl Acad Sci USA 2000;97:10113–10119.
6. Raap AK. Advances in fluorescence in situ hybridization. Mutat Res 1998;400:287–298.
7. Zhong X, Lizardi PM, Huang X et al. Visualization of oligonucleotide probes and point mutations in interphase nuclei and DNA fibers using rolling circle amplification. Proc Natl Acad Sci USA, in press.
8. Gabert J, Thuret I, Lafage M et al. Detection of residual bcr/abl translocation by polymerase chain reaction in chronic myeloid leukaemia patients after bone-marrow transplantation. Lancet 1989; 11:1125.
9. Gerry NP, Witowski NE, Day J et al. Universal DNA microarray method for multiplex detection of low abundance point mutations. J Mol Biol 1999;292:251–262.
10. Luo J, Bergstrom D, Barany F. Improving the fidelity of *Thermos thermophilus* DNA ligase. Nucleic Acids Res 1996;24:3071–3078.
11. Ladner D, Leamon JH, Hamann S et al. Generic microarray with rolling circle amplification for high throughput detection of hotspot mutations. Lab Invest (submitted).
12. Bubendorf L, Kolmer M, Kononen J et al. Hormone therapy failure in human prostate cancer: analysis by complementary DNA and tissue microarrays. J Natl Cancer Inst 1999;91:1758–1764.
13. Duggan DJ, Bittner M, Chen Y, et al. Expression profiling using cDNA microarrays. Nat Genet 1999;21[suppl]:10–14.
14. Perou C, Jeffery SS, van de Rijn M et al. Distinctive gene expression patterns in human mammary epithelial cells and breast cancers. Proc Natl Acad Sci USA 1999;96:9212–9217.
15. Yang GP, Ross DT, Kuang WW, et al. Combining SSH and cDNA microarrays for rapid identification of differentially expressed genes. Nucleic Acids Res 1999;27:1517–1523.
16. Alizadeh AA, Eisen MB, Davis RE et al. Distinct types of diffuse large B-cell lymphoma identified by gene expression profiling. Nature 2000;403:503–511.
17. Phillips J, Eberwine JH. Antisense RNA amplification: a linear amplification method for analyzing the mRNA population from single living cells. Methods 1996;10:283–288.
18. Pollack JR, Perou CM, Alizadeh AA et al. Genome-wide analysis of DNA copy-number changes using cDNA microarrays. Nat Genet 1999;23:41–46.
19. Kallioniemi A, Kallioniemi OP, Sudar D et al. Comparative genomic hybridization for molecular cytogenetic analysis of solid tumors. Science 1992;258:818–821.

20. Loveday R, Greenman J, Simcox DL et al. Genetic changes in breast cancer detected by comparative genomic hybridization. Int J Cancer 2000;86:494–500.
21. Nupponen N, Visakorpi T. Molecular biology of progression of prostate cancer. Eur Urol 1999; 35:351–354.
22. Bova GS, Isaacs WB. Review of allelic loss and gain in prostate cancer. World J Urol 1996;14: 338–346.
23. Pinkel D, Segraves R, Sudar D et al. High resolution analysis of DNA copy number variation using comparative genomic hybridization to microarrays. Nat Genet 1998;20:207–211.
24. Solinas-Toldo S, Lampel S, Stilgenbauer S et al. Matrix-based comparative genomic hybridization: biochips to screen for genomic imbalances. Genes Chromosomes Cancer 1997;20:399–407.
25. Lichter P, Joos S, Bentz M, Lampel S. Comparative genomic hybridization: uses and limitations. Semin Hematol 2000;37:348–357.
26. Wang E, Miller LD, Ohnmacht GA, et al. High-fidelity mRNA amplification for gene profiling. Nat Biotechnol 2000;18:457–459.
27. Geiss GK, Bumgarner RE, An MC et al. Large-scale monitoring of host cell gene expression during HIV-1 infection using cDNA microarrays. Virology 2000;266:8–16.
28. Aubele M, Mattis A, Zitzelsberger H et al. Extensive ductile carcinoma in situ with small foci of invasive ductal carcinoma: evidence of genetic resemblance by CGH. Int J Cancer 2000;85:82–86.
29. Telenius H, Carter NP, Bebb CE. Degenerate oligonucleotide-primed PCR: general amplification of target DNA by a single degenerate primer. Genomics 1992;13:718–725.
30. Zhang L, Cui X, Schmitt K et al. Whole genome amplification from a single cell: implications for genetic analysis. Proc Natl Acad Sci USA 1992;89:5847–5851.
31. Barrett MT, Reid BJ, Joslyn G. Genotypic analysis of multiple loci in somatic cells by whole genome amplification. Nucleic Acids Res 1995;23:3488–3492.
32. Thomas D, Nardone G, Randall S. Amplification of padlock probes for DNA diagnostics by cascade rolling circle amplification or the polymerase chain reaction. Arch Pathol Lab Med 1999;123: 1170–1176.
33. Clark Z, Pickering J. Sniper: A fully automated, fluorescence platform incorporating rolling circle amplification for scalable, high-throughput SNP scoring. Amersham Pharmacia Biotech Life Science News 2000;6:18–21.
34. Catalona WJ, Smith DS, Wolfert RL et al. Evaluation of percentage of free serum prostate-specific antigen to improve specificity of prostate cancer screening. JAMA 1995;274:1214–1220.
35. Lu-Yao GL, McLerran D, Wasson J, Wennberg JE. An assessment of radical prostatectomy. Time trends, geographic variation, and outcomes. The Prostate Patient Outcomes Research Team. JAMA 1993;269:2633–2636.
36. Beckett ML, Cazares LH, Vlahou A et al. Prostate-specific membrane antigen levels in sera from healthy men and patients with benign prostate hyperplasia or prostate cancer. Clin Cancer Res 1999;5:4034–4040.
37. Werther K, Normark M, Hansen BF et al. The use of the CELLection kit in the isolation of carcinoma cells from mononuclear cell suspensions. J Immunol Methods 2000;238:133–141.
38. Nilsson M, Barbany G, Antson DO et al. Enhanced detection and distinction of RNA by enzymatic probe ligation. Nat Biotechnol 2000;18:791–793.
39. Bonner RF, Emmert-Buck M, Cole K et al. Laser capture microdissection: molecular analysis of tissue. Science 1997;278:1481–1483.
40. Ekins RP. Ligand assays: from electrophoresis to miniaturized microarrays. Clin Chem 1998;44: 2015–2030.

41. MacBeath G, Schreiber S. Printing proteins as microarrays for high-throughput function determination. Science 2000;289:1760–1763.
42. Wiltshire S, O'Malley S, Lambert J et al. Detection of multiple allergen-specific IgEs on microarrays by immunoassays with rolling circle amplification. Clin Chem 2000;46:1990–1993.
43. Pallisgaard N, Clausen N, Schroder H, Hokland P. Rapid and sensitive minimal residual disease detection in acute leukemia by quantitative real-time RT-PCR exemplified by t(12;21) TEL-AML1 fusion transcript. Genes Chromosomes Cancer 1999;26:355–365.
44. Koller E, Karlic H, Krieger O et al. Early detection of minimal residual disease by reverse transcriptase polymerase chain reaction predicts relapse in acute promyelocytic leukemia. Ann Hematol 1995;70:75–78.
45. Drobyski WR, Baxter-Lowe LA, Truitt RL. Detection of residual leukemia by the polymerase chain reaction and sequence-specific oligonucleotide probe hybridization after allogeneic bone marrow transplantation for AKR leukemia: a murine model for minimal residual disease. Blood 1993;81:551–559.
46. Martinelli G, Montefusco V, Testoni N et al. Clinical value of quantitative long-term assessment of bcr-abl chimeric transcript in chronic myelogenous leukemia patients after allogeneic bone marrow transplantation. Haematologica 2000;85:653–658.
47. Hoon DS, Bostick P, Kuo C et al. Molecular markers in blood as surrogate prognostic indicators of melanoma recurrence. Cancer Res 2000;60:2253–2257.
48. Dahiya R, Deng G. Molecular prognostic markers in breast cancer. Breast Cancer Res Treat 1998;52:185–200.
49. Fabian CJ, Kimler BF, Zalles CM et al. Short-term breast cancer prediction by random periareolar fine-needle aspiration cytology and the Gail risk model. J Natl Cancer Inst 2000;2:1217–1227.

Influencing the Apoptotic Mechanism in Cancer Treatment

Rebecca L. Elstrom

Craig B. Thompson

In just over a decade, our understanding of the role of cell death regulation in cancer pathogenesis has progressed dramatically. Although studies initially focused on understanding unregulated growth in cancer cells, researchers have come to understand that abnormal control of cell death also plays a critical role in the development of malignancies.

The idea that genes involved in regulating cell death might play a role in carcinogenesis first arose from studies to characterize a particular chromosomal translocation found in follicular lymphoma.[1] This translocation juxtaposed the B-cell lymphoma-2 (*Bcl-2*) gene on chromosome 18 with the immunoglobulin heavy-chain enhancer on chromosome 14. This translocation results in the overexpression of the Bcl-2 protein in B cells. Subsequent identification of the function of the Bcl-2 gene product as an inhibitor of programmed cell death,[2,3] rather than of proliferation, suggested a novel mechanism of tumorigenesis. A universal problem for multicellular organisms is the requirement for a mechanism by which to maintain appropriate balance between cell types.

Programmed cell death, or apoptosis, allows the loss of cells that either are not needed during development or may be dangerous to the organism because of mutation or other damage. Inhibition of the normal processes that control cell death may result in retention of damaged or mutated cells, contributing to tumor development. Apoptosis control mechanisms appear to be impaired in virtually all tumors, suggesting that it is imperative to cancer development to disengage the apoptotic machinery. Reactivating latent apoptotic pathways could result in the development of novel forms of cancer therapy.

MECHANISMS

The final common events in apoptosis involve activation of caspases, a family of proteins that act in a cascade to cleave cellular substrates, resulting in the characteristic morphology of apoptotic cells, including cell shrinkage, membrane bleb formation, nuclear condensation, and DNA fragmentation. Caspases are cysteine proteases with aspartate specificity and normally exist in the cell in an inactive zymogen form. The proximal procaspases 8 and 9 become activated by cellular signals (discussed later) and subsequently cleave and activate downstream effector caspases, including caspases 3, 6, and 7. These active effector caspases then cleave a variety of substrates, including structural proteins, proteins involved in signal transduction, components of the cell cycle machinery, and DNA repair proteins.

Cell Death by Murder

Two major pathways are involved in the induction of apoptosis, the first involving cell surface receptor–ligand interaction. Receptors responsible for mediating programmed cell death belong to the tumor necrosis factor receptor (TNFR) family. Members of this family contain intracellular "death domains," which are critical for transduction of the apoptotic signal. The best-studied examples of this family include TNFR1 and Fas, which are activated by binding of their respective ligands, TNF and FasL. On activation, these receptors associate with intracellular adaptor molecules via each molecule's respective death domain, allowing the N-terminal effector domain of the adaptor to interact with proximal caspases or other downstream signaling molecules. Fas-associated death domain (FADD) protein binds to the Fas molecule[4] and subsequently recruits caspase 8, resulting in its oligomerization, self-processing, and activation. FADD also plays a role in TNFR1 activation, binding through the TNFR-associated death domain (TRADD) protein[5] and, again, allowing for activation of caspase 8 (Fig. 5.1). The importance of this pathway in physiologic circumstances is demonstrated by the finding that caspase 8 is deleted or silenced by methylation in many childhood neuroblastomas.[6] These cells are resistant to receptor-mediated cell death, and replacement of caspase 8 in these cells with a retroviral expression vector restored sensitivity to TNF-α-induced apoptosis.

In addition to the caspase-mediated death signal induced by this molecule, TNFR1 can also activate downstream signaling and gene transcription via binding of tumor necrosis factor receptor-associated factors (TRAFs). TRAF1 and TRAF2

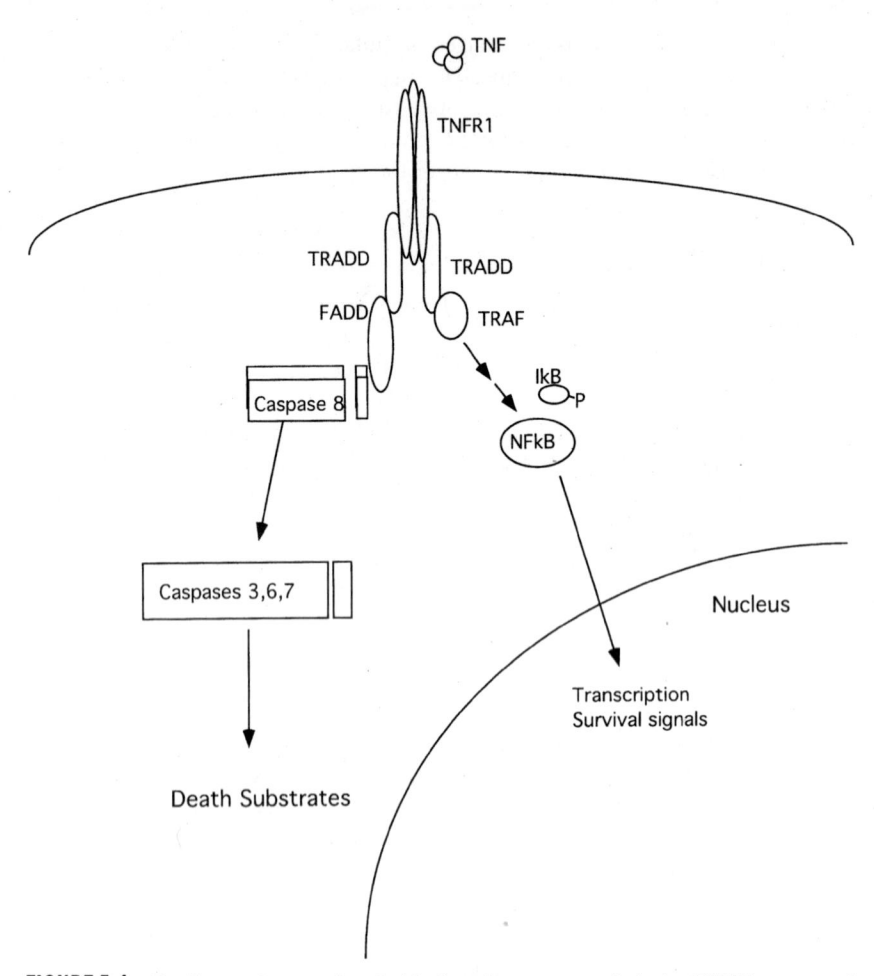

FIGURE 5.1 Death receptor complex. On binding of tumor necrosis factor, TNFR1 can associate with FADD via the adaptor TRADD. FADD subsequently binds caspase 8, leading to its oligomerization, cleavage, and activation. Activated caspase 8 then activates downstream effector caspases. Alternatively, TRADD may bind a TRAF molecule, initiating a signaling cascade that ultimately results in phosphorylation of IκB with release and translocation of NF-κB to the nucleus, activating transcription of survival promoting genes.

can bind to TRADD in place of FADD, resulting in downstream activation of Jun N-terminal kinase (JNK) and nuclear factor κB (NF-κB).[7,8] In most cell types, JNK promotes and amplifies the proapoptotic signal. NF-κB, on the other hand, is able to counteract the apoptotic action of caspases and JNK. Inhibition of transcription or protein synthesis has been shown to enhance TNF-induced cell death, and this effect is mediated by blocking NF-κB-induced up-regulation of apoptosis inhibitors such as TRAFs[9] and inhibitor-of-apoptosis proteins (IAPs).[10]

This suggests that the end result for the cell of TNF signaling depends on a complex balance of proapoptotic and antiapoptotic factors.

The TNF-related apoptosis inducing ligand (TRAIL) is a third TNF family member that induces apoptosis in many cell types.[11,12] TRAIL binds to its receptors, DR4 and DR5, and also induces cell death via a caspase cascade. The interaction of TRAIL with these ligands is, under certain circumstances, antagonized by a group of decoy receptors that are able to bind TRAIL but do not activate an apoptotic response.[13,14] These decoy receptors are expressed in many normal tissues and have been found to be overexpressed in some tumor types, including a subset of lung and colon tumors.[15] Loss of death receptors or their associated signaling adapters can render cells resistant to mechanisms imposed by neighboring cells or by immune cells that would limit cell accumulation. Furthermore, it has been proposed that once a cancer cell line has sustained a mutation in these pathways, production of the ligand may be selected, inducing death of neighboring cells and promoting invasion and metastasis.[16]

Cell Death by Suicide

The second major pathway of apoptosis involves the mitochondria (Fig. 5.2). Release of cytochrome c from mitochondria to the cytoplasm has been shown to result in caspase activation[17] and, in experimental models, introduction of exogenous cytochrome c will induce the same effect, demonstrating the importance of this molecule in the pathway. Once released, cytochrome c binds to apoptotic protease activating factor-1 (Apaf-1),[18] a molecule that contains a domain homologous to caspase prodomains, known as a *caspase recruitment domain*. In conjunction with adenosine triphosphate, the cytochrome c–Apaf-1 complex binds to and stimulates activation of caspase 9,[19] which subsequently cleaves caspase 3 to its active form, initiating the downstream caspase cascade.

The mechanism by which cytochrome c, a protein that normally resides in the mitochondrial intermembrane space, is released into the cytosol is controversial. One possible mechanism involves outer membrane rupture in response to matrix swelling. This swelling could occur because of disruption of mitochondrial metabolism and failure of electron transport due to substrate limitations, as may be seen in hypoxic cells or those lacking growth factor signals.[20,21] Alternatively, cytochrome c release could occur through alterations in membrane permeability induced by proapoptotic molecules, such as the Bcl-2-related molecule Bax (discussed later). Whatever the exact mechanism, the end result is that large molecules that normally reside in the intermembrane space are nonspecifically released into the cytoplasm, initiating an apoptotic cascade within the cell. Irradiation, ultraviolet light, and p53 activation have all been shown to initiate apoptosis through this mitochondrion-dependent mechanism.

Multiple factors have been identified that contribute to regulation of the death process. Bcl-2 family members are among the first identified and best studied of

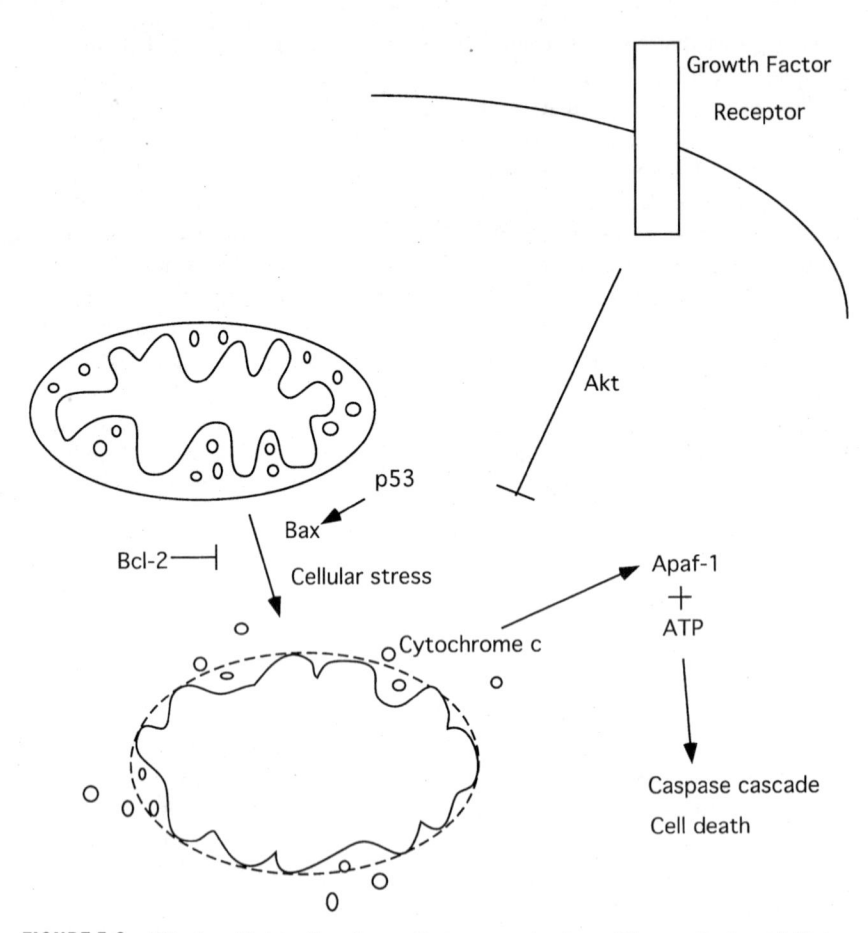

FIGURE 5.2 Mitochondrial death pathway. Under normal cell conditions, mitochondrial integrity is maintained with active respiration. Under conditions of cellular stress, homeostasis may be maintained by antiapoptotic Bcl-2 proteins such as Bcl-x$_L$ or through activity of Akt. Mitochondrial homeostasis may be disrupted either by compromise of oxidative phosphorylation or by activity of proapoptotic molecules such as Bax or Bad. Under these circumstances, outer membrane integrity is lost and cytochrome c is released into the cytoplasm, initiating the apoptotic cascade.

these factors and can be divided into two groups: those that inhibit apoptosis and those that promote it. Bcl-2 was identified first as a molecule that promoted survival in follicular lymphoma cells, and a related protein, Bcl-x$_L$, has a similar function.[22] Although the mechanism by which these molecules protect cells from apoptosis has not been fully elucidated, several characteristics are clear. Some members of the Bcl-2 family are able to form channels in lipid bilayers,[23] suggesting a potential role in regulating mitochondrial membrane permeability and, therefore, mitochondrial homeostasis. One proposal suggests that Bcl-2 proteins regulate the exchange of cytoplasmic adenosine diphosphate for mitochondrial adenosine triphosphate, maintaining homeostasis in periods of metabolic stress.

Proapoptotic Bcl-2 family members, on the other hand, promote cell death by destabilizing mitochondria. One of these molecules, Bax, is able also to form membrane channels.[24] Bax normally resides in the cell cytoplasm but, under conditions of cellular stress, can be translocated to the outer mitochondrial membrane.[25] Whether Bax acts by changing membrane permeability in a destructive fashion, forms part of a channel allowing release of cytochrome c and other intermembrane space components directly, or acts by some other mechanism is not clear. Other proapoptotic members of this family have been proposed to contribute to death by binding Bcl-2 or Bcl-xL and compromising their function. Bad, for example, is thought to regulate apoptosis in this fashion. Bad is inactivated through phosphorylation by Akt,[26] a key negative regulator of cell death that is discussed later.

Other factors have been identified that regulate programmed cell death downstream of the mitochondria. IAPs were identified initially in the *Baculovirus* genome as inhibitors of host apoptosis,[27,28] and endogenous cellular homologs have since been described.[29-31] These IAPs act by binding to and inhibiting activation of caspase 9 and may be capable of inhibiting already activated caspases. Experiments in *Drosophila melanogaster* demonstrated the presence of yet another class of regulatory molecules, members of which were able to promote cell death by antagonizing the effect of IAPs. Mammalian homologs of these proteins, termed Smac[32,33] or DIABLO, have recently been described, and it was shown that they act by binding IAPs, thus preventing IAPs from inhibiting caspases.

REGULATION OF APOPTOSIS

Akt/Protein Kinase B

To date, no one has identified a cell, including a cancer cell, that lacks caspases entirely, suggesting that activation of the cell's intrinsic apoptotic pathway must be constantly suppressed. Nearly all cells appear to require extrinsic signals, and signaling by survival factors such as growth factor promotes cell survival through suppression of apoptosis. Several signaling pathways effecting this suppression have been elucidated. The serine-threonine kinase Akt, or protein kinase B, appears to play a key role in regulating survival. Akt promotes cell survival by acting in a pathway initiated by cell surface signaling of growth factors such as insulin-like growth factor (IGF-1) and platelet-derived growth factor, which in turn activate phosphatidylinositol 3-OH kinase (PI3K). PI3K phosphorylates inositol substrates at the 3 position, producing phosphatidylinositol-3,4,5-triphosphate (PIP3). PIP3, in turn, promotes activation of Akt through phosphatidylinositol-dependent kinases, including 3-phosphoinositide-dependent kinase 1

(PDK-1) and integrin-linked kinase (ILK).[34,35] Activated Akt exerts antiapoptotic activity through multiple mechanisms. It is able to inhibit cytochrome c release from the mitochondria through a still unclear mechanism.[36] In addition, Akt phosphorylates and inactivates the proapoptotic Bcl-2 family member Bad,[26] as well as caspase 9.[37] Forkhead transcription factors have been shown to activate genes important in apoptosis, such as Fas ligand. Recently, Akt was found to phosphorylate and inactivate a member of this transcription factor family, FKHRL1,[38] suggesting yet another target of its prosurvival function.

Given its central role in promoting cell survival, regulation of Akt itself would be expected to play an important role in control of cell death. Phosphatase and tensin homolog deleted from chromosome 10 (PTEN) is a critical mediator of this regulation. PTEN is a phosphatase that acts on both protein and lipid substrates. PIP3 appears to be among the key in vivo substrates of this phosphatase, placing PTEN at a critical regulatory point in Akt activation.[39] In this context, PTEN's function is to control levels of PIP3. Loss of PTEN function allows excessive activation of Akt and resistance of the cell to death stimuli. *PTEN resides on the long arm of chromosome 10, a region that has been shown to suffer loss of heterozygosity in many human cancers.* This gene frequently is mutated or deleted in many human tumors, particularly glioblastoma multiforme, in which its tumor suppressor function was first described.[40,41] Multiple other tumor types, including prostate cancer, breast cancer, and melanoma, frequently lack normal PTEN function. Restoration of wild-type PTEN expression in tumor cell lines restores sensitivity to apoptosis.[42] Homozygous loss of PTEN function usually is a late event in tumorigenesis, but loss of one allele is frequent even in early-stage cancers. In this context it is interesting that, in a mouse model, heterozygotes show abnormal apoptosis and severe autoimmunity,[43] suggesting that PTEN function within a cell may be dose-dependent and that haploinsufficiency of this molecule may play an important role in tumor development.

The importance of unregulated Akt activity in oncogenesis was further suggested recently by the finding that *TCL-1*, a gene frequently activated in T-cell prolymphocytic leukemia by translocation into proximity with components of the T-cell receptor, associates with and facilitates Akt activation.[44]

p53 and Apoptosis

p53 is one of the most extensively studied components of programmed cell death. That it plays a central role in tumorigenesis has been clear since the realization that more than half of human tumors contain mutations in the *p53* gene. p53 is a transcription factor that, under normal circumstances, is held at low concentration in the cell. p53 levels are controlled in large part by MDM2, a protein that binds to and promotes degradation of p53 through ubiquitin-mediated proteolysis.[45,46] It has also been suggested recently that MDM2 binding may lead to the export of p53 from the nucleus, abrogating its ability to transactivate its targets.[47]

p53 activation must be induced through the sensing of various situations of cellular stress, such as DNA damage, hypoxia, or limited nucleic acid substrates. The mechanism by which p53 becomes activated appears to be related to phosphorylation, which destabilizes its interaction with MDM2,[48] but the details of this process remain under investigation. On activation, however, p53 transactivates a set of genes that are involved in cell cycle arrest,[49] including *p21 (WAF1/Cip1)* and *GADD45*. p53 also promotes activation of genes involved in apoptosis, including *Bax, Fas, Noxa* (a novel Bcl-2-related proapoptotic protein),[50] *DR5*, and *IGF-BP3*. IGF-BP3 blocks the signaling pathway induced by IGF by binding to its receptor and therefore lowers the threshold for apoptosis. In addition to its activity in transcriptional activation, p53 has been shown to participate in protein-protein interactions, but the significance of these interactions in regulation of cell death remains unclear.

In addition to MDM2, the tumor suppressor p14ARF plays a critical role in regulation of the p53 pathway. p14ARF is encoded by the *INK4a* gene,[51] which also codes for the p16INK4a cell cycle–regulating protein. p14ARF exerts its tumor suppressor effect by regulating the inhibitory activity of MDM2 on p53.[52-54] p14ARF binds directly to MDM2 and blocks its effects on p53, including ubiquitination of p53, transport of p53 out of the nucleus, and inhibition of p53 transcriptional activation. Transcription of p14ARF appears to be repressed by p53, whereas MDM2 transcription is directly activated by p53, suggesting a negative-feedback regulatory mechanism. Overexpression or activation of oncogenes, such as *c-myc*, induces apoptosis via increased levels of p53. The mechanism by which p53 is increased in this situation appears to be related to activation of p14ARF expression[55] by the inappropriate mitogenic signals seen by the cell in the presence of the activated oncogene.

p53 inactivation is well documented in many human tumors. The most common mutation involves a point mutation in the DNA-binding domain of p53, and this results in stabilization and accumulation of the mutant protein. Deletions also are commonly seen. The effects of p53 can be disrupted in the absence of its mutation by disruption of other components of the pathway. For example, *MDM2* amplification has been demonstrated in a significant subset of sarcomas.[56] Mutation or deletion of the *INK4a* locus is a frequent occurrence, particularly in human tumors in which p53 inactivation is less commonly seen, such as mesothelioma.[57] Loss of p14ARF expression would lead to uncontrolled MDM2 activity and functional inactivation of p53.

DNA Damage and Apoptosis: Beyond *p53*

For p53 to carry out its role of cell cycle arrest and apoptosis in response to DNA damage, that damage must be sensed by the cell and a signal relayed to activate p53. Several factors involved in this DNA damage checkpoint have been identified, including products of genes that are seen mutated in primary tumors.

These include the ataxia telangiectasia mutated (*ATM*)[58] and *ATM*-related (*ATR*) genes.[59] The hereditary disorder ataxia-telangiectasia is associated with a predisposition to cancer, particularly in the lymphoid lineage, which is related to the lack of a functional *ATM* gene product. The ATM protein is a serine–threonine kinase that is activated by DNA damage, subsequently leading to phosphorylation and derepression of p53. Although initial studies suggested direct phosphorylation of p53 by ATM, more recent investigations have raised the likelihood that ATM acts indirectly, through an intermediary kinase. One potential candidate for this role is Chk2, which has been shown to be necessary for p53 activation in vivo and can directly phosphorylate p53 in vitro.[60]

Another key component of the apoptotic response to DNA damage is *BRCA1*. *BRCA1* is the most common gene implicated in hereditary breast cancer, with approximately 50% of inherited mutations that predispose to breast cancer mapping to the *BRCA1* locus. The product of the *BRCA1* gene is a nuclear protein that is phosphorylated in response to DNA damage. Although the mechanisms by which BRCA1 functions are not completely clear, it appears to play a role in induction of apoptosis through transcriptional activation. Like p53, BRCA1 activation appears to depend on functional ATM.[61]

CANCER THERAPY: DISRUPTION AND RESTORATION OF APOPTOTIC MECHANISMS

The presence of multiple pathways for induction of programmed cell death in response to perturbation of normal growth and cell cycle, along with the fact that these pathways must be disabled in parallel for productive tumorigenesis, suggests that therapies directed at influencing or restoring the cancer cells' innate death pathways could play a role in anticancer therapy. The disruption of key factors involved in apoptosis in various tumor types has led many investigators to pursue this issue.

Chemotherapy Response and Resistance

Cancer chemotherapeutic agents have traditionally been believed to exert their antitumor effect through toxicity leading to necrosis. More recently, however, our understanding of the importance of programmed cell death in tumorigenesis, as well as further understanding of the mechanisms of chemotherapeutic agents, has led to the proposal that these drugs function by activating the cell's own apoptotic pathways. Glucocorticoids, for example, play a central role in the treatment of lymphoma, and they act by inducing apoptosis in both normal and malignant lymphocytes. The mechanism by which glucocorticoids act, however, has remained a mystery. A recent report described the translocation of a type of steroid hormone receptor to the mitochondria, with resultant direct release of cytochrome c,[62] but the physiologic relevance of this pathway remains to be determined.

Loss of apoptotic pathways in cancer cells can be associated not only with tumor progression but also with resistance to therapy. For example, topoisomerase inhibitors, such as etoposide, cause the topoisomerase molecule to become covalently bound to the DNA strand, resulting in a double-strand break in the DNA. With an intact DNA damage–sensing and –response mechanism, this modification will induce apoptosis in the cell. In a cell with a mutated or inactive *p53*, however, the cell may succeed in completing the cell cycle and continue growing in the presence of the break, thereby introducing more replication infidelity and perhaps even gross chromosomal abnormalities. Other antineoplastic chemotherapeutic agents also depend on apoptosis to achieve their full benefits. Loss of p14ARF has been shown to make cells resistant to the effects of ionizing radiation and doxorubicin, for example. Similarly, in a mouse model of *Myc*-induced lymphoma, mutation of *p53* or *p14ARF* made tumors dramatically less responsive to cyclophosphamide.[63]

Fas/FasL interaction may be important in tumor response to some chemotherapeutic agents. For example, paclitaxel treatment has been suggested to kill cells at least partially through a Fas/FasL mechanism,[64] and other drugs such as doxorubicin, methotrexate, and cisplatin have been shown in some systems to induce FasL expression.[65,66] The mechanism by which FasL expression is induced is not clear, but correlation between decreased FasL response and drug resistance has been seen.

Given the importance of Bcl-2 and Bcl-x_L in preventing apoptosis, it is not surprising that these molecules have an effect on the susceptibility of cancer cells to chemotherapy. This resistance has been demonstrated in multiple cases. For example, a study correlating response of ovarian cancer to cisplatin-based chemotherapy revealed a significantly poorer initial response to therapy and overall survival in women with tumors that overexpressed Bcl-2.[67] In addition, a mouse model evaluating the effect of Bcl-x_L overexpression on mammary tumors showed marked resistance of the tumors to methotrexate and 5-fluorouracil.[68] Strategies to overcome the effects of these molecules or to bypass their activity in apoptotic pathways represent an important focus of investigation.

One tactic that has been used to address this issue is the use of antisense oligonucleotides. Leech et al[69] showed inhibition of Bcl-x_L expression using an antisense oligonucleotide, and an increase in apoptosis accompanied this inhibition in non–small cell lung cancer (NSCLC) cell lines studied in vitro. Clinical studies evaluating a Bcl-2 antisense oligonucleotide in acute myeloid leukemia and acute lymphoblastic leukemia are currently being initiated.

Another component of the death pathway that can affect the susceptibility of cancer cells to chemotherapy involves the transcription factor NF-κB. As previously discussed, NF-κB activation promotes antideath mechanisms in cells. Treatment with some chemotherapeutic agents, such as irinotecan (CPT-11), daunorubicin, and mitoxantrone,[70] results in activation of NF-κB-mediated transcription, correlating with reduced sensitivity of cancer cells to therapy. The importance of NF-κB-mediated resistance was emphasized in a recent study revealing abrogation of resistance to CPT-11 by adenoviral transfer of the NF-κB repressor IκB.[71]

The importance of apoptosis in the response of cancer cells to therapy is not universally accepted. Some argue that tumor cell death is the result of a toxic insult that compromises the viability of the cell directly, without engaging apoptosis. Evidence for this direct effect has been derived from the fact that, particularly in radiation therapy, death is not always instantaneous, but rather cells lose the ability to divide over several generations. This loss of clonogenicity is believed to demonstrate the effect of damage that compromises viability over time rather than resulting in abrupt cell suicide. Furthermore, mechanisms of resistance to therapy have long been proposed that are not related to loss of apoptotic mechanisms. For example, changes in drug metabolism, cellular uptake and excretion of drug, and cellular targets are believed to be important in at least some cases of chemotherapeutic drug resistance. Probably both apoptotic and nonapoptotic mechanisms can be involved in response and resistance of tumors to therapy.

Influencing the Apoptotic Mechanism in Cancer Treatment

Given the critical importance of programmed cell death in the response of tumors to therapy, researchers are actively investigating means by which to reactivate apoptotic pathways in cancer cells. These strategies could be used as primary therapy or in combination with traditional anticancer therapies to induce sensitization.

Death Receptor Activation The receptor-ligand pathway presents a straightforward target for activating apoptosis. TNF and FasL have been investigated as systemic therapy, but the toxicity profiles of these cytokines are unacceptable, causing massive immune activation and hemorrhagic lesions in various organs, particularly the liver. TRAIL, on the other hand, has been investigated as an anticancer agent in mice and primates and appears to have a much more tolerable side effect profile, inducing apoptosis in cancer cells and regression of tumors while exerting minimal effect on normal cells.[72,73] This specificity has been attributed to the presence of decoy receptors in normal but not most neoplastic tissues or, alternatively, to intracellular caspase inhibitors.[74] However, a recent study of the effects of TRAIL on human hepatocytes, which showed significant killing, has raised the concern that humans may be more susceptible to TRAIL-induced liver damage than were previously studied species.[75] Further investigation will be required to evaluate the safety of this potentially important anticancer agent.

Targeting Mitochondria Other investigators have focused on the mitochondrion as a target of therapy. Lonidamine, a derivative of indazole-3-carboxylic acid, has recently been used in combination regimens in metastatic breast cancer[76,77] and advanced NSCLC,[78] demonstrating improved response rates for both tumor types and improved survival in NSCLC. It has been suggested that this drug acts directly on mitochondria to effect a loss of mitochondrial membrane potential and cytochrome c release.[79] However, with the release of recent data that loss of mitochondrial membrane potential is a late event in apoptosis,[20,36,80] the possibility of this being a secondary effect remains. The synthetic retinoid CD437, which shows activity against multiple types of cancer cell lines in vitro, has also been described to induce apoptosis, in part via a direct interaction with mitochondria,[81,82] but the exact mechanism by which this occurs is unclear.

Another strategy targeting mitochondria in therapy involves gene transfer of the proapoptotic molecule Bax via an adenoviral vector. Overexpression of Bax was found, in ovarian cancer cells, both to induce apoptosis directly and to sensitize the cells to chemotherapy.[83] Questions of safety and specificity will need to be addressed before this tactic achieves clinical relevance, however.

Modulation of the PTEN/Akt Pathway The common finding of PTEN disruption in many tumors has suggested the PTEN/Akt pathway as another potentially valuable therapeutic target. Again, gene therapy strategies are under investigation to replace PTEN in cancers in which its function has been lost. Persad et al[84] have taken a novel approach to this issue by investigating inhibition of ILK in PTEN-mutant prostate cancer cells. They demonstrated that introduction of a dominant-negative ILK suppressed Akt phosphorylation and stimulated cell cycle arrest and subsequent apoptosis in these cells.[84] This result suggests that pharmacologic kinase inhibition may demonstrate success as a therapeutic approach.

Strategies to inhibit PI3K also are under investigation. Razzini et al[85] have investigated the use of synthetic inositol phosphates on PI3K and its downstream targets. They found that inositol 1,3,4,5,6-pentakiphosphate and inositol 1,4,5,6-tetrakiphosphate effectively antagonized PI3K and inhibited Akt by competing with PIP3, and these drugs can inhibit colony formation and proliferation in breast cancer and small cell lung cancer cell lines. Using another approach, Hu et al[86] targeted PI3K directly using the kinase inhibitor LY294002. They found marked inhibition of ovarian cancer progression in athymic mice treated intraperitoneally, and this was correlated with significant apoptosis of the carcinoma cells.

The p53 Pathway in Treatment The *p53* pathway has presented a potentially useful target of therapy, given its almost uniform disruption in cancer. In cancers with disruption or mutation of the p53 molecule itself, gene therapy has been under active investigation. In theory, a cell whose survival depends on a loss of p53 would be easily disposed of if the molecule could be replaced. The difficulties inherent in gene therapy are well illustrated in this context, however. To be effective in eradicating a tumor, the vector would have to reach all of the involved cells. In addition, the safety of gene therapy, especially using viral vectors (which have been most commonly studied), has yet to be demonstrated. Although still an intriguing possibility, this type of replacement therapy requires significant optimization.

Another interesting strategy that is under investigation and targets *p53*-mutant tumors is direct adenoviral cytotoxicity. The adenovirus depends for its pathogenicity on binding of p53 by the viral protein E1B, which allows viral replication. An adenovirus strain lacking the E1B molecule could be expected to infect productively and lyse only those cells lacking wild-type p53, such as many cancer cells, and preliminary in vitro studies have shown promising results.[87] The theoretic objection may be raised that normal cells expressing p53 may be induced to undergo apoptosis by viral infection in the absence of E1B, resulting in significant potential toxicity. Preliminary studies have shown contradictory results,[87,88] and clarification of this matter will require further investigation. Intralesional therapy with this adenovirus construct has shown promising results in accessible tumors.[89] The directed intralesional delivery makes systemic toxicity much less of a concern. The difficulties of delivering virus to every tumor cell may limit the curative potential of this therapy, but significant palliation may be accomplished.

A unique characteristic of p53 mutations in many cancers is that the inactivating point mutation inhibits ubiquitin-mediated proteolysis, resulting in accumulation of the p53 protein in cancer cells. These mutations also reduce the thermodynamic stability of the DNA-binding domain of p53, destabilizing the active conformation of the molecule. Recently, investigators have studied the possibility of pharmacologically stabilizing the active conformation of the DNA-binding domain. Foster et al[90] identified a group of small molecules, typified by the compound CP-31398, that is able to stabilize mutant p53 in its active conformation, and they have shown tumor responsiveness in a nude mouse model using *p53*-mutant human tumor xenografts (Fig. 5.3). The safety and clinical utility of this type of molecule in human cancers is being evaluated.

The other key components of the p53 pathway, MDM2 and p14ARF, have also presented targets of anticancer therapy. Antisense RNA has been evaluated in inhibiting MDM2 protein expression, and several investigators have found this strategy to induce apoptosis effectively in MDM2-overexpressing tumor cells.[91,92] Although antisense as a therapy in vivo presents significant logistic difficulties, its success in vitro raises hopes that the identification of a pharmacologic inhibitor of MDM2 could also be of significant interest. It can be imagined that this strategy would be useful also in tumors demonstrating a loss of p14ARF.

CONCLUSION

Our growing understanding of the processes required for a cell to become malignant has provided increasing insight into potential tools to combat cancer. Although much is understood about the mechanisms of programmed cell death and the significance of their disruption in cancer, clearly further research is

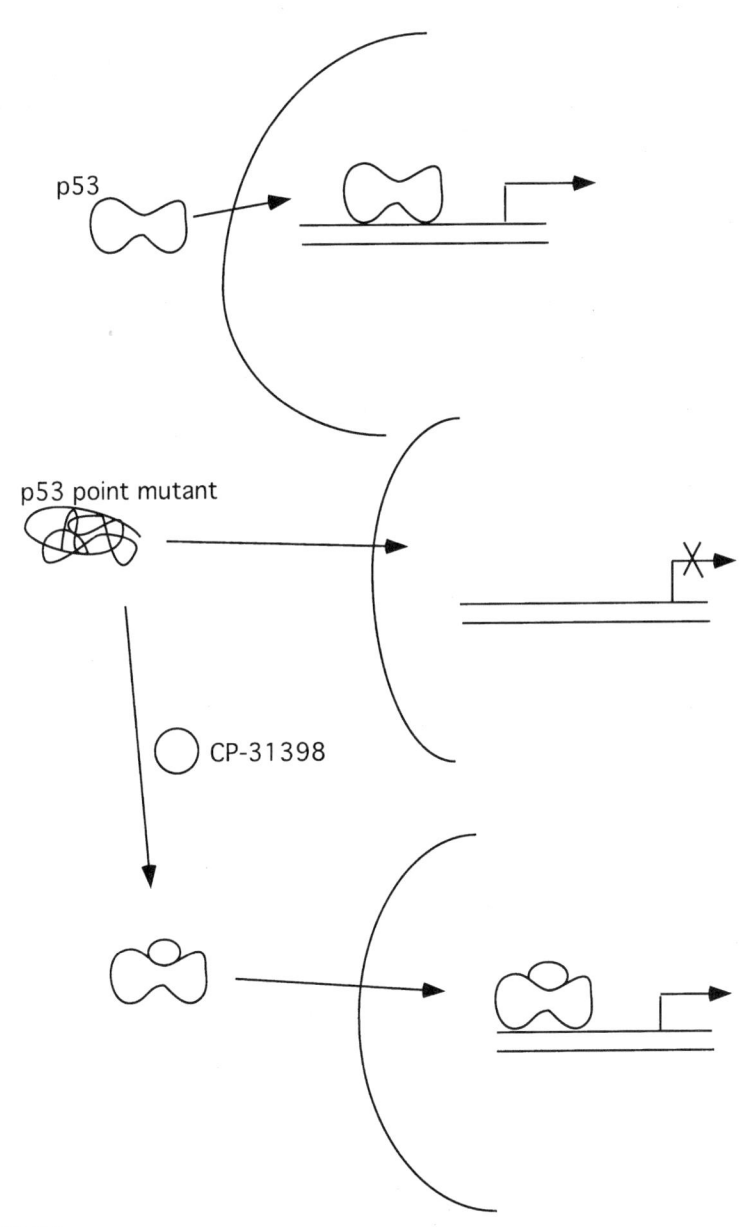

FIGURE 5.3 Pharmacologic rescue of mutant *p53*. When activated by DNA damage or other cellular stress, p53 enters the nucleus and activates transcription of cell cycle arrest and proapoptotic genes. Point mutations in *p53* may destabilize its active conformation, resulting in accumulation of a nonfunctional molecule. Drugs such as CP31398 can bind to and stabilize the conformation of p53, allowing normal transcriptional activity and control of cell growth and proliferation.

necessary if we are to understand fully the many missing pieces of this story. Future subjects of study will include determining the balance between receptor-mediated death and survival signals and the details of the ways in which DNA damage and other nuclear events induce genes such as *ATM* and *p53* to regulate cell cycle arrest or apoptosis. Using this increasing understanding to design creative therapeutic strategies may dramatically change our approach to fighting cancer in the future.

REFERENCES

1. Tsujimoto Y, Cossman J, Jaffe E, Croce CM. Involvement of the bcl-2 gene in human follicular lymphoma. Science 1985;228:1440–1443.
2. McDonnell TJ, Deane N, Platt FM et al. bcl-2-immunoglobulin transgenic mice demonstrate extended B cell survival and follicular lymphoproliferation. Cell 1989;57:79–88.
3. Vaux DL, Cory S, Adams JM. Bcl-2 gene promotes haemopoietic cell survival and cooperates with c-*myc* to immortalize pre-B cells. Nature 1988;335:440–442.
4. Chinnaiyan AM, O'Rourke K, Tewari M, Dixit VM. FADD, a novel death domain–containing protein, interacts with the death domain of Fas and initiates apoptosis. Cell 1995;81:505–512.
5. Hsu H, Xiong J, Goeddel DV. The TNF receptor 1–associated protein TRADD signals cell death and NF-κB activation. Cell 1995;81:495–504.
6. Teitz T, Wei T, Valentine MB et al. Caspase 8 is deleted or silenced preferentially in childhood neuroblastomas with amplification of MYCN [see comments]. Nat Med 2000;6:529–535.
7. Sheikh MS, Fornace AJ Jr. Death and decoy receptors and p53-mediated apoptosis. Leukemia 2000;14:1509-1513.
8. Ashkenazi A, Dixit VM. Apoptosis control by death and decoy receptors. Curr Opin Cell Biol 1999;11:255–260.
9. Bertrand F, Desbois-Mouthon C, Cadoret A et al. Insulin antiapoptotic signaling involves insulin activation of the nuclear factor κB-dependent survival genes encoding tumor necrosis factor receptor-associated factor 2 and manganese-superoxide dismutase. J Biol Chem 1999;274: 30596–30602.
10. Wang CY, Mayo MW, Korneluk RG et al. NF-kappaB antiapoptosis: induction of TRAF1 and TRAF2 and c-IAP1 and c-IAP2 to suppress caspase-8 activation. Science 1998;281:1680–1683.
11. Wiley SR, Schooley K, Smolak PJ et al. Identification and characterization of a new member of the TNF family that induces apoptosis. Immunity 1995;3:673–682.
12. Pitti RM, Marsters SA, Ruppert S et al. Induction of apoptosis by Apo-2 ligand, a new member of the tumor necrosis factor cytokine family. J Biol Chem 1996;271:12687–12690.
13. Sheridan JP, Marsters SA, Pitti RM et al. Control of TRAIL-induced apoptosis by a family of signaling and decoy receptors [see comments]. Science 1997;277:818–821.
14. Pan G, Ni J, Wei YF et al. An antagonist decoy receptor and a death domain-containing receptor for TRAIL [see comments]. Science 1997;277:815–818.
15. Pitti RM, Marsters SA, Lawrence DA et al. Genomic amplification of a decoy receptor for Fas ligand in lung and colon cancer. Nature 1998;396:699–703.
16. Owen-Schaub LB, van Golen KL, Hill LL, Price JE. Fas and Fas ligand interactions suppress melanoma lung metastasis. J Exp Med 1998;188:1717–1723.
17. Liu X, Kim CN, Yang J et al. Induction of apoptotic program in cell-free extracts: requirement for dATP and cytochrome c. Cell 1996;86:147–157.

18. Zou H, Henzel WJ, Liu X et al. Apaf-1, a human protein homologous to *C. elegans* CED-4, participates in cytochrome c-dependent activation of caspase-3 [see comments]. Cell 1997;90: 405–413.
19. Li P, Nijhawan D, Budihardjo I et al. Cytochrome c and dATP-dependent formation of Apaf-1/caspase-9 complex initiates an apoptotic protease cascade. Cell 1997;91:479–489.
20. Vander Heiden MG, Chandel NS, Williamson EK et al. Bcl-xL regulates the membrane potential and volume homeostasis of mitochondria [see comments]. Cell 1997;91:627–637.
21. Heffner RR, Barron SA. The early effects of ischemia upon skeletal muscle mitochondria. J Neurol Sci 1978;38:295–315.
22. Boise LH, Gonzalez-Garcia M, Postema CE et al. bcl-x, a bcl-2-related gene that functions as a dominant regulator of apoptotic cell death. Cell 1993;74;597–608.
23. Minn AJ, Velez P, Schendel SL et al. Bcl-x(L) forms an ion channel in synthetic lipid membranes. Nature 1997;385:353–357.
24. Schlesinger PH, Gross A, Yin XM et al. Comparison of the ion channel characteristics of proapoptotic BAX and antiapoptotic BCL-2. Proc Natl Acad Sci USA 1997;94:11357–11362.
25. Khaled AR, Kim K, Hofmeister R et al. Withdrawal of IL-7 induces Bax translocation from cytosol to mitochondria through a rise in intracellular pH [see comments]. Proc Natl Acad Sci USA 1999; 96:14476–14481.
26. Datta SR, Dudek H, Tao X et al. Akt phosphorylation of BAD couples survival signals to the cell-intrinsic death machinery. Cell 1997;91:231–241.
27. Crook NE, Clem RJ, Miller LK. An apoptosis-inhibiting baculovirus gene with a zinc finger-like motif. J Virol 1993;67:2168–2174.
28. Clem RJ, Miller LK. Control of programmed cell death by the baculovirus genes p35 and iap. Mol Cell Biol 1994;14:5212–5222.
29. Liston P, Roy N, Tamai K et al. Suppression of apoptosis in mammalian cells by NAIP and a related family of IAP genes. Nature 1996;379:349–353.
30. Rothe M, Pan MG, Henzel WJ et al. The TNFR2-TRAF signaling complex contains two novel proteins related to baculoviral inhibitor of apoptosis proteins. Cell 1995;83:1243–1252.
31. Uren AG, Pakusch M, Hawkins CJ et al. Cloning and expression of apoptosis inhibitory protein homologs that function to inhibit apoptosis and/or bind tumor necrosis factor receptor-associated factors. Proc Natl Acad Sci USA 1996;93:4974–4978.
32. Du C, Fang M, Li Y et al. Smac, a mitochondrial protein that promotes cytochrome c–dependent caspase activation by eliminating IAP inhibition. Cell 2000;102:33–42.
33. Verhagen AM, Ekert PG, Pakusch M et al. Identification of DIABLO, a mammalian protein that promotes apoptosis by binding to and antagonizing IAP proteins. Cell 2000;102:43–53.
34. Balendran A, Casamayor A, Deak M, et al. PDK1 acquires PDK2 activity in the presence of a synthetic peptide derived from the carboxyl terminus of PRK2. Curr Biol 1999;9:393–404.
35. Delcommenne M, Tan C, Gray V et al. Phosphoinositide-3-OH kinase-dependent regulation of glycogen synthase kinase 3 and protein kinase B/AKT by the integrin-linked kinase. Proc Natl Acad Sci USA 1998;95:11211–11216.
36. Kennedy SG, Kandel ES, Cross TK, Hay N. Akt/Protein kinase B inhibits cell death by preventing the release of cytochrome c from mitochondria. Mol Cell Biol 1999;19:5800–5810.
37. Cardone MH, Roy N, Stennicke HR et al. Regulation of cell death protease caspase-9 by phosphorylation [see comments]. Science 1998;282:1318–1321.
38. Brunet A, Bonni A, Zigmond MJ et al. Akt promotes cell survival by phosphorylating and inhibiting a Forkhead transcription factor. Cell 1999;96:857–868.

39. Di Cristofano A, Pandolfi PP. The multiple roles of PTEN in tumor suppression. Cell 2000;100: 387–390.
40. Li J, Yen C, Liaw D et al. PTEN, a putative protein tyrosine phosphatase gene mutated in human brain, breast, and prostate cancer [see comments]. Science 1997;275:1943–1947.
41. Steck PA, Pershouse MA, Jasser SA et al. Identification of a candidate tumour suppressor gene, MMAC1, at chromosome 10q23.3 that is mutated in multiple advanced cancers. Nat Genet 1997; 15:356–362.
42. Cheney IW, Johnson DE, Vaillancourt MT et al. Suppression of tumorigenicity of glioblastoma cells by adenovirus-mediated MMAC1/PTEN gene transfer. Cancer Res 1998;58:2331–2334.
43. Di Cristofano A, Kotsi P, Peng YF et al. Impaired Fas response and autoimmunity in Pten+/– mice. Science 1999;285:2122–2125.
44. Laine J, Kunstle G, Obata T et al. The protooncogene TCL1 is an Akt kinase coactivator. Mol Cell 2000;6:395-407.
45. Haupt Y, Maya R, Kazaz A, Oren M. Mdm2 promotes the rapid degradation of p53. Nature 1997; 387:296–299.
46. Kubbutat MH, Jones SN, Vousden KH. Regulation of p53 stability by Mdm2. Nature 1997;387: 299–303.
47. Geyer RK, Yu ZK, Maki CG. The MDM2 RING-finger domain is required to promote p53 nuclear export. Nat Cell Biol 2000;2:569–573.
48. Unger T, Juven-Gershon T, Moallem E et al. Critical role for Ser20 of human p53 in the negative regulation of p53 by Mdm2. EMBO J 1999;18:1805–1814.
49. Levine AJ. p53, the cellular gatekeeper for growth and division. Cell 1997;88:323–331.
50. Oda E, Ohki R, Murasawa H et al. Noxa, a BH3-only member of the Bcl-2 family and candidate mediator of p53-induced apoptosis. Science 2000;288:1053–1058.
51. Kamijo T, Zindy F, Roussel MF et al. Tumor suppression at the mouse INK4a locus mediated by the alternative reading frame product p19ARF. Cell 1997;91:649–659.
52. Pomerantz J, Schreiber-Agus N, Liegeois NJ et al. The Ink4a tumor suppressor gene product, p19Arf, interacts with MDM2 and neutralizes MDM2's inhibition of p53. Cell 1998;92:713–723.
53. Zhang Y, Xiong Y, Yarbrough WG. ARF promotes MDM2 degradation and stabilizes p53: ARF-INK4a locus deletion impairs both the Rb and p53 tumor suppression pathways. Cell 1998;92: 725–734.
54. Kamijo T, Weber JD, Zambetti G et al. Functional and physical interactions of the ARF tumor suppressor with p53 and Mdm2. Proc Natl Acad Sci USA 1998;95:8292–8297.
55. Zindy F, Eischen CM, Randle DH et al. Myc signaling via the ARF tumor suppressor regulates p53-dependent apoptosis and immortalization. Genes Dev 1998;12:2424–2433.
56. Oliner JD, Kinzler KW, Meltzer PS et al. Amplification of a gene encoding a p53-associated protein in human sarcomas [see comments]. Nature 1992;358:80–83.
57. Cheng JQ, Jhanwar SC, Klein WM et al. p16 alterations and deletion mapping of 9p21–p22 in malignant mesothelioma. Cancer Res 1994;54:5547–5551.
58. Savitsky K, Bar-Shira A, Gilad S et al. A single ataxia telangiectasia gene with a product similar to PI-3 kinase [see comments]. Science 1995;268:1749–1753.
59. Tibbetts RS, Brumbaugh KM, Williams JM et al. A role for ATR in the DNA damage-induced phosphorylation of p53. Genes Dev 1999;13:152–157.
60. Hirao A, Kong YY, Matsuoka S et al. DNA damage–induced activation of p53 by the checkpoint kinase Chk2 [see comments]. Science 2000;287:1824–1827.
61. Li S, Ting NS, Zheng L et al. Functional link of BRCA1 and ataxia telangiectasia gene product in DNA damage response. Nature 2000;406:210–215.

62. Li H, Kolluri SK, Gu J et al. Cytochrome c release and apoptosis induced by mitochondrial targeting of nuclear orphan receptor TR3 [see comments]. Science 2000;289:1159–1164.
63. Schmitt CA, McCurrach ME, de Stanchina E et al. INK4a/ARF mutations accelerate lymphomagenesis and promote chemoresistance by disabling p53. Genes Dev 1999;13:2670–2677.
64. Srivastava RK, Sasaki CY, Hardwick JM, Longo DL. Bcl-2-mediated drug resistance: inhibition of apoptosis by blocking nuclear factor of activated T lymphocytes (NFAT)–induced Fas ligand transcription. J Exp Med 1999;190:253–265.
65. Friesen C, Herr I, Krammer PH, Debatin KM. Involvement of the CD95 (APO-1/FAS) receptor/ligand system in drug-induced apoptosis in leukemia cells. Nat Med 1996;2:574–577.
66. Fulda S, Strauss G, Meyer E, Debatin KM. Functional CD95 ligand and CD95 death-inducing signaling complex in activation-induced cell death and doxorubicin-induced apoptosis in leukemic T cells. Blood 2000;95:301–308.
67. Mano Y, Kikuchi Y, Yamamoto K et al. Bcl-2 as a predictor of chemosensitivity and prognosis in primary epithelial ovarian cancer. Eur J Cancer 1999;35:1214–1219.
68. Liu R, Page C, Beidler DR et al. Overexpression of Bcl-x(L) promotes chemotherapy resistance of mammary tumors in a syngeneic mouse model. Am J Pathol 1999;155:1861–1867.
69. Leech SH, Olie RA, Gautschi O et al. Induction of apoptosis in lung-cancer cells following bcl-xL antisense treatment. Int J Cancer 2000;86:570–576.
70. Boland MP, Foster SJ, O'Neill LA. Daunorubicin activates NFκB and induces κB-dependent gene expression in HL-60 promyelocytic and Jurkat T lymphoma cells. J Biol Chem 1997;272:12952–12960.
71. Cusack JC Jr, Liu R, Baldwin AS Jr. Inducible chemoresistance to 7-ethyl-10-[4-(1-piperidino)-1-piperidino]-carbonyloxycamptothecin (CPT-11) in colorectal cancer cells and a xenograft model is overcome by inhibition of nuclear factor-κB activation. Cancer Res 2000;60:2323–2330.
72. Walczak H, Miller RE, Ariail K et al. Tumoricidal activity of tumor necrosis factor–related apoptosis-inducing ligand in vivo [see comments]. Nat Med 1999;5:157–163.
73. Ashkenazi A, Pai RC, Fong S et al. Safety and antitumor activity of recombinant soluble Apo2 ligand. J Clin Invest 1999;104:155–162.
74. Griffith TS, Chin WA, Jackson GC et al. Intracellular regulation of TRAIL-induced apoptosis in human melanoma cells. J Immunol 1998;161:2833–2840.
75. Jo M, Kim TH, Seol DW et al. Apoptosis induced in normal human hepatocytes by tumor necrosis factor–related apoptosis-inducing ligand [see comments]. Nat Med 2000;6:564–567.
76. Pacini P, Rinaldini M, Algeri R et al. FEC (5-fluorouracil, epidoxorubicin and cyclophosphamide) versus EM (epidoxorubicin and mitomycin-C) with or without lonidamine as first-line treatment for advanced breast cancer. A multicentric randomised study. Final results. Eur J Cancer 2000;36:966–975.
77. Amadori D, Frassineti GL, De Matteis A et al. Modulating effect of lonidamine on response to doxorubicin in metastatic breast cancer patients: results from a multicenter prospective randomized trial. Breast Cancer Res Treat 1998;49:209–217.
78. Ianniello GP, de Cataldis G, Comella P, et al. Cisplatin, epirubicin, and vindesine with or without lonidamine in the treatment of inoperable nonsmall cell lung carcinoma: a multicenter randomized clinical trial. Cancer 1996;78:63–69.
79. Ravagnan L, Marzo I, Costantini P et al. Lonidamine triggers apoptosis via a direct, Bcl-2-inhibited effect on the mitochondrial permeability transition pore. Oncogene 1999;18:2537–2546.
80. Banki K, Hutter E, Gonchoroff NJ, Perl A. Elevation of mitochondrial transmembrane potential and reactive oxygen intermediate levels are early events and occur independently from activation of caspases in Fas signaling. J Immunol 1999;162:1466–1479.

81. Marchetti P, Zamzami N, Joseph B et al. The novel retinoid 6-[3-(1-adamantyl)-4-hydroxyphenyl]-2-naphthalene carboxylic acid can trigger apoptosis through a mitochondrial pathway independent of the nucleus. Cancer Res 1999;59:6257–6266.
82. Sun SY, Yue P, Chandraratna RA et al. Dual mechanisms of action of the retinoid CD437: nuclear retinoic acid receptor–mediated suppression of squamous differentiation and receptor-independent induction of apoptosis in UMSCC22B human head and neck squamous cell carcinoma cells. Mol Pharmacol 2000;58:508–514.
83. Xiang J, Gomez-Navarro J, Arafat W et al. Pro-apoptotic treatment with an adenovirus encoding Bax enhances the effect of chemotherapy in ovarian cancer. J Gene Med 2000;2:97–106.
84. Persad S, Attwell S, Gray V et al. Inhibition of integrin-linked kinase (ILK) suppresses activation of protein kinase B/Akt and induces cell cycle arrest and apoptosis of PTEN-mutant prostate cancer cells. Proc Natl Acad Sci USA 2000;97:3207–3212.
85. Razzini G, Berrie CP, Vignati S et al. Novel functional PI 3-kinase antagonists inhibit cell growth and tumorigenicity in human cancer cell lines. FASEB J 2000;14:1179–1187.
86. Hu L, Zaloudek C, Mills GB et al. In vivo and in vitro ovarian carcinoma growth inhibition by a phosphatidylinositol 3-kinase inhibitor (LY294002). Clin Cancer Res 2000;6:880–886.
87. You L, Yang CT, Jablons DM. ONYX-015 works synergistically with chemotherapy in lung cancer cell lines and primary cultures freshly made from lung cancer patients. Cancer Res 2000;60:1009–1013.
88. Dix BR, O'Carroll SJ, Myers CJ et al. Efficient induction of cell death by adenoviruses requires binding of E1B55k and p53. Cancer Res 2000;60:2666–2672.
89. Khuri FR, Nemunaitis J, Ganly I et al. A controlled trial of intratumoral ONYX-015, a selectively replicating adenovirus, in combination with cisplatin and 5-fluorouracil in patients with recurrent head and neck cancer [see comments]. Nat Med 2000;6:879–885.
90. Foster BA, Coffey HA, Morin MJ, Rastinejad F. Pharmacological rescue of mutant p53 conformation and function [see comments]. Science 1999;286:2507–2510.
91. Meye A, Wurl P, Bache M et al. Colony formation of soft tissue sarcoma cells is inhibited by lipid-mediated antisense oligodeoxynucleotides targeting the human mdm2 oncogene. Cancer Lett 2000;149:181–188.
92. Wang H, Zeng X, Oliver P et al. MDM2 oncogene as a target for cancer therapy: an antisense approach. Int J Oncol 1999;15:653–660.

Genetic Susceptibility to Tobacco Carcinogenesis

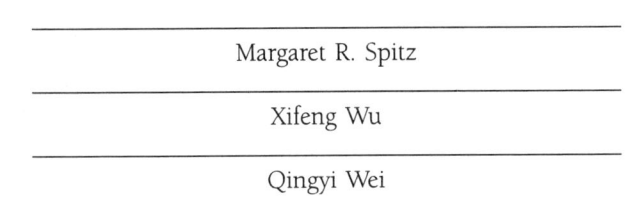

Margaret R. Spitz

Xifeng Wu

Qingyi Wei

Individuals differ in their susceptibility to environmental insults in general and to tobacco exposure specifically. More than 80% of lung cancers are attributed to tobacco. However, only a fraction of smokers will develop lung cancer in their lifetime. The molecular epidemiology approach, with the confluence of sophisticated advances in molecular biology and field-tested epidemiologic methodology, has enhanced tobacco exposure assessment and has furthered knowledge on tobacco carcinogenesis and susceptibility. However, even from classic epidemiologic studies, indirect indicators of host susceptibility to tobacco carcinogenesis are identifiable.

CLASSIC EPIDEMIOLOGIC STUDIES

Gender

Whether women are more susceptible to the carcinogenic effects of cigarettes than are men remains controversial. Risch et al[1] found that the association between smoking and lung cancer was considerably stronger for women than for men, with higher odds ratios (ORs) for women within each of the major histologic subtypes at various strata of tobacco exposure. Zang and Wynder[2] reported similar findings based on a case-control study of 1889 cases and 2070 controls. McDuffie[3] evaluated questionnaire data on 730 men and 197 women with lung cancer and noted that the disease was more frequently diagnosed at an earlier age in women and that a higher percentage were in the lower pack-year category. In a registry-based case-control study of 14,956 cases and 36,438 controls, relative risks were consistently higher in women than men for all histologic types except adenocarcinoma.[4] Muscat et al[5] reported a similar gender differential in oral cancer. However, more recent studies have failed to confirm these findings. A multicenter case-control study showed comparable risks in men and women.[6] Three prospective population-based studies that included 867 lung cancer cases did not confirm these previous reports of a higher relative risk in women than in men.[7]

Diet

The relationship between diet and lung cancer has been extensively explored in ecologic, case-control, and prospective studies and therefore is not reviewed in this chapter. Of relevance to this topic, however, is the issue of diet-exposure and diet-gene interactions. An example of the latter, (i.e., differential responses to variation in diet by genotype) will be reviewed in the section Metabolic Polymorphisms. Two examples of diet-exposure interactions are noteworthy. Recently, Sinha et al[8] reported that specific heterocyclic amines in the diet were associated with significantly increased risk of lung cancer in nonsmokers and in light to moderate smokers. In the Netherlands cohort study of 939 male lung cancer cases, protective effects were noted for folate, vitamin C, and β-cryptoxanthin, mainly in current smokers.[9]

Familial Aggregation of Tobacco-Related Cancers

Familial aggregation studies of lung cancer provide indirect evidence for the role of genetic predisposition. Tokuhata and Lilienfeld[10] and Ooi et al[11] found increased risks for lung cancer in both smoking and nonsmoking relatives of lung cancer patients. In men, but not women, the effect from smoking appeared to be stronger than the familial effect. Smoking was found to interact synergistically with a family history of lung cancer and to increase lung cancer risk substantially above that for nonsmokers without a family history of lung cancer.[10,12,13] Sellers et al[14] performed segregation analyses and reported results compatible with Mendelian codominant inheritance of a rare major autosomal gene for lung cancer predisposition. More recently, Yang and Schwartz[15] confirmed these findings. These patterns of inheritance studies suggest that a small proportion of lung cancer is due to "lung cancer genes" that are likely to be of low frequency but high penetrance.[16]

DNA REPAIR CAPACITY

Defective repair of genetic damage is one of the factors responsible for initiation of carcinogenesis and, therefore, is an important determinant of susceptibility to tobacco carcinogenesis. Maintenance of genomic integrity requires intact DNA repair and cell cycle control systems. A defect in either of these systems will lead to genomic instability. For instance, in response to DNA damage, normal cells increase their p53 levels,[17] thereby promoting cell-cycle arrest or inducing apoptosis and allowing the cell sufficient time to repair its DNA and thus prevent the transmission of genetic errors to its daughter cells. The pathways of various tumor suppressor genes have been discussed extensively elsewhere, and therefore we will concentrate on reviewing the DNA repair system.

Several pathways exist for repairing genomic damage induced by tobacco exposure (Table 6.1). Many human genes involved in DNA repair have been cloned and their functions intensively investigated, including those responsible for base excision repair (BER), nucleotide excision repair (NER), mismatch repair (MMR), and recombinational repair (RCR).

TABLE 1 Human DNA Repair Pathways

Type	Genes Involved	Damage Involved
Base excision	DNA ligase (LIG1, LIG3), DNA glycosylase (hOGG1, hMYH, hNTG1, AAG, TDG, UDG1), FEN1, PCNA, RFC, XRCC1	Single-base damage repair
Nucleotide excision repair	XPA, XPB/ERCC3, XPC, XPD/ERCC2, XPE, XPF, XPG/ERCC5, TFIIH, ERCC1, p34, p38, p41, p44, p62, hssL1, HHR23A, HHR23B, hSSB, ERCC4, CSB/ERCC6, PCNA, DNA polymerase, DNA ligase	Bulky nucleotide damage including UV photoproducts and chemical carcinogen-induced adducts
Mismatch repair	hMLH1, hPMS1, hPMS2, hMSH2, hMSH3, hMSH6/hGTBP	Base mismatch
Recombinational repair	HsRAD51, HsRAD52, HsRAD54, ERCC1, XPF, XRCC1, XRCC2, XRCC3, XRCC4, XRCC5, XRCC6, XRCC7, XRCC8	Double-strand breaks V(D)J recombination

Note: See references 20–22, 27, 28, 50, and 51 for further details.

DNA REPAIR SYSTEMS AND PATHWAYS

Base Excision Repair Pathway

Exposure to tobacco carcinogens generates reactive oxygen species that cause DNA base damage.[18] It has been estimated from the urine excretion and the leukocyte levels of 8-hydroxyguanine that such exposure increases the oxidative DNA damage rate by 35%–50%.[18] This type of DNA damage, causing only relatively minor changes in the helical DNA structure, is removed by one of the most highly conserved DNA repair mechanisms, BER,[19] and has been comprehensively reviewed.[20,21] In the first step of repair, DNA glycosylates catalyze the cleavage of the glycosidic bond between the damaged base and the sugar moiety, leaving an abasic site in DNA. Subsequently, the repair of DNA is completed by successive actions of other enzymes.[22] Impaired BER leads to an increased rate of oxidative DNA damage.

Although vitamin C intake[23] and a diet including brussels sprouts[24] are shown to reduce the rate of urinary 8-hydroxyguanine excretion by up to 28%, supplementation of other antioxidants such as vitamin E and β-carotene has failed to alter the estimated rate of oxidative DNA damage in smokers.[25,26] Although overwhelming evidence exists from experimental studies, there is a lack of evidence, particularly from prospective studies, for a causal relationship between oxidative DNA damage and its mutagenic and carcinogenic effect in humans.[18]

Nucleotide Excision Repair Pathway

The NER pathway removes bulky adducts and may be the most active mechanism of repair, especially when the other pathways are overloaded with damage. The function of the NER genes has been comprehensively reviewed[27–29] and includes damage site recognition followed by incision, excision, elongation, and ligation.[22] Deficiencies in the NER pathway lead to various syndromes that share sensitivity to sunlight and certain developmental disorders, including Cockayne dystrophy and trichothiodystrophy.[27,30] The classic excision repair deficiency syndrome is xeroderma pigmentosum (XP), which involves extreme sun sensitivity and a cutaneous malignancy rate 2000 times that of the general population.[29] XP is an autosomal recessive disorder involving mutations in one of the XP genes (*XPA, XPB, XPC, XPD, XPE, XPF,* and *XPG*). Heterozygotes have only a slightly increased risk of nonmelanoma skin cancers.[31] However, neither homozygotes nor heterozygotes exhibit the significantly increased rates of tobacco-induced cancers that one might predict, given the nature of their repair problem,[27,30–32] in part because most XP patients do not live sufficiently long to develop such cancers. Even so, XP patients clearly are sensitive to the exogenous mutagen ultraviolet radiation and, consequently, excision repair is an intriguing area for investigation of susceptibility to other common environmentally induced malignancies.

The relevance of NER in tobacco carcinogenesis is best illustrated in studies of DNA damage induced by the well-characterized tobacco carcinogen benzo[a]-

pyrene [B(a)P], a polycyclic aromatic hydrocarbon (PAH) compound. B(a)P is a classic DNA-damaging carcinogen found in tobacco smoke and the environment as a result of fuel combustion.[33] B(a)P bioactivation in vivo by cytochrome P450 and epoxide hydrolase generates highly toxic electrophilic and free-radical reactive intermediates, such as B(a)P diol epoxide (BPDE). These compounds can damage DNA irreversibly by covalent binding or oxidation and form BPDE-DNA adducts.[34,35] The NER pathway is responsible for removal of such adducts and for the restoration of normal DNA structure.[36] Unrepaired BPDE adducts probably also cause chromosomal aberrations, as evidenced in the BPDE mutagen sensitivity assay described later.

Smokers have higher PAH-DNA adduct levels than do nonsmokers[37,38] and levels of DNA adducts in nonneoplastic surgical lung parenchymal samples[39] and in alveolar macrophages[40] also are higher in current than in former smokers. These adducts can block the transcription of an essential gene,[36] if not repaired efficiently by the NER pathway.[27] BPDE-DNA adducts are repaired more efficiently in the transcribed than in the untranscribed strand[41,42]; thus mutations occur more frequently in the untranscribed strand. In addition, BPDE has been found to bind preferentially to mutational hot spots, resulting in G→T transversions in the *p53* tumor suppressor gene in cells deficient in NER.[43] Therefore, a high frequency of G→T transversion mutations in the *p53* gene in tobacco-related cancers[44,45] strongly suggests an etiologic link between exposure to tobacco carcinogens such as B(a)P, inefficient DNA repair capacity (DRC), and lung cancer risk.

Mismatch Repair Pathway

The enzymes of the MMR pathway recognize normal nucleotides that are either unpaired or paired with noncomplementary nucleotides. Such defects occur as a result of incorporation errors by polymerase during chromosome replication, as a result of chemically induced damage, or from the formation of heteroduplex intermediates during genetic recombination.[46] In vitro studies of misincorporation errors by normal DNA polymerase have revealed an incorrect nucleotide insertion rate of once every 1 million base pairs, which equals 3000 new mutations every time a human cell divides.[47] The actual number of mutations is much lower than this due to postreplication MMR.[46] Physical or chemical damage can result in conversion of one nucleotide to another or alterations in base pairings. For example, a G-T mispairing can result from deamination with a guanine.[48] Oxidative damage to guanine can produce 8-oxo-guanine which pairs incorrectly with adenine.[49] Our current understanding of MMR has come chiefly from studying this system in bacteria and yeast and, interestingly, the basic processes of correcting mispairing seems to have been conserved in higher eukaryotes. The functions of each MMR gene have been comprehensively reviewed.[50,51]

Two-thirds of replication error–positive sporadic tumors have somatic mutations in MMR genes.[52] A number of types of sporadic tumors have microsatellite instability, including lung and upper aerodigestive tract cancers.[53,54] Consequently, the MMR pathway is an area of keen interest in tobacco carcinogenesis. One study reported that approximately half of lung tumor specimens had reduced expression levels of hMLH1 or hMSH2 protein,[55] with reduced expression levels of both proteins observed in 34% of specimens. In adenocarcinomas, the reduction of hMSH2 expression was more frequent, whereas in squamous cell carcinoma, hMLH1 expression was more frequently reduced. hMLH1 reduced expression was more frequently associated with heavy smoking and higher pack-years.

Chang et al,[56] using eight dinucleotide repeat markers, reported that 28 of 68 patients with non–small cell lung cancer (41.2%) were defined as being positive for microsatellite instability (MI). MI occurred more frequently in squamous cell carcinoma. Three-fourths of MI-positive patients (76.9%) expressed no hMLH1 protein. Although an increase in MI has been observed at certain tetranucleotide repeat markers (AAAGn) in smoking-related cancers such as lung, bladder, and head and neck, the genetic mechanism underlying these elevated microsatellite alterations at selected tetranucleotide repeats in tumors is still unknown.[57]

Using a multiplex reverse transcriptase–polymerase chain reaction (RT-PCR) assay, Wei et al[58] simultaneously evaluated the relative expression levels of five MMR genes (*hMSH2, hMLH1, hPMS1, hPMS2,* and *hGTBP/hMSH6*) in the peripheral lymphocytes of 78 patients with head and neck cancer and 86 controls. The relative MMR gene expression was not correlated with disease stage or tumor site in the cases or with smoking and alcohol use in the controls, but increased with age in both cases and controls. The mean messenger RNA expression levels of *hMLH1, hPMS1,* and *hGTBP/hMSH6* were statistically significantly lower in cases than controls. Significantly increased ORs were associated only with low expression of *hMLH1* (OR = 4.4) and *hGTBP/hMSH6* (OR = 2.1), suggesting that low *hMLH1* and *hGTBP/hMSH6* expression may be associated with cancer risk.

Recombination Repair Pathway

Strand breaks require RCR. Interstrand cross-links are repaired by NER and also, in part, by RCR. Although radon, a naturally occurring radioactive gas, can cause DNA strand breaks and overwhelming evidence exists that exposure to radon, at levels found in mines, leads to lung cancer,[59] no evidence exists that a defective RCR pathway is linked to tobacco carcinogenesis.

MEASUREMENT OF DNA REPAIR CAPACITY

Host Cell Reactivation Assay

Assays that measure cellular DNA repair are now being applied in population studies to investigate the association between DNA repair and susceptibility to cancer. Generally, cellular responses to DNA damage fall into three major categories: direct reversal of damage (e.g., enzymatic photoreactivation), excision of damage by BER or NER, and postreplication repair.[27] The presence of only one unrepaired DNA lesion can block the transcription of an essential gene.[60] A wide range of repair ability exists in the general population, with XP patients representing the extreme end of the repair spectrum.[28]

Although many assays are available that measure the efficiency of multiple steps of excision repair individually,[61] the ability to test the entire pathway is needed for population studies, in which time, cost, and repeatability of measurements are major concerns. Therefore, measuring the expression level of damaged reporter genes (host cell reactivation assay) is the assay of choice. This assay uses undamaged cells, is relatively rapid, and is an objective way of measuring repair.[61] In the assay, a damaged nonreplicating recombinant plasmid (pCMV*cat*) harboring a chloramphenicol acetyltransferase reporter gene is introduced by transfection into lymphocytes. Reactivated chloramphenicol acetyltransferase enzyme activity is measured as a function of excision repair of the damaged bacterial gene.[61] Both lymphocytes and skin fibroblasts from patients who have basal cell carcinoma but not XP demonstrate lower excision-repair rates than individuals without cancer.[62] Consequently, the repair capacity of lymphocytes can be considered a reflection of an individual's overall repair capacity.

Wei et al[63,64] investigated whether differences in DRC for repairing tobacco carcinogen-induced DNA damage are associated with differential susceptibility to lung cancer. In both the initial pilot study[63] (51 patients and 56 frequency-matched controls) and a subsequent, large, hospital-based case-control study[64] (316 each of lung cancer patients and controls), statistically significantly lower DRC was observed in cases as compared with controls and was associated with a greater than twofold increased risk of lung cancer. As compared to the highest DRC quartile in the controls, suboptimal DRC was associated with adjusted risks for lung cancer of 1.8, 2.0, and 4.3 for the second, third, and fourth quartiles of DRC, respectively ($P_{trend} < .001$). Case subjects who were younger at diagnosis (< 60 years), female, or lighter smokers or who reported a family history of cancer exhibited the lowest DRC and the highest lung cancer risk among their subgroups, suggesting that these subgroups may be especially susceptible to lung cancer.[64] Cheng et al[65] investigated the role of DRC in head and neck cancer and, again, DRC was significantly lower in cases (8.6%) than in controls (12.4%) with a similar dose-response trend.

Mutagen Sensitivity

Another functional assay that gauges host susceptibility is the mutagen sensitivity assay that quantifies chromatid breaks induced by in vitro mutagen exposure in short-term cultures of peripheral blood lymphocytes.[66] Several case-control[67,68] and cohort studies[69,70] have suggested that bleomycin-induced and baseline lymphocytic chromosomal aberrations can be used as cancer predictors. Bleomycin is considered to be radiomimetic (i.e., causing the generation of free oxygen radicals), a fact relevant to tobacco-induced carcinogenesis because numerous compounds in tobacco condensate may generate free oxygen radicals that can induce single- and double-stranded breaks. In case-control studies, mutagen sensitivity has consistently been shown to be a significant independent predictor of the risk for lung and upper aerodigestive tract cancers.[66-68,71-74] Lighter smokers and former smokers appear to be at higher risk (OR = 5.7) than heavier smokers (OR = 3.2), as are younger patients (OR = 7.8). In upper aerodigestive tract cancer, bleomycin sensitivity was highest in subjects younger than 30.[75] These findings are consistent with the hypothesis that cancer is more likely to develop at younger ages in people who have the sensitive phenotype. The relative risk for second primary tumors among patients with an initial primary head and neck tumor was 2.67 for mutagen-sensitive subjects.[76]

The bleomycin assay has been modified using BPDE as the challenge mutagen. BPDE sensitivity has also been associated with a significantly elevated risk for lung cancer, with an OR of 7.26,[12] as compared with an OR of 4.56 for bleomycin sensitivity in the same subjects. As with bleomycin sensitivity, risks were higher for lighter smokers and younger patients. There was also a dose-response relationship between the quartiles of numbers of BPDE-induced breaks and lung cancer risk, with ORs of 2.39, 3.12, and 15.03, respectively. Age, gender, and smoking status do not appear to modify the sensitivity profile.[68] Risk was highest in subjects who were sensitive to both BPDE and bleomycin.[12] Defects in both BER and NER mechanisms may therefore dramatically increase the risk of smoking-related cancer.

Hsu[71] has suggested that the mutagen sensitivity assay indirectly measures the effectiveness of one or more DNA repair mechanisms. A correlation between the cellular DRC measured by the host cell reactivation assay and the frequency of mutagen-induced in vitro chromatid breaks has been reported.[77] Mutagen sensitivity may also involve an inherent chromatin alteration that permits more efficient translation of DNA damage into chromosome damage after exposure to a mutagen.[78]

^{32}P-Postlabeling Assay of DNA Adducts

A relatively large variation is observed in the level of persistent DNA adducts in vivo.[39,79] This variation could also be a valid phenotypic marker for the joint effect of host metabolic activities and DNA repair in response to carcinogen exposure.[80] Using the ^{32}P-postlabeling assay,[81] Phillips et al[82] noted a linear relationship between the levels of aromatic DNA adducts in human lung and the number of cigarettes smoked per day. Although some studies have failed to find a correlation between lymphocyte adduct levels and smoking habits,[83-85] one study reported a significant difference between the levels in smokers and nonsmokers.[85] Importantly, this difference was not observed in DNA isolated from the granulocytes of the same individuals, suggesting that lymphocytes may be a more appropriate cell type for analysis.

A new assay of in vitro induction of carcinogen-DNA adducts has been developed[80] by treating stimulated lymphocytes with BPDE, which does not need bioactivation because it is an ultimate carcinogen. Therefore, the levels of BPDE-induced DNA adducts reflect not exposure but genetic variation in phase II enzymes and DRC. However, phase II enzymes have little, if any, effect on the in vitro formation of adducts in this assay, because of the relatively large dose (4 μM) of BPDE used and the rapid binding of BPDE to DNA, which peaks within 15 minutes.[86] Because the ultimate carcinogen is exactly the same, the observed variation in the measured adduct levels is a hundredfold rather than a thousandfold, as is often seen in smoking-related adducts in vivo. The levels of total BPDE-induced DNA adducts were significantly higher in case subjects (median, 50.7 per 10^7 nt) than in controls (median, 17.2 per 10^7 nt). Nonsmokers and individuals younger than 65 years had higher adduct levels than did older case subjects and subjects who were former smokers, suggesting that predisposed individuals have a higher risk because of an inherited sensitivity to carcinogens, even at lower doses.[80] This finding was recently confirmed in 221 lung cancer cases and 229 controls.[87]

DNA Repair Gene Transcript (Messenger RNA) Levels

The multiplex RT-PCR assay has been used to measure the levels of several DNA repair gene transcripts relative to those of a ubiquitous housekeeping gene.[88] In this technique, transcripts from five MMR genes and the β-actin gene are simultaneously amplified, and the transcript levels are quantified in relation to the β-actin level by computerized densitometry analysis of gel electrophoresis of the multiplex RT-PCR products. Head and neck cancer patients expressed lower transcript levels of MMR genes (*hGTB/hMSH6, hPMS1,* and *hMLH1*) as compared to controls. After adjusting for confounding variables, lower expression levels of *hGTBP/hMSH6* and *hMLH1* were found to be significant risk factors for cancer, with ORs of 2.1 and 4.4, respectively.[58]

POLYMORPHISMS IN DNA REPAIR GENES

Genetic polymorphisms of DNA repair genes may also contribute to variation in DRC. Clearly, functional (phenotypic) studies of DNA repair in individuals with various genotypes of these polymorphisms are needed. However, detecting subtle differences in DRC due to a single polymorphism of a single gene in a very complex pathway will be very difficult. Recently, the entire coding regions of several DNA repair genes on chromosome 19 [i.e., three NER genes (*ERCC1, XPD/ERCC2,* and *XPF/ERCC4*), one RCR gene (*XRCC3*), and one BER gene (*XRCC1*)] were resequenced in 12 normal individuals.[89] Of these, 7 variants of

ERCC1, 17 of XPD/ERCC2, 6 of XPF/ERCC4, 4 of XRCC3, and 12 of XRCC1 were identified. Among these variants, four variants of XPD/ERCC2, three variants of XRCC1, one variant of XRCC3, and one variant of XPF/ERCC4 resulted in an amino acid changes. Later, another six variants of XPF/ERCC4 were identified in 38 individuals,[90] two variants of XPA and two XPB/ERCC3 were identified in 35 individuals, and one variant of XPC was identified.[91] Although the significance of these variants is largely unknown, the implication is that variants that cause amino acid substitutions may have an impact on the function of the proteins and, therefore, on efficiency of DNA repair. Those variants that do not cause an amino acid change may also have an impact on the DNA repair function because they may cause messenger RNA instability or may be linked to genetic changes in other unknown genes.[92]

XPD/ERCC2

XPD protein is an evolutionarily conserved helicase, a subunit of transcription factor IIH (TFIIH) that is essential for transcription and NER.[93] Mutations in XPD prevent its protein from interacting with p44, another subunit of TFIIH,[94] and cause decreased helicase activity, resulting in a defect in NER. Mutations at different sites result in distinct clinical phenotypes.[95] XPD is also thought to be involved in repairing genetic damage induced by tobacco carcinogens.[96]

Patients with basal cell carcinomas and the 35931 AA+AC or 22541 AA+AC genotypes exhibited increased levels of DNA strand breaks after ultraviolet-C irradiation.[97] The nucleotide variation at A35931C is located approximately 50 bases upstream from the poly(A) signal, and may alter XPD protein function. Similarly, in another study of 31 women, those with the XPD 35931 AA genotype also had higher levels of chromatid aberrations induced by x-irradiation.[98] However, this finding was not confirmed in another study that measured the frequency of smoking-induced sister chromatid exchanges and polyphenol DNA adducts (n = 61).[99] The discrepancy in the effect of the A35931C polymorphism in these three studies may be due to either the difference in DNA damage induced by different carcinogens or to the relatively small sample sizes analyzed.

In a case-control study of 189 head and neck patients and 496 cancer-free controls, Sturgis et al[100] found that the frequency of the 22541 AA homozygous genotype was lower in cases (15.9%) than in controls (20.4%), but this difference was not statistically significant. The frequency of the 35931 CC homozygous genotype was higher in cases (16.4%) than in controls (11.5%) and was associated with a borderline increased risk (OR = 1.55). The risk was higher in older subjects (OR = 2.22), current smokers (OR = 1.83), and current drinkers (OR = 2.59). The reported polymorphic site causes an amino acid substitution[89] and may affect protein function.[101] The XPD C22541A polymorphism is silent, resulting in no amino acid substitution.[89] It is possible, however, that such a sequence variation could affect RNA stability or otherwise disturb protein synthesis.[92]

XRCC1

A polymorphism at the *XRCC1* 28152 site (G→A) of codon 399 in exon 10 results in a nonconservative amino acid substitution of arginine for glutamine; the polymorphism at the *XRCC1* 26304 site (C→T) of codon 194 in exon 6 results in a nonconservative amino acid substitution of arginine for tryptophan. Although the functional relevance of these variants is unknown, codon 399 is within the *XRCC1* BRCT domain (codons 314–402),[102] which is highly homologous to *BRCA1* (a gene also involved in DNA repair), containing a binding site for poly(adenosine diphosphate–ribose) polymerase.[103] Because the role of *XRCC1* in BER brings together DNA polymerase β, DNA ligase III, and poly(adenosine diphosphate–ribose) polymerase at the site of DNA damage,[104–106] the codon 399 variant could have an altered repair activity. The codon 194 polymorphism resides in the linker regions of the *XRCC1* N-terminal domain separating the helix 3 and DNA polymerase β involved in binding a single-nucleotide gap DNA substrate.[107] Therefore, it is less likely to cause a significant change in the repair function. However, very few studies have examined the associations between polymorphisms of the DNA repair gene *XRCC1* and the risk of cancer. Lunn et al[108] reported that the *XRCC1* 28152 A allele (G→A at codon 399 Gln) was associated with higher levels of both aflatoxin B1–DNA adducts and glycophorin A variants in a normal population, suggesting that the *XRCC1* 28152 AA genotype may be an adverse genotype.

Sturgis et al[109] reported that 88.7% of 203 head and neck cancer cases and 85.6% of 424 controls lacked the *XRCC1* 26304 T allele, with a significant OR for oral cavity and pharyngeal cancers of 2.46. Thirty-two case subjects (15.8%) and 46 controls (10.8%) were homozygous for the *XRCC1* 28152 A allele (adjusted OR = 1.59 for all cases). Furthermore, when the two genotypes were combined, the adjusted OR was 1.51 for either risk genotype and 2.02 for both risk genotypes.

MMH/OGG1

The *hOGG1* gene is localized on chromosome 3p25 and encodes two forms of protein that result from an alternative splicing of a single messenger RNA.[110] The α-hOGG1 protein has a nuclear localization, whereas the β-hOGG1 is targeted to the mitochondrion. The α-hOGG1 protein is a DNA glycosylase/AP lyase that excises 8-hydroxyguanine and Fapy-G from gamma-irradiated DNA. Both somatic and polymorphic mutations of the *hOGG1* gene exist in lung and kidney tumors.[111,112] The mutant forms α-hOGG1-Gln46 and α-hOGG1-His154 are defective in their catalytic capacities, especially for 8-hydroxyguanine.[113] A polymorphism at codon 326 (Ser326Cys) leads to hOGG1-Ser326 and hOGG1-Cys326 proteins.[111] Activity in the repair of 8-hydroxyguanine appears to be greater with Ser326 protein than with the Cys326 protein. Because tobacco carcinogens produce 8-hydroxyguanine residues, the capacity to repair these lesions can be involved in cancer susceptibility.

Sugimura et al[114] found that those with the *hOGG1* (Cys/Cys) of codon 326 were at an increased risk of squamous cell and nonadenocarcinoma lung cancer, as compared to those with the Ser/Cys or those with the Ser/Ser genotypes combined (ORs of 3.0 and 2.2, respectively). The distributions of this polymorphism varied for different populations (Chinese, Japanese, Micronesians, Melanesians, Hungarians, and Australian whites), with much lower prevalence of the Cys allele in the latter three populations. Another population-based study of 128 lung cancer cases and 268 controls identified a polymorphic allele 3 in *hMMH/ OGG1* exon 1 and found it to be significantly related to risk of adenocarcinoma of the lung (OR = 3.2) among Japanese.[115] European patients with head and neck or kidney cancer were shown to possess a similar polymorphism.[116] Polymorphisms involving intron 4 and exon 7 were present in 30% of 33 patients. Loss of heterozygosity at the *hOGG1* gene locus was found to be a very common occurrence in lung tumorigenesis.[117] However, the *hOGG1* polymorphisms studied were not found to be major contributors to individual lung cancer susceptibility in whites.

METABOLIC POLYMORPHISMS

Most chemical carcinogens require metabolic activation before they can interact with cellular macromolecules. The internal dose of tobacco carcinogens to which lung tissue is exposed is therefore modulated by genetic polymorphisms in the enzymes responsible for activation and detoxification of these carcinogens. These polymorphisms, although generally associated with low risks for cancer, are frequent in the population and, therefore, the attributable risks are high. In this chapter, we focus on select genes that are involved in the metabolism of tobacco carcinogens such as arylamines, *N*-nitrosamines, PAHs, and B(a)P. A comprehensive review is beyond the scope of this chapter.

CYP1A1

The *CYP1A1* gene codes for aryl hydrocarbon hydroxylase, which initiates a multienzyme pathway that activates both PAHs and B(a)P into highly electrophilic metabolites and also catabolizes arylamines. Aryl hydrocarbon hydroxylase activity varies up to several thousandfold among subjects, is highly inducible, and is much more inducible in patients with lung cancer than in controls.[118] However, these findings are equivocal, and the evidence that the CYP1A1 protein plays a critical role in tobacco-induced carcinogenesis remains meager. Three polymorphisms at the *CYP1A1* gene locus have been identified. The first is the *Ile462Val* polymorphism in which isoleucine is substituted by valine at codon 462 in exon 7, thereby affecting the encoded protein's function. Japanese persons in Okinawa with this homozygous polymorphism were reported to have a significant risk of lung cancer (OR = 3.32), especially for squamous cell carcinoma (OR = 4.85) and small cell carcinoma (OR = 9.35).[119] The second polymorphism, *Msp1*–restriction fragment length polymorphism, is a T→C transition downstream of the polyadenylation site. The presence of at least one copy of the *CYP1A1 Msp1* variant allele was reported to be associated with a 2.4-fold increased risk of squamous cell lung carcinoma in subjects of white, Japanese, or Hawaiian origin[120] but not in a Finnish population.[121] A third polymorphism is the *Msp*1 restriction fragment length polymorphism, located at the 3'-noncoding region of the *CYP1A1* gene and found only in African Americans.[122] A recent metaanalysis of 15 case-control studies indicated a positive but not statistically significant association between two *CYP1A1* polymorphisms (*Ile462Val* and *Msp*1) and lung cancer risk.[123] The ORs (nonsignificant) for one or two copies of the variant Msp1 allele were 1.09 and 1.27, respectively. For *Ile462Val*, the respective ORs were 1.16 and 1.62.

CYP1A2

CYP1A2 protein is involved in the metabolic activation of heterocyclic and aromatic amines and certain nitroaromatic compounds. Substantial interindividual variability in *CYP1A2* activity has been reported,[124] and a genetic basis for these differences has been suggested. Recently, two genetic polymorphisms were identified in the *CYP1A2* gene.[125,126] The first polymorphism is a C→A point mutation in intron 1 of the *CYP1A2* gene.[125] The variant A allele is associated with high enzyme activity in individuals exposed to tobacco smoke.[125,126] Sachse et al[127] further showed that smokers homozygous for the variant A allele had a 1.6-fold higher metabolic activity as compared to smokers who displayed other genotypes. The second polymorphism is in the 5'-flanking region of the gene, where G is replaced by A at position −2964.[126] This point mutation resulted in a significant decrease in enzymatic activity in Japanese smokers. To date, no major epidemiologic study has investigated the role of *CYP1A2* as a risk factor in cancer. However, Landi et al[128] reported that subjects with rapid *CYP1A2* activity (or rapid oxidizers) showed the highest 4-aminobiphenyl-hemoglobin adduct levels at a low smoking dose.

CYP2E1

CYP2E1 enzyme is important in the metabolic activation of various N-nitrosamines, including the potent tobacco-specific procarcinogen 4-(methylnitrosamino)-1-(3-pyridyl)-butanone, and is highly inducible. Restriction fragment length polymorphisms detected by PstI or RsaI digestion have been associated with transcriptional regulation of gene expression.[129] Another genetic polymorphism was identified in intron 6 with restriction endonuclease DraI.[130] A Swedish study suggested that people with the *CYP2E1* RsaI or PstI c2 allele might be at lower risk for lung cancer.[131] Consistent with this finding, Wu et al[132] reported that individuals who were homozygous for the c1 *CYP2E1* allele (c1/c1) had a higher lung cancer risk than did those who were heterozygous or carried the rare homozygous c2/c2 genotype. Furthermore, cases displaying the c1/c1 genotype developed cancer at an earlier age and with lower cigarette pack-years of exposure than did patients displaying the c1/c2 or c2/c2 genotypes. A Japanese case-control study of lung cancer showed a significant association between the *CYP2E1 DraI* polymorphism and lung cancer.[130] A joint effect between c1/c1 genotype and mutagen sensitivity was also noted in lung cancer risk.[132,133] Other enzymes (not reviewed here) related to tobacco carcinogen metabolism include *CYP2A6, CYP3A4, CYP1B1, CYP2C9,* and *CYP2C19.*

GLUTATHIONE-*S*-TRANSFERASES

The glutathione-S-transferase (*GST*) supergene family of enzymes catalyzes the detoxification of electrophilic compounds by glutathione conjugation. The cytosolic *GST* enzyme family consists of six gene classes, classified according to their primary structure, termed α, μ, π, σ, τ, and ζ. The *GST* genes demonstrate varying levels of enzyme activity that are genetically controlled and may affect cancer risk. *GSTM1*, from the μ subfamily, and *GSTT1*, from the τ subfamily of *GSTs*, both possess polymorphic variants that result in greatly reduced enzyme activity, possibly conferring an increased risk for cancer. Genetic polymorphisms have been identified for *GSTM1, GSTP1,* and *GSTT1.*

GSTM1

The *GSTM1* gene product is important for detoxifying epoxides of the carcinogenic compounds, PAHs. *GSTM1* has four possible phenotypes that result from homozygous and heterozygous combinations of three alleles, *GSTM1*0* (null), *GSTM1*A*, and *GSTM1*B*. The homozygous null genotype results in deletion of the gene and lack of enzyme expression and has been correlated with a higher risk for smoking-related cancers. This genotype occurs in approximately 50% of white populations. A recent meta-analysis of 19 case-control genotype studies reported an overall lung cancer risk of only 1.14 associated with the *GSTM1* null genotype.[134] Meta-analysis of 15 case-control studies found a positive association between *GSTM1* and bladder cancer risk (pooled OR = 1.53).[135] Thus, it appears that the *GSTM1* null genotype is consistently, but modestly, associated with smoking-related cancer risk.

GSTT1

Because the GSTT1 enzyme is involved in both detoxification and activation reactions, predicting the biological consequences of its polymorphism is somewhat difficult. Significant differences in the prevalence of the null genotype exist among various ethnic groups, ranging from 10% to 65%. Brockmoller et al[136] showed a 2.6-fold increased risk of bladder cancer in nonsmokers with the *GSTT1* null genotype. However, the published data on the association between this polymorphism and cancer risk are limited. In this regard, however, recent published studies have shown that people with the *GSTT1* null genotype alone have a slight, but not significant, increased risk of cancer, whereas those with both *GSTM1* null and *GSTT1* null genotypes are at higher risk of both lung[137] and head and neck cancers.[138]

The role of dietary factors in inducing or inhibiting metabolic enzyme activity is also relevant. Isothiocyanates are nonnutrient compounds in cruciferous vegetables with anticarcinogenic properties. One proposed mechanism for their protective action is through down-regulation of cytochrome P450 enzyme levels and induction of phase II detoxifying enzymes. In a study of 503 lung cancer cases and 465 controls, no main effect was associated with the *GSTM1* null genotype (OR = 1.09), but a statistically significant OR of 1.41 was associated with the *GSTT1* null genotype.[139] On stratified analysis, risks were elevated for low isothiocyanate intake and either null genotype in current smokers. The comparable OR in the presence of both null genotypes was 5.45.[139] Similarly, in a cohort of Chinese men, individuals without detectable levels of a urinary biomarker of total isothiocyanates who also were *GSTM1* or *GSTT1* null were shown to be at increased lung cancer risk.[140] Some of the inconsistencies reported in the role of GST genotypes in lung cancer risk could be due to unexpected confounding from dietary factors.

GSTP1

The *GSTP1* gene is located at 11q13. GSTP1 enzyme is abundant in the lung, esophagus, and placenta. Considerable interindividual variation in enzymatic activity exists in both normal and tumor tissue. Currently, two allelic variants based on single nucleotide base changes are known. One polymorphism is on exon 5 (Ile105Val) and the second on exon 6 (Ala114Val). Although, Ryberg et al[141] suggested that the mutant exon 5 allele is more efficient in catalyzing aromatic epoxides, Johansson et al[142] reported that subjects with the variant genotype have a higher lung cancer risk than do those with the normal gene (Ile105Ile).

NAT

The *NAT* gene is located on 8p. Two isozymes, involved in the acetylation of arylamines, are encoded by the *NAT1* and *NAT2* genes. Epidemiologic studies have shown an association between smoking-related cancers (e.g., bladder, colorectal, lung, and head and neck cancers) and *NAT* polymorphisms.

NAT2 NAT2 is known to be polymorphic, with rapid, intermediate, or slow acetylator phenotypes. Twenty-six different *NAT2** allelic variants are known; of these, *NAT2*4* is a fast-acetylating phenotype, whereas *NAT2*5*, *NAT2*6*, and *NAT2*7* are slow-acetylating phenotypes.[133] Hepatic N-acetylation of aromatic amines catalyzed by NATs is a competing pathway that leads to detoxification of the amines in tobacco smoke. Thus, high activity of these enzymes should be associated with decreased risk for smoking-related cancer.[143] In a review of NAT2 phenotype studies, Vine and McFarland[144] found slightly increased risks (OR = 1.3–1.7) for slow NAT2 acetylators. The slow NAT2 acetylator was reported to be associated with head and neck cancer,[145] esophageal cancer,[146] and laryngeal cancer.[147] The most consistently reported association is between bladder cancer and slow NAT2 acetylators.[148,149] Higher levels of 4-aminobiphenyl hemoglobin adducts have been noted in smokers with slow acetylator genotypes as compared to rapid acetylators.[150] Hirvonen et al,[137] however, did not find any difference in the level of urinary mutagenicity between slow acetylators and fast acetylators and suggested that the role of the NAT2 polymorphism in the development of bladder cancer may have been overestimated. The association between lung cancer and NAT2 polymorphisms is inconclusive. Wu et al[151] suggested that NAT2 slow acetylation, together with mutagen sensitivity, is associated with increased lung cancer risk. In contrast, two other studies reported an increased risk of lung cancer in smokers who were rapid acetylators.[152,153]

NAT1 O-acetylation of the N-hydroxy arylamine by bladder NAT1 is a another activation step leading to the formation of aromatic amine-DNA adducts. Twenty-four different allelic variants have been identified. A mutation in NAT1*10 involves a T→A change at position 1088 of the consensus polyadenylation signal. Individuals with heterozygous NAT1*10 showed two times more enzyme activity and higher DNA adduct levels in the mucosa of the urinary bladder than those with wild-type alleles.[154] Taylor et al[155] reported a 12.9- to 26-fold increased risk for bladder cancer in smokers with NAT1*10. Badawi et al[156] suggested that subjects with the combined slow NAT2 and rapid NAT1 (NAT*10) genotypes exhibited the highest adduct levels and the highest NAT activity among all other combined NAT1-NAT2 genotypes. However, Okkels et al[148] did not find such a relationship. One study reported an association between the slow NAT1 (NAT*10) allele and lung cancer risk,[157] whereas another study did not.[158] NAT1*11 variant involves a 9 base pair deletion in the trinucleotide repeat sequence (nucleotides 1065–1088) of the 3' untranslated region. It is not clear whether the NAT1*11 mutation alters the enzyme activity.[156]

mEPHX

The microsomal epoxide hydrolase (mEPHX) gene, located on chromosome 1q, is involved in detoxification of B(a)P by the addition of water to a range of alkenes and arene oxides to form *trans*-dihydrodiols.[159] Two mEPHX variants modulate enzyme activity. In the first variant, termed the *slow allele*, tyrosine is replaced by histidine at residue 113, in exon 3, due to T→C substitution. As a result of the substitution, enzyme activity decreases by 40% to 50%.[160] In the second variant, termed the *fast allele*, arginine replaces histidine at residue 139, in exon 4, due to an A→G substitution. The resulting substitution leads to a 25% increase in enzyme activity. Seven additional polymorphisms have been identified in non-coding regions, some of which are reported to affect weakly the transcriptional regulation of the *mEPHX* gene.[161]

Individuals with particularly slow mEPHX activity (homozygotes) may be more susceptible to chronic obstructive pulmonary disease and emphysema than those with more rapid enzyme activity.[162] London et al[163] reported that African Americans (but not whites) with the homozygous slow allele were at lower risk of lung cancer (adjusted OR = 0.08). However, Benhamou et al[164] noted increased risk of squamous and small cell lung cancer with high enzyme activity in French smokers.

Myeloperoxidase

Myeloperoxidase (MPO) is a lysosomal phase I metabolic enzyme located in monocytes and macrophages and primary granules of neutrophils.[165] Acute inflammation of lung tissue, such as that from tobacco smoke, results in an immune response, local recruitment of neutrophils at the sites of pulmonary inflammation, and release of this enzyme.[166] MPO has been shown to convert metabolites of the tobacco smoke procarcinogen B(a)P to the highly reactive and carcinogenic BPDE.[167,168] A polymorphic G→A nucleotide base shift occurs in a hormone response element region 463 base pairs upstream of the *MPO* gene,[169,170] which destroys the binding region for the general transcription factor SP1. Piedrafita et al[170] demonstrated that individuals with the A allele had overall weaker transcriptional activity of the *MPO* gene due to the reduced binding of the SP1 transcription factor. Because overall transcriptional activity is decreased in individuals with the variant allele (A allele), ultimately less enzyme would be available for the conversion of the B(a)P intermediate to the highly carcinogenic BPDE. London et al[171] were the first to report a protective association between the variant allele of *MPO* and lung cancer risk (OR = 0.30). Schabath et al[172] and others[173,174] have confirmed this finding in a range of ethnic populations.

CONCLUSION

Study of tobacco-induced cancers provides many opportunities for teasing out the intricacies of genetic susceptibility. Most likely, multiple susceptibility factors must be taken into account to represent the true dimensions of gene-environment interactions. We need to capitalize on technologic advances in high-throughput, automated approaches for rapid, large-scale genotyping in order to identify and evaluate biological markers that are more selectively predictive of individual risk, in adequately-powered population-based studies. Emerging technology uses automated work stations capable of extracting DNA from blood samples and performing DNA amplification, hybridization, and detection. Although initially a high-cost endeavor, the utility of such instrumentation to acquire hundreds more genotypes, 1000-fold faster, with less sample ultimately will reduce the cost of existing assays some 100-fold while conserving precious resources. A concomitant need exists for state-of-the-art archiving laboratories for long-term storage and tracking of human samples using individualized bar-coding and tracking systems. The ethical, educational, social, and informatics considerations that will result are challenging.

ACKNOWLEDGMENT

This study was supported by grants CA55769 (M.R.S.), CA 86390 (M.R.S.), R01 CA74851 (Q.W.), R29 70334 (Q.W.), and CA74880 (X.W.) from the National Cancer Institute.

REFERENCES

1. Risch HA, Howe GR, Jain M et al. Are female smokers at higher risk for lung cancer than male smokers? A case-control analysis by histologic type. Am J Epidemiol 1993;138:281–293.
2. Zang EA, Wynder EL. Differences in lung cancer risk between men and women: examination of the evidence. J Natl Cancer Inst 1996;88:183–192.
3. McDuffie HH, Klaassen DJ, Dosman JA. Men, women and primary lung cancer—a Saskatchewan personal interview study. J Clin Epidemiol 1991;44:537–544.
4. Brownson RC, Chang JC, Davis JR. Gender and histologic type variations in smoking-related risk of lung cancer. Epidemiology 1992;3:61–64.
5. Muscat JE, Richie JP Jr, Thompson S, Wynder EL. Gender differences in smoking and risk of oral cancer. Cancer Res 1996;56:5192–5197.
6. Kreuzer M, Boffetta P, Whitley E et al. Gender differences in lung cancer risk by smoking: a multicentre case-control study in Germany and Italy. Br J Cancer 2000;82:227–233.
7. Prescott E, Osler M, Hein HO et al. Gender and smoking-related risk of lung cancer. The Copenhagen Center for Prospective Population Studies. Epidemiology 1998;91:79–83.
8. Sinha R, Kulldorff M, Swanson CA et al. Dietary heterocyclic amines and the risk of lung cancer among Missouri women. Cancer Res 2000;60:3753–3756.
9. Voorrips LE, Goldbohm RA, Brants HA et al. A prospective cohort study on antioxidant and folate intake and male lung cancer risk. Cancer Epidemiol Biomarkers Prev 2000;9:357–365.
10. Tokuhata GK, Lilienfeld AM. Familial aggregation of lung cancer in humans. J Natl Cancer Inst 1963;30:289–312.
11. Ooi WL, Elston RC, Chen VW et al. Increased familial risk for lung cancer. J Natl Cancer Inst 1986;76:217–222.
12. Wu AH, Fontham ET, Reynolds P et al. Family history of cancer and risk of lung cancer among lifetime nonsmoking women in the United States. Am J Epidemiol 1996;143:535–542.
13. Osann KE. Lung cancer in women: the importance of smoking, family history of cancer, and medical history of respiratory disease. Cancer Res 1991;51:4893–4897.
14. Sellers TA, Bailey-Wilson JE, Elston RC et al. Evidence for Mendelian inheritance in the pathogenesis of lung cancer. J Natl Cancer Inst 1990;82:1272–1279.
15. Yang P, Schwartz AG. Genetic epidemiology of lung cancer: II. Control segregation analysis of families of non-smoking lung cancer probands. Genet Epidemiol 1993;10:344.

16. Amos CI, Caporaso NE, Weston A. Host factors in lung cancer risk: a review of interdisciplinary studies. Cancer Epidemiol Biomarkers Prev 1992;1:505–513.
17. Khanna KK, Lavin MF. Ionizing radiation and UV induction of p53 protein by different pathways in ataxia-telangiectasia cells. Oncogene 1993;8:3307–3312.
18. Loft S, Poulsen HE. Cancer risk and oxidative DNA damage in man. J Mol Med 1996;74:297–312.
19. Eisen JA, Hanawalt PC. A phylogenomic study of DNA repair genes, proteins, and processes. Mutat Res 1999;435:171–213.
20. Memisoglul A, Samson L. Base excision repair in yeast and mammals. Mutat Res 2000;451:39–51.
21. Krokan HE, Nilsen H, Skorpen F et al. Base excision repair of DNA in mammalian cells. FEBS Lett 2000;476:73–77.
22. Friedberg EC, Walker GC, Siede W. DNA Repair and Mutagenesis. Washington, DC: ASM Press, 1995.
23. Witt EH, Reznick AZ, Viguie CA et al. Exercise, oxidative damage and effects of antioxidant manipulation. J Nutr 1992;122[suppl 3]:766–773.
24. Verhagen H, Poulsen HE, Loft S et al. Reduction of oxidative DNA-damage in humans by Brussels sprouts. Carcinogenesis 1995;16:969–970.
25. The Alpha-Tocopherol, Beta Carotene Cancer Prevention Study Group. The effect of vitamin E and betacarotene on the incidence of lung cancer and other cancers in male smokers. N Engl J Med 1994;330:1029–1035.
26. van Poppel G, Poulsen H, Loft S, Verhagen H. No influence of betacarotene on oxidative DNA damage in male smokers. J Natl Cancer Inst 1995;87:310–311.
27. Sancer A. DNA repair in humans. Annu Rev Genet 1995;29:69–105.
28. Hoeijmakers JHJ. Human nucleotide excision repair syndromes: molecular clues to unexpected intricacies. Eur J Cancer 1994;30:1912–1921.
29. Cleaver JE, Kraemer K, Scriver CR et al, eds. The Metabolic Basis of Inherited Diseases II. New York: McGraw-Hill, 1989:2949.
30. Cleaver JE. Common pathways for ultraviolet skin carcinogenesis in the repair and replication defective groups of xeroderma pigmentosum. J Dermatol Sci 2000;23:1–11.
31. Swift M, Chase C. Cancer in families with xeroderma pigmentosum. J Natl Cancer Inst 1979;62:1415–1421.
32. Kraemer KH, Lee MM, Andrews AD, Lambert WC. The role of sunlight and DNA repair in melanoma and nonmelanoma skin cancer. The xeroderma pigmentosum paradigm. Arch Dermatol 1994;130:1018–1021.
33. Phillips DH. Fifty years of B(a)P. Nature 1983;303:468–472.
34. Gelboin HV. Benzo[a]pyrene metabolism, activation, and carcinogenesis: role and regulation of mixed function oxidases and related enzymes. Physiol Rev 1980;60:1107–1166.
35. MacLeod MC, Tang MS. Interaction of benzo[a]pyrene-diol-epoxides with linear and supercoiled DNA. Cancer Res 1985;45:51–56.
36. Tang MS, Pierce JR, Doisy RP et al. Differences and similarities in the repair of two benzo[a]pyrene diol epoxide isomers induced DNA adducts by *uvrA*, *uvrB*, and *uvrC* gene products. Biochemistry 1992;31:8429–8436.
37. Everson RB, Randerath E, Santella RM et al. Detection of smoking-related covalent DNA adducts in human placenta. Science 1986;231:54–57.
38. Perera FP, Santella RM, Brenner D et al. DNA adducts, protein adducts, and sister chromatid exchange in cigarette smokers and nonsmokers. J Natl Cancer Inst 1987;79:449–456.

39. Geneste O, Camus AM, Castegaro M et al. Comparison of pulmonary DNA adduct levels, measured by 32P-postlabelling and aryl hydrocarbon hydroxylase activity in lung parenchyma of smokers and ex-smokers. Carcinogenesis 1991;12:1301–1305.
40. Izzotti A, Rossi GA, Bagnasco M, Flora SD. Benzo[a]pyrene diol epoxide-DNA adducts in alveolar macrophages. Carcinogenesis 1991;12:1281–1285.
41. Chen RH, Maher VM, Brouwer J et al. Preferential repair and strand-specific repair of benzo[a]pyrene diol epoxide adducts in HPRT gene of diploid human fibroblasts. Proc Natl Acad Sci USA 1992;89:5413–5417.
42. Denissenko MF, Pao A, Pfeifer GP, Tang M. Slow repair of bulky DNA adducts along the nontranscribed strand of the human p53 gene may explain the strand bias of transversion mutations in cancers. Oncogene 1998;16:1241–1247.
43. Denissenko MF, Pao A, Tang M, Pfeifer GP. Preferential formation of benzo[a]pyrene adducts at lung cancer mutational hotspots in p53. Science 1996;274:430–432.
44. Hollstein M, Sidransky D, Vogelstein B, Harris CC. p53 mutations in human cancers. Science 1991;253:49–53.
45. Bennett WP, Hussain SP, Vahakangas KH et al. Molecular epidemiology of human cancer risk: gene-environment interactions and p53 mutation spectrum in human lung cancer. J Pathol 1999;187:8–18.
46. Fishel R, Kolodner RD. Identification of mismatch repair genes and their role in the development of cancer. Curr Opin Genet Dev 1995;5:382–395.
47. Loeb LA, Kunkel TA. Fidelity of DNA synthesis. Annu Rev Biochem 1982;51:429–457.
48. Lieb M. Bacterial genes mutL, mutS, and dcm participate in repair of mismatches at 5-methylcytosine sites. J Bacteriol 1987;169:5241–5246.
49. Michaels ML, Miller JH. The GO system protects organisms from the mutagenic effect of the spontaneous lesion 8-hydroxyguanine (7,8-dihydro-8-oxoguanine). J Bacteriol 1992;174:6321–6325.
50. Modrich P. Mismatch repair, genetic stability, and cancer. Science 1994;266:1959–1960.
51. Kolodner RD. Mismatch repair: mechanisms and relationship to cancer susceptibility. Trends Biochem Sci 1995;20:397–401.
52. Kinzler KW, Vogelstein B. Lessons from hereditary colon cancer. Cell 1996;87:159–170.
53. Dutrillaux, B. Pathways of chromosome alteration in human epithelial cancers. Adv Cancer Res 1995;67:59–82.
54. Field JK. Genomic instability in squamous cell carcinoma of the head and neck. Anticancer Res 1996;16:2421–2431.
55. Xinarianos G, Liloglou T, Prime W et al. HMLH1 and hMSH2 expression correlates with allelic imbalance on chromosome 3p in non-small cell lung carcinomas. Cancer Res 2000;60:4216–4221.
56. Chang JW, Chen YC, Chen CY et al. Correlation of genetic instability with mismatch repair protein expression and p53 mutations in non-small cell lung cancer. Clin Cancer Res 2000;6:1639–1646.
57. Ahrendt SA, Decker PA, Doffek K et al. Microsatellite instability at selected tetranucleotide repeats is associated with p53 mutations in non-small cell lung cancer. Cancer Res 2000;60:2488–2491.
58. Wei Q, Eicher SA, Guan Y et al. Reduced expression of hMLH1 and hGTBP/hMSH6: a risk factor for head and neck cancer. Cancer Epidemiol Biomarkers Prev 1998;7:309–314.
59. Phillips PS, Denman AR. Radon: a human carcinogen. Sci Prog 1997;80:317–336.
60. Protic-Sabljic M, Kraemer KH. One pyrimidine dimer inactivates expression of a transfected gene in xeroderma pigmentosum cells. Proc Natl Acad Sci USA 1985;82:6622–6626.

61. Athas WF, Hedayati M, Matanoski GM et al. Development and field-test validation of an assay for DNA repair in circulating lymphocytes. Cancer Res 1991;51:5786–5793.
62. Wei Q, Matanoski GM, Farmer ER et al. DNA repair and aging in basal cell carcinoma: a molecular epidemiology study. Proc Natl Acad Sci USA 1993;90:1614–1618.
63. Wei Q, Cheng L, Hong WK et al. Reduced DNA repair capacity in lung cancer patients. Cancer Res 1996;56:4103–4107.
64. Wei Q, Cheng L, Amos CI et al. Repair of tobacco carcinogen-induced DNA adducts and lung cancer risk: a molecular epidemiological study. J Natl Cancer Inst 2000;92:1764–1772.
65. Cheng L, Eicher SA, Guo Z et al. Reduced DNA repair capacity in head and neck cancer patients. Cancer Epidemiol Biomarkers Prev 1998;7,465–468.
66. Hsu TC, Johnston DA, Cherry LM et al. Sensitivity to genotoxic effects of bleomycin in humans: possible relationship to environmental carcinogenesis. Int J Cancer 1989;43:403–409.
67. Strom SS, Wu X, Sigurdson AJ et al. Lung cancer, smoking patterns, and mutagen sensitivity in Mexican-Americans. Monogr Natl Cancer Inst 1995;18:29–33.
68. Wu X, Delclos GL, Annegers FJ et al. A case-control study of wood-dust exposure, mutagen sensitivity, and lung-cancer risk. Cancer Epidemiol Biomarkers Prev 1995;4:583–588.
69. Hagmar L, Brogger A, Hansteen I et al. Cancer risk in humans predicted by increased levels of chromosome aberrations in lymphocytes: Nordic study group on the health risk of chromosome damage. Cancer Res 1994;54:2919–2922.
70. Bonassi S, Abbondandolo A, Camurri L et al. Are chromosome aberrations in circulating lymphocytes predictive of future cancer onset in humans? Preliminary results of an Italian cohort study. Cancer Genet Cytogenet 1995;79:133–135.
71. Hsu TC. Genetic instability in the human population: a working hypothesis. Hereditas 1983; 98:1–9.
72. Spitz MR, Hsu TC, Wu XF et al. Mutagen sensitivity as a biologic marker of lung cancer risk in African Americans. Cancer Epidemiol Biomarkers Prev 1995;4:99–103.
73. Hsu TC, Spitz MR, Schantz SP. Mutagen sensitivity: a biologic marker of cancer susceptibility. Cancer Epidemiol Biomarkers Prev 1991;1:83–89.
74. Spitz MR, Fueger JJ, Beddingfield NA et al. Chromosome sensitivity to bleomycin-induced mutagenesis, an independent risk factor for upper aerodigestive tract cancers. Cancer Res 1989; 49:4626–4628.
75. Schantz SP, Hsu TC, Ainslie N, Moser RP. Young adults with head and neck cancer express increased susceptibility to mutagen-induced chromosome damage. JAMA 1989;262:3313–3315.
76. Spitz MR, Hoque A, Trizna Z et al. Mutagen sensitivity as a risk factor for second malignant tumors following upper aerodigestive tract malignancies. J Natl Cancer Inst 1994;86:1681–1684.
77. Wei Q, Spitz MR, Gu J et al. DNA repair capacity correlates with mutagen sensitivity in lymphoblastoid cell lines. Cancer Epidemiol Biomarkers Prev 1996;5:199–204.
78. Pandita TK, Hittelman WN. Evidence of a chromatin basis for increased mutagen sensitivity associated with multiple primary malignancies of the head and neck. Int J Cancer 1995;61:738–743.
79. Everson RB, Randerath E, Santella RM et al. Detection of smoking-related covalent DNA adducts in human placenta. Science 1986;231:54–57.
80. Li D, Wang M, Cheng L et al. In vitro induction of benzo(a)pyrene diol epoxide–DNA adducts in peripheral lymphocytes as a susceptibility marker for human lung cancer. Cancer Res 1996; 56:3638–3641.
81. Reddy MV, Randerath K. Nuclease P1-mediated enhancement of sensitivity of 32P-postlabeling test for structurally diverse DNA adducts. Carcinogenesis 1986;7:1543–1551.

82. Phillips DH, Hewer A, Grover PL. Aromatic DNA adducts in human bone marrow and peripheral blood leukocytes. Carcinogenesis 1986;7:2071–2075.
83. van Schooten FJ, Hillebrand MJ, van Leeuwen FE et al. Polycyclic aromatic hydrocarbon–DNA adducts in white blood cells from lung cancer patients: no correlation with adduct levels in lung. Carcinogenesis 1992;13:987–993.
84. Savela K, Hemminki K. DNA adducts in lymphocytes and granulocytes of smokers and nonsmokers detected by the 32P-postlabelling assay. Carcinogenesis 1991;12:503–508.
85. Gupta RC, Earley K, Sharma S. Use of human peripheral blood lymphocytes to measure DNA binding capacity of chemical carcinogens. Proc Natl Acad Sci USA 1988;85:3513.
86. Krolewski B, Little JB, Reynolds RJ. Effect of duration of exposure to benzo(a)pyrene diol-epoxide on neoplastic transformation, mutagenesis, cytotoxicity, and total covalent binding to DNA of rodent cells. Teratog Carcinog Mutagen 1988;8:127–136.
87. Li D, Firozi PF, Wang L et al. Sensitivity to DNA damage induced by benzo(a)pyrene diol epoxide and risk of lung cancer—a case-control analysis. Cancer Res (in press).
88. Wei Q, Xu X, Cheng L et al. Simultaneous amplification of four DNA repair genes and beta-actin in human lymphocytes by multiplex reverse transcriptase-PCR. Cancer Res 1995;55:5025–5029.
89. Shen MR, Jones IM, Mohrenweiser H. Nonconservative amino acid substitution variants exist at polymorphic frequency in DNA repair genes in healthy humans. Cancer Res 1998;58:604–608.
90. Fan F, Liu C, Tavare S, Arnheim N. Polymorphisms in the human DNA repair gene XPF. Mutat Res 1999;406:115–120.
91. Khan SG, Metter EJ, Tarone RE et al. A new xeroderma pigmentosum group C poly(AT) insertion/deletion polymorphism. Carcinogenesis 2000;21:1821–1825.
92. Dybdahl M, Vogel U, Frentz G et al. Polymorphisms in the DNA repair gene *XPD*: correlations with risk and age at onset of basal cell carcinoma. Cancer Epidemiol Biomarkers Prev 1999;8:77–81.
93. Coin F, Marinoni JC, Rodolfo C, et al. Mutations in the XPD helicase gene result in XP and TTD phenotypes, preventing interaction between XPD and the p44 subunit of TFIIH. Nat Genet 1998;20:184–188.
94. Taylor EM, Broughton BC, Botta E et al. Xeroderma pigmentosum and trichothiodystrophy are associated with different mutations in the XPD (ERCC2) repair/transcription gene. Proc Natl Acad Sci USA 1997;94:8658–8663.
95. Reardon JT, Ge H, Gibbs E, Sancar A, Hurwitz J, Pan ZQ. Isolation and characterization of two human transcription factor IIH (TFIIH)–related complexes: ERCC2/CAK and TFIIH. Proc Natl Acad Sci USA 1996;93:6482–6487.
96. Sturgis EM, Spitz MR, Wei Q. DNA repair and genomic instability in tobacco induced malignancies of the lung and upper aerodigestive tract. Environ Carcinogen Ecol 1998;C16:1–30.
97. Moller P, Wallin H, Dybdahl M et al. Psoriasis patients with basal cell carcinoma have more repair-mediated DNA strand-breaks after UVC damage in lymphocytes than psoriasis patients without basal cell carcinoma. Cancer Lett 2000;151:187–192.
98. Lunn RM, Helzlsouer KJ, Parshad R et al. XPD polymorphisms: effects on DNA repair proficiency. Carcinogenesis 2000;21:551–555.
99. Duell EJ, Wiencke JK, Cheng TJ et al. Polymorphisms in the DNA repair genes XRCC1 and ERCC2 and biomarkers of DNA damage in human blood mononuclear cells. Carcinogenesis 2000;21:965–971.
100. Sturgis EM, Zheng R, Li L et al. XPD/ERCC2 polymorphisms and risk of head and neck cancer: A case-control analysis. Carcinogenesis 2000;21:2219–2223.
101. Broughton BC, Steingrimsdottir H, Lehmann AR. Five polymorphisms in the coding sequence of the xeroderma pigmentosum group D gene. Mutat Res 1996;362:209–211.

102. Zhang X, Morera S, Bates PA et al. Structure of an XRCC1 BCRT domain: a new protein-protein interaction module. EMBO J 1998;17:6404–6411.
103. Masson M, Niedergang C, Schreiber V et al. XRCC1 is specifically associated with PARP polymerase and negatively regulates its activity following DNA damage. Mol Cell Biol 1998;18:3563–3571.
104. Caldecott KW, McKeown CK, Tucker JD et al. An interaction between the mammalian DNA repair protein XRCC1 and DNA ligase III. Mol Cell Biol 1994;14:68–76.
105. Kubota Y, Nash RA, Klungland A et al. Reconstitution of DNA base excision-repair with purified human proteins: interaction between DNA polymerase beta and the XRCC1 protein. EMBO J 1996;15:6662–6670.
106. Cappelli E, Taylor R, Cevasco M et al. Involvement of XRCC1 and DNA ligase gene products in DNA base excision repair. J Biol Chem 1997;272:23970–23975.
107. Marintchev A, Mullen MA, Maciejewski MW et al. Solution structure of the single-strand break repair protein XRCC1 N-terminal domain. Nat Struct Biol 1999;6:884–893.
108. Lunn RM, Langlois RG, Hsieh LL et al. XRCC1 polymorphisms: effects on aflatoxin B1-DNA adducts and glycophorin A variant frequency. Cancer Res 1999;59:2557–2561.
109. Sturgis EM, Castillo EJ, Li L et al. Polymorphisms of DNA repair gene XRCC1 in squamous cell carcinoma of the head and neck. Carcinogenesis 1999;20:2125–2129.
110. Boiteux S, Radicella JP. The human OGG1 gene: structure, functions, and its implication in the process of carcinogenesis. Arch Biochem Biophys 2000;377:1–8.
111. Kohno T, Shinmura K, Tosaka M et al. Genetic polymorphisms and alternative splicing of the hOGG1 gene, that is involved in the repair of 8-hydroxyguanine in damaged DNA. Oncogene 1998;16:3219–3225.
112. Chevillard S, Radicella JP, Levalois C et al. Mutations in OGG1, a gene involved in the repair of oxidative DNA damage, are found in human lung and kidney tumours. Oncogene 1998;16:3083–3086.
113. Audebert M, Radicella JP, Dizdaroglu M. Effect of single mutations in the OGG1 gene found in human tumors on the substrate specificity of the OGG1 protein. Nucleic Acids Res 2000;28:2672–2678.
114. Sugimura H, Kohno T, Wakai K et al. hOGG1 Ser326Cys polymorphism and lung cancer susceptibility. Cancer Epidemiol Biomarkers Prev 1999;8:669–674.
115. Ishida T, Takashima R, Fukayama M et al. New DNA polymorphisms of human MMH/OGG1 gene: prevalence of one polymorphism among lung-adenocarcinoma patients in Japanese. Int J Cancer 1999;80:18–21.
116. Blons H, Radicella JP, Laccoureye O et al. Frequent allelic loss at chromosome 3p distinct from genetic alterations of the 8-oxoguanine DNA glycosylase 1 gene in head and neck cancer. Mol Carcinog 1999;26:254–260.
117. Wikman H, Risch A, Klimek F et al. hOGG1 polymorphism and loss of heterozygosity (LOH): significance for lung cancer susceptibility in a Caucasian population. Int J Cancer 2000;88:932–937.
118. Shields PG, Caporaso NE, Falk RT et al. Lung cancer, race and a CYP1A1 genetic polymorphism. Cancer Epidemiol Biomarkers Prev 1993;2:481–485.
119. Sugimura H, Wakai K, Genka K et al. Association of Ile462Val (Exon 7) polymorphism of cytochrome P450 IA1 with lung cancer in the Asian population: further evidence from a case-control study in Okinawa. Cancer Epidemiol Biomarkers Prev 1998;7:413–417.
120. Le Marchand L, Sivaraman L, Pierce L et al. Associations of CYP1A1, GSTM1, and CYP2E1 polymorphisms with lung cancer suggest cell type specificities to tobacco carcinogens. Cancer Res 1998;58:4858–4863.

121. Hirvonen A, Hugsgatvel-Pursiainen K, Karjalainen A et al. Point-mutational Msp1 and Ile-Val polymorphisms closely linked in the CYP1A1 gene: lack of association with susceptibility to lung cancer in a Finnish study population. Cancer Epidemiol Biomarkers Prev 1992;1:485–489.
122. London SJ, Daly AK, Fairbrother KS et al. Lung cancer risk in African-Americans in relation to a race-specific CYP1A1 polymorphism. Cancer Res 1995;55:6035–6037.
123. Houlston, RS. CYP1A1 polymorphisms and lung cancer risk: a meta-analysis. Pharmacogenetics 2000;10:105–114.
124. Eaton DL, Gallagher EP, Bammler TK, Kunze KL. Role of cytochrome P4501A2 in chemical carcinogenesis: implications for human variability in expression and enzyme activity. Pharmacogenetics 1995;5:259–274.
125. MacLeod S, Tand Y-M, Yokoi T et al. The role of recently discovered genetic polymorphism in the regulation of the human CYP1A2 gene. Proc Am Assoc Cancer Res 1998;39:396.
126. Nakajima M, Yokoi T, Mizutani M et al. Genetic polymorphism in the 5'-flanking region of human CYP1A2 gene: effect on the CYP1A2 inducibility in humans. J Biochem (Tokyo) 1999;125:803–808.
127. Sachse C, Brockmoller J, Bauer S, Roots I. Functional significance of a C→A polymorphism in intron 1 of the cytochrome P450 CYP1A2 gene tested with caffeine. Br J Clin Pharmacol 1999;47:445–449.
128. Landi MT, Zocchetti C, Bernucci I et al. Cytochrome P4501A2: enzyme induction and genetic control in determining 4-aminobiphenyl-hemoglobin adduct levels. Cancer Epidemiol Biomarkers Prev 1996;5:693–698.
129. Hayashi SI, Watanabe J, Kawajiri K. Genetic polymorphisms in the 5'-flanking region change transcriptional regulation of the human cytochrome P450IIEI gene. J Biochem 1991;111:559–565.
130. Uematsu F, Kikuchi H, Motomiya M et al. Association between restriction fragment length polymorphism of the human cytochrome P450IIEI gene and susceptibility to lung cancer. Jpn J Cancer Res 1991;82:254–256.
131. Persson I, Johansson I, Bergling H et al. Genetic polymorphism of cytochrome P4502E1 in a Swedish population: relationship to incidence of lung cancer. FEBS Lett 1993;319:207–211.
132. Wu X, Shi H, Jiang H et al. Associations between cytochrome P4502E1 genotype, mutagen sensitivity, cigarette smoking and susceptibility to lung cancer. Carcinogenesis 1997;18:967–973.
133. Autrup H. Genetic polymorphisms in human xenobiotic metabolizing enzymes as susceptibility factors in toxic response. Mutat Res 2000;464:65–76.
134. Houlston RS. Glutathione S-transferase M1 status and lung cancer risk: a meta-analysis. Cancer Epidemiol Biomarkers Prev 1999;8:675–682.
135. Johns LE, Houlston RS. Glutathione S-transferase 1(GSTM1) status and bladder cancer risk: a meta-analysis. Mutagenesis 2000;15:399–404.
136. Brockmoller J, Cascorbi I, Kerb R, Roots I. Combined analysis of inherited polymorphisms in arylamine N-acetyltransferase 2, glutathione S-transferase M1 and T1, microsomal epoxide hydrolase, and cytochrome P450 enzymes as modulators of bladder cancer risk. Cancer Res 1996;56:3915–3925.
137. Hirvonen A, Nylund L, Kociba P et al. Modulation of urinary mutagenicity by genetically determined carcinogen metabolism in smokers. Carcinogenesis 1994;15:813–815.
138. Cheng L, Sturgis EM, Eicher SA et al. Glutathione-S-transferase polymorphisms and risk of squamous cell carcinoma of the head and neck. Int J Cancer 1999;84:220–224.
139. Spitz MR, Duphorne CM, Detry MA et al. Dietary intake of isothiocyanates: evidence of a joint effect with glutathione S-transferase polymorphisms in lung cancer risk. Cancer Epidemiol Biomarkers Prev 2000;9:1017–1020.

140. London SJ, Yuan JM, Chung FL et al. Isothiocyanates, glutathione S-transferase M1 and T1 polymorphisms and lung cancer risk: a prospective study of men in Shanghai, China. Lancet 2000;356:724–729.
141. Ryberg D, Skaug V, Hewer A et al. Genotypes of glutathione transferase M1 and P1 and their significance for lung DNA adduct levels and cancer risk. Carcinogenesis 1997;18:1285–1289.
142. Johansson AS, Stenberg G, Widersten M, Mannervik B. Structure-activity relationships and thermal stability of human glutathione transferase P1-1 governed by the H-site residue 105. J Mol Biol 1998;278:687–698.
143. Vineis P, Bartsch H, Caporaso N et al. Genetically based N-acetyltransferase metabolic polymorphism and low-level environmental exposure to carcinogens. Nature 1994;369:154–156.
144. Vine MF, McFarland LT. Markers of susceptibility. In: Hulka BS, Wilcosky TC, Griffith JD, eds. Biological Markers in Epidemiology. New York: Oxford University Press, 1990:196–213.
145. Gonzalez MV, Alvarez V, Pello MF et al. Genetic polymorphism of N-acetyltransferase-2, glutathione S-transferase-M1, and cytochromes P450IIE1 and P450IID6 in the susceptibility to head and neck cancer. J Clin Pathol 1998;51:294–298.
146. Morita S, Yano M, Tsujinaka T et al. Association between genetic polymorphisms of glutathione S-transferase P1 and N-acetyltransferase 2 and susceptibility to squamous-cell carcinoma of the esophagus. Int J Cancer 1998;79:517–520.
147. Morita S, Yano M, Tsujinaka T et al. Genetic polymorphisms of drug-metabolizing enzymes and susceptibility to head-and-neck squamous-cell carcinoma. Int J Cancer 1999;80:685–688.
148. Okkels H, Sigsgaard T, Wolf H, Autrup H. Arylamine N-acetyltransferase 1 (NAT1) and 2 (NAT2) polymorphisms in susceptibility to bladder cancer: the influence of smoking. Cancer Epidemiol Biomarkers Prev 1997;6:225–231.
149. Filiadis IF, Georgiou I, Alamanos Y et al. Genotypes of N-acetyltransferase-2 and risk of bladder cancer: a case-control study. J Urol 1999;161:1672–1675.
150. Yu MC, Skipper PL, Taghizadeh K et al. Acetylator phenotype, aminobiphenyl-hemoglobin adduct levels, and bladder cancer risk in white, black, and Asian men in Los Angeles, California. J Natl Cancer Inst 1994;86:712–716.
151. Wu X, Liu JH, Trizna Z, Spitz MR. The association of N-acetylator, mutagen sensitivity and lung cancer risk. Proc Am Assoc Cancer Res 1996;37:263.
152. Cascorbi I, Brockmoller J, Mrozikiewicz PM et al. Homozygous rapid arylamine N-acetyltransferase (NAT2) genotype as a susceptibility factor for lung cancer. Cancer Res 1996;56:3961–3966.
153. Nyberg F, Hou SM, Hemminki K et al. Glutathione S-transferase mu1 and N-acetyltransferase 2 genetic polymorphisms and exposure to tobacco smoke in nonsmoking and smoking lung cancer patients and population controls. Cancer Epidemiol Biomarkers Prev 1998;7:875–883.
154. Bell DA, Badawi AF, Lang NP et al. Polymorphism in the N-acetyltransferase 1 (NAT1) polyadenylation signal: association of NAT110 allele with higher N-acetylation activity in bladder and colon tissue. Cancer Res 1995;55:5226–5229.
155. Taylor JA, Umbach DM, Stephens E et al. The role of N-acetylation polymorphisms in smoking-associated bladder cancer: evidence of a gene-gene-exposure three-way interaction. Cancer Res 1998;58:3603–3610.
156. Badawi A, Hirvonen A, Bell DA et al. Role of aromatic amine acetyltransferases, NAT1 and NAT2, in carcinogen-DNA adduct formation in the human urinary bladder. Cancer Res 1995;55:5230–5237.
157. Bouchardy C, Mitrunen K, Wikman H et al. N-acetyltransferase NAT1 and NAT2 enotypes and lung cancer risk. Pharmacogenetics 1998;8:291–298.
158. Ishibe N, Wiencke JK, Zuo Z et al. Polymorphisms in the N-acetyltransferase 1 (NAT1) gene and lung cancer risk in a minority population. Biomarkers 1998;3:219–226.

159. Lancaster JM, Brownlee HA, Bell DA et al. Microsomal epoxide hydrolase polymorphism as a risk factor for ovarian cancer. Mol Carcinog 1996;17:160–162.
160. Hassett C, Aicher L, Sidhu JS, Omiecinski CJ. Human microsomal epoxide hydrolase: genetic polymorphism and functional expression in vitro of amino acid variants. Hum Mol Genet 1994; 3:421–428.
161. Raaka S, Hassett C, Omiencinski CJ. Human microsomal epoxide hydrolase: 5' flanking region genetic polymorphisms. Carcinogenesis 1998;19:387–393.
162. Smith CAD, Harrison D. Association between polymorphisms in gene for microsomal epoxide hydrolase and susceptibility to emphysema. Lancet 1997;350:630–633.
163. London SJ, Smart J, Daly AK. Lung cancer risk in relation to genetic polymorphisms of microsomal epoxide hydrolase among African-Americans and Caucasians in Los Angeles County. Lung Cancer 2000;28:147–155.
164. Benhamou S, Reinikainen M, Bouchardy C et al. Association between lung cancer and microsomal epoxide hydrolase genotypes. Cancer Res 1998;58:5291–5293.
165. Klebanoff SJ. Myeloperoxidase: occurrence and biological function. In: Everse J, Everse KE, Grisham MB, eds. Peroxidases in Chemistry and Biology. Boca Raton: CRC Press, 1991:1–35.
166. Schmekel B, Karlsson SE, Linden M et al. Myeloperoxidase in human lung lavage: I. A marker of local neutrophil activity. Inflammation 1990;14:447–454.
167. Mallet WG, Mosebrook DR, Trush MA. Activation of (+/–)-*trans*-7,8-dihydroxy-7,8-dihydrobenzo[a]pyrene to diolepoxides by human polymorphonuclear leukocytes or myeloperoxidase. Carcinogenesis 1991;12:521–524.
168. Petruska JM, Mosebrook DR, Jakab GJ, Trush MA. Myeloperoxidase-enhanced formation of (+/–)-*trans*-7,8-dihydroxy-7,8-dihydrobenzo[a]pyrene-DNA adducts in lung tissue in vitro: a role of pulmonary inflammation in the bioactivation of a procarcinogen. Carcinogenesis 1992;13: 1075–1081.
169. Austin GE, Lam L, Zaki SR et al. Sequence comparison of putative regulatory DNA of the 5' flanking region of the myeloperoxidase gene in normal and leukemic bone marrow cells. Leukemia 1993;7:1445–1450.
170. Piedrafita FJ, Molander RB, Vansant G et al. An Alu element in the myeloperoxidase promoter contains a composite SP1-thyroid hormone-retinoic acid response element. J Biol Chem 1996; 271:14412–14420.
171. London SJ, Lehman TA, Taylor JA. Myeloperoxidase genetic polymorphism and lung cancer risk. Cancer Res 1997;57:5001–5003.
172. Schabath MB, Spitz MR, Zhang X et al. Genetic variants of myeloperoxidase and lung cancer risk. Carcinogenesis 2000;21:1163–1166.
173. Le Marchand L, Seifried A, Lum A, Wilkens LR. Association of the myeloperoxidases-463G→A polymorphism with lung cancer risk. Cancer Epidemiol Biomarkers Prev 2000;9:181–184.
174. Cascorbi I, Henning S, Brockmoller J et al. Substantially reduced risk of cancer of the aerodigestive tract in subjects with variant-463A of the myeloperoxidase gene. Cancer Res 2000;60:644–649.

Thalidomide for Cancer Therapy

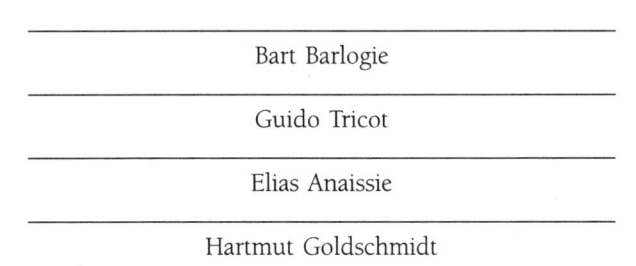

Bart Barlogie
Guido Tricot
Elias Anaissie
Hartmut Goldschmidt

Tumor angiogenesis has emerged as an interesting novel target of cancer therapy owing to the seminal work by Folkman et al.[1] Ongoing neoangiogenesis has been recognized as a critical requirement of not only solid but hematologic tumor growth.[2] During the last 5 years, many reports have noted an adverse prognosis for patients who have a variety of clinical malignancies and increased microvessel density in tumor lesions.[3–5] The initiation and sustenance of neoangiogenesis is complex and involves multiple cytokine loops. These loops typically involve proangiogenic vascular endothelial growth factor (VEGF) and basic fibroblast growth factor (bFGF), which are released by either neoplastic cells or through interaction of malignant cells with the microenvironment. The proangiogenic factors in turn promote survival and proliferation signals in tumor-associated stromal cells and in endothelial cells, which also receive proliferative and migration signals.[6,7]

Data from preclinical experiments with pharmacologic doses of endostatin and angiostatin demonstrated regression in established tumors and prevention of tumor development in the case of tumor cell inoculation after such therapy.[8–10]

Two of the exciting facets of antiangiogenic therapy for tumor growth control are the lack of development of drug resistance with repeated administration and the recognition that tumors may not be completely eradicated but are rendered dormant for extended periods.[11]

The public excitement about antiangiogenic tumor therapy—generated by the endostatin and angiostatin preclinical experiments—led to a single-patient compassionate-therapy trial with the teratogenic agent thalidomide,[12] which, in the rabbit cornea model, possessed marked antiangiogenic properties[13] and was the only drug available for clinical studies at that time. Though this first patient derived only marginal clinical benefit, the awareness of thalidomide's multitargeted mechanisms[14–16] prompted an additional accrual of a patient with multiple myeloma. The second patient unexpectedly experienced the induction of nearly complete remission (CR), despite presenting with advanced disease that was resistant to high-dose alkylating agent therapy and allogeneic transplantation. This clinical anecdote prompted a formal, large, phase II trial of dose-escalating thalidomide in advanced and refractory multiple myeloma.[17] Study results showed objective responses in one-third of patients treated, with complete or near-CRs in more than 10% of the patients with cytotoxic therapy-refractory myeloma. These observations provided compelling evidence that more than three decades after the initial introduction of melphalan and glucocorticoids,[18,19] thalidomide represented a new class of agents with independent antitumor activity in this disease. These single-institution results have since been confirmed by investigators in the United States and around the world.[20] Based on these encouraging data in multiple myeloma, phase II trials have also been initiated in other hematologic malignancies with increased microvessel density (e.g., myelodysplastic syndromes) and in solid tumors.[21] This chapter summarizes the currently available clinical and, where available, translational research data on thalidomide used to treat neoplastic diseases.

MULTIPLE MYELOMA: THE ARKANSAS EXPERIENCE

Thalidomide was administered at 200 mg as a single-agent evening dose with dose escalation of 200 mg every 2 weeks up to a maximum dose of 800 mg according to each patient's tolerance.[22] The characteristics of the 169 patients treated are summarized in Table 7.1. Importantly, 67% had cytogenetic abnormalities, including 37% with the high-risk chromosome 13 deletion. Among the patients, 76% received one cycle and 53% had two or more cycles of high-dose melphalan with peripheral blood stem cell support. Responses were usually obtained within a median of less than 2 months and were accompanied by improvement in disease-associated laboratory abnormalities, such as recovery from anemia and reduction in bone marrow plasmacytosis and a reduction or even resolution of focal plasmacytoma lesions recognized on magnetic resonance imaging (Fig. 7.1). Using serial paraprotein measurements in serum and urine

TABLE 7.1 Phase II Study of Thalidomide

Regimen	Characteristics	Percentage
200 mg	Age > 60 yr	44
↓	β_2-Microglobulin > 6 mg/L	22
400 mg	Abnormal cytogenetics	67
↓ q2wk	Deletion 13	37
600 mg	Prior therapy > 60 mo	20
↓	Prior high-dose therapy	76
800 mg	> 1 cycle	53

Notes: University of Arkansas for Medical Sciences UARK98-003; $N = 169$. Therapy consists of melphalan, 200 mg/m^2, and peripheral blood stem cell support.

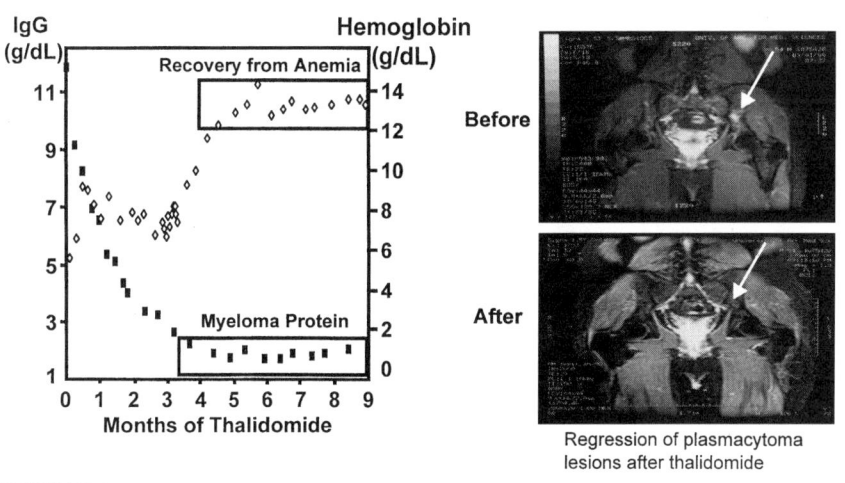

FIGURE 7.1 Example of thalidomide response. Rapid and marked myeloma response is accompanied by recovery of hemoglobin (*left panel*). Disappearance of hyperintense plasmacytoma lesion on magnetic resonance imaging (sort tau inversion recovery image; *right panel*).

to assess treatment efficacy, 37% achieved paraprotein reduction (PPR) by at least 25%, including 30% with PPR of at least 50%; 14% achieved PPR of at least 90%, including 2% with true CR using immunofixation and bone marrow criteria (Table 7.2). Toxicities of grade 3 and higher included sedation in 25%, constipation that was difficult to manage despite laxatives in 16%, peripheral neuropathy (mainly sensory) in 9%, and deep venous thrombosis in 2%. There was no treatment-related mortality (see Table 7.2). As a result of these toxicities, only 50% of patients received the targeted maximum dose of 800 mg, but more than 90% tolerated an intermediate dose of 400 mg of thalidomide. With a median follow-up of 22 months for living patients, 2-year overall survival and event-free

TABLE 7.2 Thalidomide in Advanced Myeloma

	Percentage
Response[a]	
CR	2
90% ≤ rate < CR	12
75% ≤ rate < 90%	6
50% ≤ rate < 75%	10
25% ≤ rate < 50%	7
Total	37
Toxicity ≥ grade 3	
Treatment-related mortality	0
Sedation	25
Constipation	16
Neuropathy	9
Deep venous thrombosis	2

CR, complete remission.
[a]Paraprotein reduction.

survival rates were approximately 60% and 15%, respectively (Fig. 7.2). PPR was associated with improvement in other laboratory features, especially reduction in bone marrow plasmacytosis and β_2-microglobulin (β_2M) and increases in hemoglobin and levels of uninvolved immunoglobulins (Table 7.3).

A prognostic factor analysis of baseline laboratory variables revealed that both event-free and overall survival were inferior in the presence of abnormal cytogenetics, plasma cell-labeling index (PCLI) greater than the median of 0.5%, and

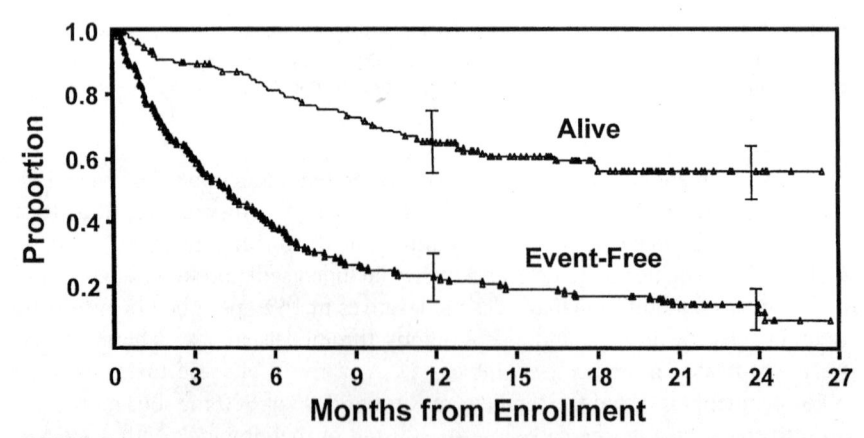

FIGURE 7.2 Phase II study of thalidomide. Kaplan-Meier plots of event-free and overall survival.

TABLE 7.3 Myeloma Protein Response and Associated Laboratory Changes

| | | M-Protein Response | | | | | |
| | | ≥ 50% | | | < 50% | | |
Parameter	N	Median % Change	Interquartile Range	N	Median % Change	Interquartile Range	P Value
Bone marrow plasma cells	41	−20	75	78	+13	183	< 0.0001
β₂-Microglobulin	42	−7	35	86	+22	55	< 0.0001
Immunoglobulin M	29	+58	107	56	−9	48	.002
Hemoglobin	44	+9	15	89	0	24	.003

elevation of β_2M or C-reactive protein (CRP; Table 7.4). In the absence of information about cytogenetics and PCLI, which was frequently not routinely available, patients' risk could be defined on the basis of β_2M and CRP. Using these prognostic criteria, different risk groups could be defined, either on the basis of β_2M, PCLI, and cytogenetics or solely on the basis of β_2M and CRP (Fig. 7.3).

TABLE 7.4 Prognostic Variables with Thalidomide

	Event-Free Survival		Overall Survival	
	HR	P Value	HR	P Value
With PCLI and cytogenetics				
Abnormal cytogenetics	2.2	<0.001	2.5	0.002
PCLI > 0.5%	1.9	0.002	1.8	0.009
β_2M > 3 mg/L	1.5	0.02	3.0	<0.001
CRP > 7 mg/L	N/A	—	1.8	0.01
Without PCLI and cytogenetics				
β_2M > 3 mg/L	1.6	0.009	3.3	<0.001
CRP > 7 mg/L	1.4	0.08	1.9	0.005

β_2M, β_2-microglobulin; CRP, C-reactive protein; HR, hazard ratio; N/A, not available; PCLI, plasma cell–labeling index.

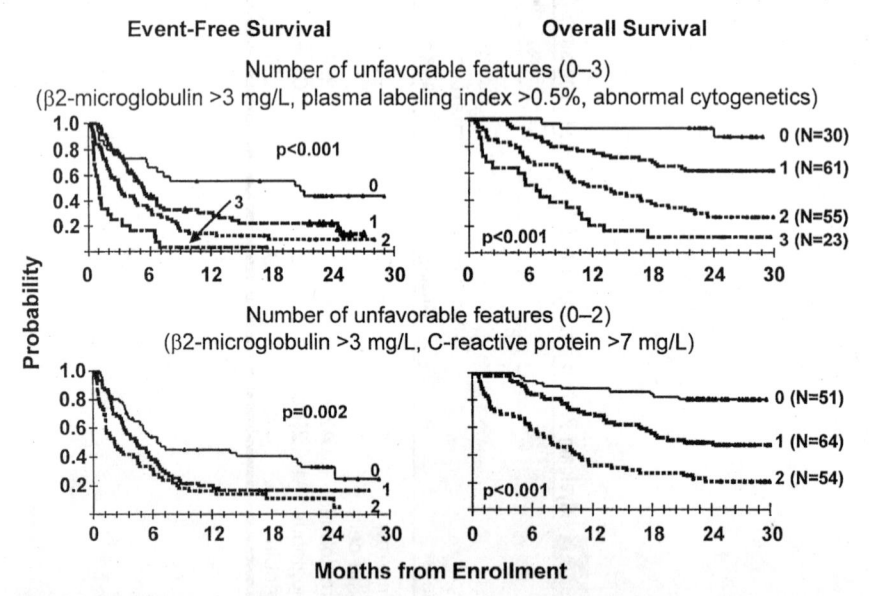

FIGURE 7.3 Clinical outcome according to prognostic factors. Risk discrimination for event-free survival (*left*) and overall survival (*right*) on the basis of β_2-microglobulin, plasma cell–labeling index, and cytogenetics (*top*) or β_2-microglobulin and C-reactive protein (*bottom*).

The study was not designed to evaluate the presence of a dose-response relationship formally but was predicated clearly on such an assumption. A 3-month landmark analysis was conducted to determine whether patients who received more than the median dose of 42 g in the first 3 months of treatment experienced a higher response rate and longer survival. Indeed, response rates were significantly higher (at all PPR levels) among the 83 patients receiving the higher dose as compared with the 66 patients receiving at least 42 g over a period of 3 months ($P < 0.001$); likewise, a higher 3-month cumulative dose of thalidomide was associated with superior overall survival but not event-free survival (Fig. 7.4). This dose effect on survival originated in the patient cohort displaying more than one risk factor (Table 7.5). As a result, the 2-year survival was 42% for patients receiving more than 42 g thalidomide versus 20% for those receiving no more than 42 g over a period of 3 months ($P = 0.01$).

Ancillary measurements of bone marrow microvessel density using CD34 monoclonal antibody staining failed to reveal a correlation between clinical response and either baseline level or reduction of microvessel density. Patients' sera have not yet been analyzed to correlate clinical outcome with reduction in serum or plasma concentrations of VEGF and bFGF.

OTHER THALIDOMIDE STUDIES IN MULTIPLE MYELOMA

Refractory Myeloma

Single-Agent Thalidomide A recent Swedish report essentially confirmed the Arkansas data, citing its response rate of 43% in 20 patients with advanced and

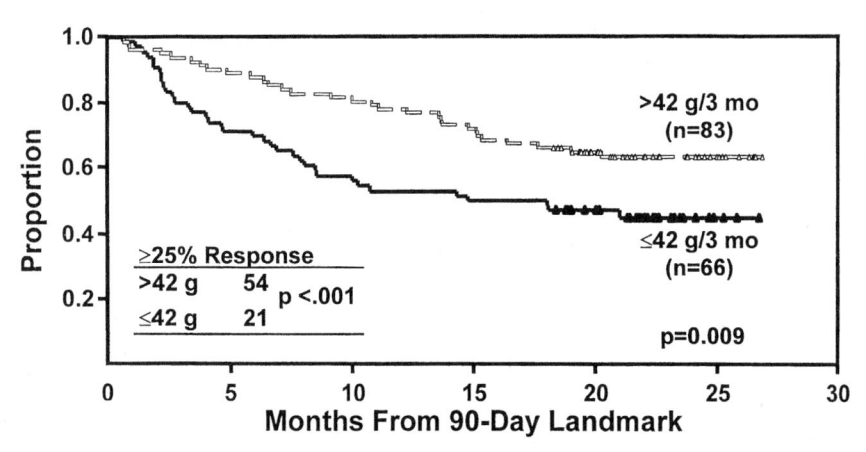

FIGURE 7.4 Higher response rate and longer overall survival with higher thalidomide dose. Of 149 patients surviving a 3-month landmark, those receiving more than 42 g thalidomide over a period of 3 months experienced a higher response rate and superior survival (83 patients) than did the 66 patients receiving a lower cumulative dose.

TABLE 7.5 Benefits of Higher-Dose Thalidomide in Patients with High-Risk Disease

No. Risk Factors	Thalidomide Dose (> 42 g over 3 mo)	N	Response ≥ 25%	P Value	Alive at 2 yr (%)	P Value
≥ 1	Yes	55	45	0.01	74	NS
	No	36	19		66	
≥ 1	Yes	28	43	0.02	42	0.01
	No	30	13		20	

NS, not significant.
Note: Risk factors are β_2-microglobulin > 3 mg/L; plasma cell-labeling index > 0.5%; and abnormal cytogenetics.

refractory myeloma. The study suggested greater antitumor activity and possibly better tolerance when thalidomide was administered in divided doses.[23]

Six studies were presented at the recent American Society of Hematology 2000 meeting on the use of thalidomide for refractory myeloma, reporting PPR of at least 25%, of at least 50% and, in some cases, of at least 75%. Patient cohorts varied in size from 26 to 83 (Table 7.6).[22,24–28] PPR greater than 50% could be obtained in 25% to 47% of patients; the median was 35% when the Arkansas group of 169 patients was included. PPR of no less than 75% was noted in 12% and 13% of patients, respectively, in two studies, matching the 20% incidence in the Arkansas experience. The frequency of prior transplant was not always reported.

Thalidomide Plus Dexamethasone Three studies reported on the use of thalidomide in combination with dexamethasone pulsing (see Table 7.6).[29–31] One study included 12 patients with prior autologous transplant among 38 with either unresponsive relapse ($N = 14$) or resistant relapse ($N = 24$). PPR of no less than 50% were almost identical at 51% and 52%, with at least 75% PPR noted in 24% of the former study.

Combination Chemotherapy Plus Thalidomide The virtual lack of myelosuppression of single-agent thalidomide even in advanced multiple myeloma (MM) after transplantation has prompted several combination trials with cytotoxic agents (see Table 7.6). Two studies[32,33] evaluated the addition of either cyclophosphamide alone or cyclophosphamide plus etoposide to thalidomide plus dexamethasone, yielding high (i.e., $\geq 50\%$) PPR rates of 86% and 78%.

The Arkansas group currently evaluates, in a randomized fashion, the addition of thalidomide in two settings: (1) high-dose dexamethasone pulsing for patients with low tumor bulk and hypoproliferative disease and at low risk for relapse after high-dose therapy and (2) DCEP (dexamethasone, 40 mg for 4 days and 4-day continuous infusions of daily doses of cyclophosphamide, 400 mg/m^2; etoposide, 40 mg/m^2; and cisplatin, 10 mg/m^2 with subsequent G-CSF 300 mg subcutaneously) for patients with high tumor burden and hyperproliferative disease and at high risk for relapse.

For patients previously treated but not given transplants and referred to the Arkansas center, a six-drug combination of DT PACE is under investigation. DT PACE consists of high-dose dexamethasone pulsing, thalidomide (400 mg), and 4-day continuous infusions of cisplatin, doxorubicin (Adriamycin), cyclophosphamide, and etoposide (see Table 7.6).[34] The study addresses whether, in DT PACE–sensitive patients, continuation of DT PACE is as effective as a standard tandem autologous transplant with melphalan, 200 mg/m^2. One hundred thirty-five patients have currently completed the two-cycle induction phase, yielding a true CR rate of 27%, PPR of at least 75% in 44% of patients, and PPR of at least 50% in 54% of patients. In the DT PACE–unresponsive group (PPR < 50%), melphalan-based high-dose therapy was applied to 32 patients, yielding a CR

TABLE 7.6 Thalidomide in Multiple Myeloma

Treatment Regimen	Study	N	Prior Transplants	Response Rate by PPR Level ≥ 75%	≥ 50%	≥ 25%
Thalidomide alone: refractory disease						
Median thal 400 mg (range, 50–800 mg)	Yakoub-Agha et al[24]	83	58 (17 two transplants)	13%	47%	66%
Thal 200–800 mg	Raza et al[25]	26	N/A	12%	46%	69%
Thal 200 mg	Rodriguez et al[26]	40	18	N/A	N/A	75%
Thal 100–800 mg	Tosi et al[27]	27	13 (9 two transplants)	N/A	25%	45%
Thal 200–800 mg (12 wk); Thal + IFN (> 12 wk)	Prince et al[28]	27	N/A	N/A	30%	N/A
Thal 200–800 mg	Barlogie et al[22]	169	128 (90 two transplants)	20%	30%	37%
Summary		372		17% (48 of 278)	35% (117 of 332)	52% (178 of 345)
Thalidomide + dexamethasone: refractory disease						
Thal 100 mg; dex 40 mg × 4 days q28d	Palumbo et al[29]	37	0	24%	51%	73%
Thal 200–400 mg; dex 40 mg × 4 days (days 1–4, 9–12, 17–20 q35d)	Dimopoulos et al[30]	38	12	N/A	52%	N/A

Regimen	Reference	N	Grade 3/4 neuropathy	Response rate	Complete response	Survival
Thal 200–800 mg; dex 20 mg/m² (days 1–5, 8–15 in month 1; days 1–5 in following months)	Weber et al[31]	47	N/A	N/A	52%	N/A
Summary		122			52% (63 of 122)	
Thalidomide + dexamethasone + chemotherapy: refractory disease						
Thal 100–400 mg; dex 20 mg/m²; days 1–4, 9–12, 17–20; CTX 1.8 g/m²	Kropff et al[32]	20	14	N/A	86% (of 14 evaluable)	N/A
TCED: dex 40 mg; CTX 400 mg/m²; VP16 40 mg/m² (× 4 days); and thal 400 mg/day	Moehler et al[33]	42	N/A	7% (CR)	78%	N/A
DT PACE: dex 40 mg; DDP 10 mg/m²; doxorubicin 10 mg/m²; CTX 400 mg/m²; VP16 40 mg/m² (× 4 days); and thal 400 mg/day × 2 cycles	Barlogie (unpublished data)	135	0	44% (CR, 27%)	54%	
Summary		197		35% (62 of 177)	62% (118 of 191)	

TABLE 7.6 *Continued*

Treatment Regimen	Study	N	Prior Transplants	Response Rate by PPR Level ≥ 75%	≥ 50%	≥ 25%
Thalidomide: untreated myeloma						
Symptomatic disease						
Thal 200–800 mg; dex 40 mg (days 1–4, 9–12, 17–20, q35d)	Rajkumar et al[36]	26	0	N/A	77%	N/A
Smoldering disease						
Thal 200–800 mg	Rajkumar et al[36]	16	0	N/A	38%	N/A
Thal 200–600 mg	Weber et al[31]	26	0	N/A	35%	N/A
Summary		68			51% (35 of 68)	

CTX, cyclophosphamide; DDP, cisplatin; dex, dexamethasone; N/A, not available; thal, thalidomide; VP16, etoposide.

rate of 16% and PPR of no less than 75% in 44% of patients. So far, 79 responding patients have been randomly assigned to transplantation versus continuation of DT PACE, yielding CR rates of 69% and 35%, respectively. For the entire group of 180 patients enrolled prior to October 12, 2000, 64% remain event-free and 80% alive at 12 months. Twelve months after random assignment, those values are 75% and 85%, respectively, regardless of treatment arm. Further accrual and follow-up are needed to determine whether the lower CR rate with DT PACE translates into shorter disease control and poorer survival in all patients.

Biaxin Plus Thalidomide Plus Dexamethasone The Cornell group[35] treated 26 myeloma patients and 6 Waldenström's macroglobulinemia patients with the BLT-D regimen: 500 mg of clarithromycin (Biaxin) twice daily with reduction for toxicity to 250 mg, twice daily; thalidomide (50 mg) escalated every 2 weeks to a maximum of 200 mg or reduced by 50 mg for toxicity; and a single dose of dexamethasone (40 mg) every 2 weeks, reduced for toxicity to 20 or 10 mg every 2 weeks. Of 32 patients, 10 had received no prior therapy; 3 had received autologous transplants; 5 had received nonmyeloablative chemotherapy; and 14 had conventional chemotherapy. Four patients withdrew, and 4 additional patients are too early in the treatment phase for evaluation. All remaining 24 evaluable patients responded with a median follow-up of 10 months (range, 2–16 months). Responses included 3 CRs with disappearance of all disease evidence (13%); near-CR with reduction in abnormal immunoglobulin levels to normal levels in 11 (46%); major responses with more than 75% reduction in immunoglobulin levels in 6 (25%); and 4 (17%) partial responses (PRs; no less than 50% reduction in the immunoglobulin spike). Responses were accompanied by concurrent improvement in bone marrow infiltration and in hemoglobin and renal function parameters. Gastrointestinal toxicity was present in almost one-half of patients, 92% had neurologic toxicity, and 72% had endocrine toxicities. Four deaths were recorded, all occurring in responding patients. Three of the four deaths occurred suddenly in patients with severe cardiopulmonary disease. All remaining patients continue to respond. Of the 24 initially response-assessable patients, 83% remain alive and 75% on study, with a median follow-up of 10 mos. It remains to be seen whether the addition of Biaxin to dexamethasone + thalidomide is additive or synergistic.

Untreated Multiple Myeloma

Preliminary results in three trials for newly diagnosed myeloma patients are also summarized in Table 7.6. The Mayo Clinic group[36] treated 26 patients with active myeloma using thalidomide at 200 mg (initially with dose escalation to 800 mg, observing two grade IV skin toxicities) with standard dexamethasone pulsing (40 mg on days 1–4, 9–12, and 17–20), yielding a 77% incidence of PPR of no less than 50%. The same group also evaluated thalidomide alone in a 200- to 800-mg dose escalation schedule in 16 patients with smoldering disease, yielding a

38% incidence of PPR in at least 50%,[36] virtually identical to the 35% in 26 patients with indolent disease reported from the M.D. Anderson group (thalidomide, 200–600 mg).[31] It remains to be seen whether the combination of dexamethasone + thalidomide is superior to either dexamethasone or thalidomide alone in patients with newly diagnosed disease. It should also be emphasized that not a single patient attained CR, suggesting that long-term disease control with this combination is unlikely.

Total Therapy II

At the University of Arkansas, Total Therapy II evaluates the contribution of thalidomide to an intensive program with curative intent. With an accrual goal of 300 patients, 275 have been enrolled between October 13, 1998 and January 1, 2001. As delineated in Table 7.7 and Figure 7.5, CR and near-CR rates (only immunofixation positive, bone marrow negative) increased progressively to an

TABLE 7.7 Efficacy of Total Therapy II

Response	Induction (%)	Transplant 1 (%)	Transplant 2 (%)
Complete remission	26	45	53
90% ≤ rate < CR	19	18	17
75% ≤ rate < 90%	12	14	10
50% ≤ rate < 75%	27	7	4

CR, complete remission.
Note: First 100 patients eligible for second transplant.

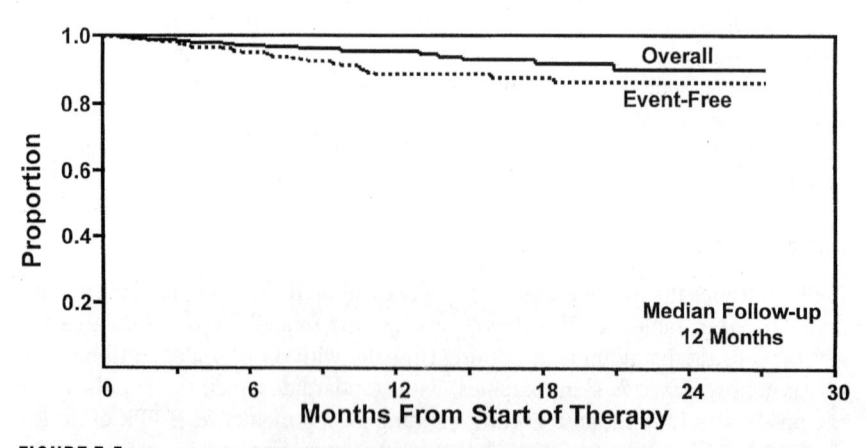

FIGURE 7.5 Survival for 275 patients enrolled in Total Therapy II. High event-free and overall survival rates at 24 months after starting Total Therapy II (for details, see text).

unprecedented 70% as patients proceeded from induction therapy to the first and second high-dose melphalan cycle (intent-to-treat). Data are given for all patients regardless of randomization to thalidomide.

THALIDOMIDE IN MULTIPLE MYELOMA: SUMMARY

Collectively, the foregoing data clearly indicate single-agent activity of thalidomide in advanced and refractory MM, even for posttransplantation relapse. Combination studies are difficult to evaluate at present, as only a few studies (from Arkansas) have taken a randomized trial design approach. The 77% PR rate (PPR ≥ 50%) reported from Mayo Clinic for an up-front combination of thalidomide and dexamethasone may be higher than the 43% response rate with single-agent dexamethasone alone (PPR ≥ 75%)[37] and thus approaches results with primary VAD (see Ref. 37). A randomized trial in the Eastern Cooperative Oncology Group will address clinical efficacy and toxicity of thalidomide plus dexamethasone versus dexamethasone alone. In the prior treatment setting of advanced and refractory MM, however, the single-agent thalidomide PR rate is near 35% and increases to more than 50% with added dexamethasone and beyond 75% with added cyclophosphamide and etoposide or cisplatin. The preliminary Total Therapy II data indicate very high CR rates overall but are blinded as to the contribution of thalidomide. One-third of 42 patients with smoldering myeloma responded to single-agent thalidomide.

MECHANISMS OF THALIDOMIDE ACTION

Mechanistically, data on the antiangiogenic activity of chemotherapy are sparse and difficult to interpret. The observation of higher response rates in the setting of high serum levels of basic fibroblast growth factor in one study and of high levels of VEGF in another study are intriguing and deserve further clarification.[36,38,39] A direct antitumor effect of thalidomide and its newer congeners (IMIDs and SELCIDs)[40] is likely in view of apoptosis and antiproliferative data reported by the Dana-Farber group[41] and based on demonstration of *myc* gene suppression by the Arkansas group.[42] Cytokine-modulated and immunomodulatory effects have also been observed.[43]

THALIDOMIDE TOXICITIES IN MYELOMA TREATMENT

Peripheral neuropathy developing with long-term administration of thalidomide is a major concern.[44] Hypercoagulability reported by the Arkansas group seems to be mainly related to combinations of thalidomide with dexamethasone and combination chemotherapy.[45] Hypothyroidism is readily treatable and has also been reported with interferon-alpha and interferon-gamma, presumably pertaining to an autoimmune mechanism.[46] Cardiac toxicities have probably been underreported but can involve serious sinus bradycardia with syncopal episodes, none of which have been fatal. Among patients with cardiac amyloid, however, this may present a serious problem. Dampening of peripheral blood stem cell (PBSC) mobilization was initially observed in the Total Therapy II program when thalidomide was given during the stem cell mobilization phase with cyclophosphamide, Adriamycin, and dexamethasone.[47] Because the CD34 target was in excess of 20 million per kilogram, thalidomide has since been discontinued after the 4 days of cytotoxic drug administration, and differences between thalidomide and no-thalidomide arms are no longer observed. DT PACE, on the other hand, has been used for PBSC mobilization without apparent negative consequences for the quality of PBSC collection. This issue requires further investigation and may relate to the bone marrow egress mechanisms of CD34 cells, which have been recently linked to modification of cell adhesion molecules such as VLA-4/VCAM-1.[48]

THALIDOMIDE USES FOR OTHER HEMATOLOGIC MALIGNANCIES

Myelodysplasia and Acute Myeloblastic Leukemia

The M.D. Anderson group compared use of liposomal daunorubicin-cytarabine (in 38 patients) with thalidomide added to this chemotherapy regimen (in 36 patients).[49] The "earliest complete remission rates" were 53% and 44%, respectively. According to study design and historical controls, it was thought that thalidomide in this setting did not deserve further evaluation, and the study was discontinued.

The Rush-Presbyterian Group in Chicago reported data about 83 patients mainly with early phases of myelodysplasia, especially refractory anemia and refractory anemia with ringed sideroblasts, noting a 41% PR rate.[50] Benefit was linked to low cytokine activity prior to thalidomide and to a lower apoptosis index of the myelodysplasia marrow. The same group also reported that thalidomide exerted effects on stromal cells of patients with myelodysplasia in vitro; "stromal cell activity" was increased, and a transition from a monoclonal to a polyclonal stromal cell population was observed in several cases, suggesting involvement of stromal cells in the disease process and a potentially favorable effect of thalidomide.

Chronic Lymphocytic Leukemia

The Rush investigators also reported on a dose- and time-dependent increase in CD22 antigen expression observed after in vitro exposure to thalidomide.[51] No clinical data are yet available.

Waldenström's Macroglobulinemia

A team from Greece reported a PPR of no less than 50% in 5 of 20 patients (3 untreated, 2 previously treated).[52] These researchers started with thalidomide,

200 mg, and escalated the dose every 2 weeks to a maximum of 600 mg. The activity of thalidomide in this disease subgroup should be further evaluated.

Miscellaneous Hematologic Malignancies

Anecdotal activity (Vescio, Cedars-Sinai Medical Center) in six cases of amyloidosis[53] and five cases of myelofibrosis[54] (in three patients, idiopathic myelofibrosis; in two patients, myeloproliferative disorders with associated myelofibrosis) require further patient accrual and follow-up.

THALIDOMIDE DOSE AND SCHEDULE

The importance of dose and schedule must be further addressed. Data from Arkansas in myeloma indicate that, in the setting of advanced and refractory myeloma, higher doses may be required, especially in the presence of such high-risk features as abnormal cytogenetics, high labeling index, or high $\beta_2 M$.[22] In view of the great potential as an effective antitumor agent in multiple myeloma and perhaps in other diseases, peripheral neuropathy is a major problem with chronic dosing. Periodic interruption of therapy to allow for recovery from toxicity may have to be considered.

THALIDOMIDE IN SOLID TUMORS

The U.S. Food and Drug Administration summarized the experience of 575 single-patient investigational new drug applications submitted for the use of thalidomide in advanced malignancies. Practitioners were surveyed with a questionnaire, and responses were received from 359 of the 540 practitioners, with data obtained for 480 patients.[55]

Demographics included median age of 52 years (range, 11–90 years) with an even male–female gender ratio. Most common diagnoses included glioblastoma multiforme; malignant melanoma; and cancers of breast, prostate, colon, pancreas, and kidney. An additional 30 diagnoses for fewer than 20 patients each were also listed.

Individual dosing varied with 33% of patients receiving 400 mg; 26% receiving 200 mg; and the remainder receiving doses in excess of 800 mg and up to 2,400 mg/day. Toxicities were similar to those reported with myeloma and included somnolence, constipation, rash, fatigue, and mental status changes whereas peripheral neuropathy was infrequent, probably because of short duration of administration. Almost one-third of patients (58) had concurrent administration of other agents, without evidence of added toxicity.

Only 36 patients (7.5%) responded to thalidomide therapy, 10 of whom received other anticancer agents concurrently. Response definitions were not provided. More than one-half of patients withdrew from therapy owing to disease progression, 10% owing to toxicity, and another 23% without documented reason.

Glioblastoma Multiforme

Thirty-seven patients with glioblastoma multiforme received 2 daily doses of thalidomide beginning at 100 mg and increasing to a maximum of 500 mg.[56] The average tolerated dose was 300 mg. Twenty-seven patients had glioblastoma multiforme at diagnosis, and 10 were upgraded from a lower grade to glioblastoma multiforme on review. The majority of patients had debulking surgery, and all had received prior radiotherapy. Seventeen received additional chemotherapy.

Of 34 patients assessable for response, 5 (15%) achieved partial remission, and 11 (32%) reached stable disease. Eighteen patients progressed. The median survival was 27 weeks. Ancillary studies documented no correlation between plasma VEGF and response or prognosis. Thalidomide was well tolerated without grade IV toxicities. Peripheral neuropathy was documented in 3 patients.

Hepatocellular Carcinoma

At M.D. Anderson Hospital, 97 patients were enrolled in a phase II trial of 400 mg thalidomide in the first week and escalation to 1,000 mg by the fifth week of treatment.[57] Of 21 evaluable patients, one PR and a minor response were noted, and 10 additional patients had stable disease for at least 2 months.

Renal Cell Carcinoma

Of 15 patients who had advanced metastatic renal cell cancer and received thalidomide in a dose escalation schedule, 1 had a PR still ongoing at more than 11 months, and 1 had a minor response of more than 3 months; 3 additional patients had stable disease, and 7 had progressive disease.[58]

Recurrent-Metastatic Squamous Cell Carcinoma of the Head and Neck

Seventeen patients were enrolled in an M.D. Anderson trial of a dose escalation schedule to 1,000 mg thalidomide daily.[59] All had received extensive prior therapy, including chemotherapy in 94% and radiation therapy in 88%, and 77% had extensive surgery. Most (94%) patients had disease progression, and responses were not noted.

CONCLUSION

Thalidomide has emerged as an active antitumor modality, with the greatest activity so far reported in multiple myeloma, both advanced and untreated, and the suggestion of synergistic antitumor activity when combined with high doses of glucocorticoids and especially combination chemotherapy. Evidence of activity also exists for single-agent thalidomide in myelodysplastic syndromes, seemingly in the more favorable subgroups of refractory anemia and refractory anemia with ringed sideroblasts with low cytokine activity and a low apoptotic rate. Continued systematic evaluations of thalidomide in other hematologic malignancies and solid tumors along with correlative laboratory investigations pertinent to angiogenesis and cytokine and immune modulation are warranted.

Of the multiplicity of thalidomide's reported mechanisms of actions, all may be operative in a single patient, considering the tumor cell heterogeneity prevalent in most malignancies. Particularly intriguing is the possibility of a direct antitumor effect, for which gene expression array studies will be of great help to pinpoint the molecular mechanisms involved.[42]

ACKNOWLEDGMENT

This study was supported in part by grant CA55819 from the National Cancer Institute.

REFERENCES

1. Folkman J. Angiogenesis in cancer, vascular, rheumatoid and other disease. Nat Med 1995;1: 27–31.
2. Perez-Atayde AR, Sallan SE, Tedrow U et al. Spectrum of tumor angiogenesis in the bone marrow of children with acute lymphoblastic leukemia. Am J Pathol 1997;150:815–821.
3. Weidner N, Semple JP, Welch WR, Folkman J. Tumor angiogenesis and metastasis-correlation in invasive breast carcinoma. N Engl J Med 1991;324:1–8.
4. Vacca A, Ribatti D, Ruco L et al. Angiogenesis extent and macrophage density increase simultaneously with pathological progression in B-cell non-Hodgkin's lymphomas. Br J Cancer 1999;79: 965–970.
5. Aguayo A, Kantarjian H, Manshouri T et al. Angiogenesis in acute and chronic leukemias and myelodysplastic syndromes. Blood 2000;96:2240–2245.
6. Shima DT, Adamis AP, Ferrara N et al. Hypoxic induction of endothelial cell growth factors in retinal cells: identification and characterization of vascular endothelial growth factor (VEGF) as the mitogen. Mol Med 1995;1:182–193.
7. Compagni A, Wilgenbus P, Impagnatiello MA et al. Fibroblast growth factors are required for efficient tumor angiogenesis. Cancer Res 2000;60:7163–7169.
8. Boehm T, Folkman J, Browder T, O'Reilly MS. Antiangiogenic therapy of experimental cancer does not induce acquired drug resistance. Nature 1997;390:404–407.
9. Yokoyama Y, Dhanabal M, Griffioen AW et al. Synergy between angiostatin and endostatin: inhibition of ovarian cancer growth. Cancer Res 2000;60:2190–2196.
10. Kirsch M, Strasser J, Allende R et al. Angiostatin suppresses malignant glioma growth in vivo. Cancer Res 1998;58:4654–4659.
11. D'Amato RJ, Loughnan MS, Flynn E, Folkman J. Thalidomide is an inhibitor of angiogenesis. Proc Natl Acad Sci USA 1994;91:4082–4085.
12. McBride WG. Thalidomide and congenital abnormalities. Lancet 1961;2:1358.

13. Kenyon BM, Browne F, D'Amato RJ. Effects of thalidomide and related metabolites in a mouse corneal model of neovascularization. Exp Eye Res 1997;64:971–978.
14. Geitz H, Handt S, Zwingenberger K. Thalidomide selectively modulates the density of cell surface molecules involved in the adhesion cascade. Immunopharmacology 1996;31:213–221.
15. Sampaio EP, Sarno EN, Galilly R et al. Thalidomide selectively inhibits tumor necrosis factor alpha production by stimulated human monocytes. J Exp Med 1991;173:699–703.
16. Haslett PA, Corral LG, Albert M, Kaplan G. Thalidomide costimulates primary human T lymphocytes, preferentially inducing proliferation, cytokine production, and cytotoxic responses in the CD8+ subset. J Exp Med 1998;187:1885–1892.
17. Singhal S, Mehta J, Desikan R et al. Antitumor activity of thalidomide in refractory multiple myeloma. N Engl J Med 1999;341:1565–1571.
18. Bergsagel DE, Griffith KM, Haut A, Stuckey WJ Jr. The treatment of plasma cell myeloma. Adv Cancer Res 1967;10:311–359.
19. Alexanian R, Haut A, Khan AU et al. Treatment for multiple myeloma. Combination chemotherapy with different melphalan dose regimens. JAMA 1969;208:1680–1685.
20. Rajkumar SV. Thalidomide in multiple myeloma. Oncology 2000;14[suppl 1]:11–16.
21. Eisen TG. Thalidomide in solid tumors: The London experience. Oncology 2000;14[suppl 1]:17–20.
22. Barlogie B, Spencer T, Tricot G et al. Long term follow up of 169 patients receiving a phase II trial of single agent thalidomide for advanced and refractory multiple myeloma (MM). Blood 2000;96[suppl 1]:514a.
23. Juliusson G, Celsing F, Turesson I et al. Frequent good partial remissions from thalidomide including best response ever in patients with advanced refractory and relapsed myeloma. Br J Haematol 2000;109:89–96.
24. Yakoub-Agha I, Attal M, Dumontet C et al. Thalidomide in patients with advanced myeloma: survival prognostic factors. Blood 2000;96[suppl 1]:167a.
25. Raza SN, Veksler Y, Sabir T et al. Durable response to thalidomide in relapsed/refractory multiple myeloma (MM). Blood 2000;96[suppl 1]:168a.
26. Rodriguez J, Oyama Y, Burt RK, Traynor AE. Achievement of maximal disease response to thalidomide is limited by patients' tolerance more often than disease resistance. Blood 2000;96[suppl 1]:294b.
27. Tosi P, Ronconi S, Zamagni E et al. Salvage therapy with thalidomide for patients with advanced relapsed/refractory multiple myeloma. Blood 2000;96[suppl 1]:296b.
28. Prince HM, Biagi JJ, Mitchell P et al. Interferon-α-2b (IF) can be combined with thalidomide (Thal) in patients with multiple myeloma (MM). Blood 2000;96[suppl 1]:293b.
29. Palumbo A, Giaccone L, Bertola A et al. Thalidomide and dexamethasone as salvage therapy for refractory and relapsed myeloma. Blood 2000;96[suppl 1]:292b.
30. Dimopoulos MA, Zervas K, Galani E et al. Thalidomide and dexamethasone combination for multiple myeloma refractory to dexamethasone-based regimens. Blood 2000;96[suppl 1]:286b.
31. Weber DM, Rankin K, Gavino M et al. Angiogenesis factors and sensitivity to thalidomide in previously untreated multiple myeloma (MM). Blood 2000;96[suppl 1]:168a.
32. Kropff MH, Innig G, Mitterer M et al. Hyperfractionated cyclophosphamide in combination with pulsed dexamethasone and thalidomide (hyper-CDT) in primary refractory or relapsed multiple myeloma. Blood 2000;96[suppl 1]:168a.
33. Moehler TM, Neben K, Hawighorst H et al. Thalidomide plus CED chemotherapy as salvage therapy in poor prognostic multiple myeloma. Blood 2000;96[suppl 1]:290b.

34. Munshi N, Desikan R, Zangari M et al. Chemotherapy with DT-PACE for previously treated multiple myeloma. Blood 1999;94[suppl 1]:123a.
35. Coleman M, Leonard JP, Nahum K, Michaeli J. Non-myelosuppressive therapy with BLT-D (Biaxin, low-dose thalidomide and dexamethasone) is highly active in Waldenström's macroglobulinemia and myeloma. Blood 2000;96[suppl 1]:167a.
36. Rajkumar SV, Hayman S, Fonseca R et al. Thalidomide plus dexamethasone (Thal/Dex) and thalidomide alone (Thal) as first line therapy for newly diagnosed myeloma (MM). Blood 2000; 96[suppl 1]:168a.
37. Alexanian R, Dimopoulos MS, Delaselle K, Barlogie B. Primary dexamethasone treatment for multiple myeloma. Blood 1992;80:887–890.
38. Kakimoto T, Hattori Y, Okamoto S et al. Thalidomide for the treatment of refractory multiple myeloma. Decreased plasma concentration of angiogenic growth factors and clinical response. Blood 2000;96[suppl 1]:289b.
39. Neben K, Moehler T, Egerer G et al. High plasma basic fibroblast growth factor concentration is associated with response to thalidomide in progressive multiple myeloma. Blood 2000;96[suppl 1]:167a.
40. Lentzsch S, Podar K, Davies FE et al. Immunomodulatory derivates (ImiDs) of thalidomide (Thal) inhibit the proliferation of multiple myeloma (MM) cell lines and block VEGF-induced activation of the MAPK-pathway. Blood 2000;96[suppl 1]:579a.
41. Payvandi F, Wu L, Gupta D et al. Effects of thalidomide analog on binding activity of transcription factors and cell cycle progression of multiple myeloma cell lines. Blood 2000;96[suppl 1]:579a.
42. Shaughnessy J, Zhan F, Tian E et al. Global gene expression analysis shows loss of c-myc and IL-6 receptor gene mRNA after exposure of myeloma to thalidomide and ImiD. Blood 2000; 96[suppl 1]:579a.
43. Davies FE, Raje N, Hideshima T et al. Thalidomide (Thal) and immunomodulatory derivates (ImiDS) augment natural killer (NK) cell cytotoxicity in multiple myeloma (MM). Blood 2000; 96[suppl 1]:837a
44. Ochonisky S, Verroust J, Bastuji-Garin S et al. Thalidomide neuropathy incidence and clinico-electrophysiologic findings in 42 patients. Arch Dermatol 1994;130:66–69.
45. Zangari M, Anaissie E, Desikan R et al. Thalidomide-induced hypercoagulability in multiple myeloma (MM). Blood 2000;96[suppl 1]:296b.
46. Badros A, Zangari M, Bodenner M et al. Hypothyroidism in patients with multiple myeloma (MM) receiving thalidomide. Blood 2000;96[suppl 1]:285b.
47. Munshi N, Desikan R, Anaissie E et al. Peripheral blood stem cell collection (PBSC) after CAD + G-CSF as part of Total Therapy II in newly diagnosed multiple myeloma (MM): influence of thalidomide (Thal) administration. Blood 2000;94[suppl 1]:578b.
48. Levesque JP, Takamatsu Y, Nilsson SK et al. Mobilization of hematopoietic cells into peripheral blood is associated with VCAM-1 proteolytic cleavage in the bone marrow. Blood 2000;96[suppl 1]:221b.
49. Estey E, Albitar M, Cortes J et al. Addition of thalidomide (T) to chemotherapy did not increase remission rate in poor prognosis AML/MDS. Blood 2000;96[suppl 1]:323a.
50. Raza A, Lisak L, Little L et al. Thalidomide as a single agent or in combination with Topotecan, Pentoxiphyllin and/or Enbrel in myelodysplastic syndromes (MDS). Blood 2000;96[suppl 1]:146a.
51. Venugopal V, Sivaraman S, Gladstone B et al. The CD22 antigen: Profile of cytokines and bioactive agents that has potential to augments its expression on tumor cells. Blood 2000;96[suppl 1]:232b.

52. Dimopoulos MA, Viniou N, Zomas A et al. Treatment of Waldenström's macroglobulinemia with thalidomide. Blood 2000;96[suppl 1]:286b.
53. Vescio RA, Berenson JR. Thalidomide is an effective agent for patients with primary amyloidosis. Blood 2000;96[suppl 1]:296b.
54. Canepa L, Ballerini F, Varaldo R et al. Myelofibrosis: Report of five cases treated with thalidomide. Blood 2000;96[suppl 1]:266b.
55. Hussein MA. Research on thalidomide in solid tumors, hematologic malignancies, and supportive care. Oncology 2000;14[suppl 12]:9–15.
56. Marx GM, McCowatt S, Boyle F et al. Phase II study of thalidomide as an anti-angiogenic agent in the treatment of recurrent glioblastoma [abst 613]. Proc Am Soc Clin Oncol 2000;19:158a.
57. Patt YZ, Hassan MM, Lozano RD et al. Phase II trial of Thalomid (thalidomide) for treatment of non-resectable hepatocellular carcinoma (HCC) [abst 1035]. Proc Am Soc Clin Oncol 2000;19:266a.
58. Minor D, Elias L. Thalidomide treatment of metastatic renal cell carcinoma [abst 1384]. Proc Am Soc Clin Oncol 2000;19:352a.
59. Tseng JE, Glisson BS, Khuri FR et al. Phase II trial of thalidomide in the treatment of recurrent and/or metastatic squamous cell carcinoma of the head and neck (SCHN) [abst 1645]. Proc Am Soc Clin Oncol 2000;19:417a.

Oxaliplatin in the Treatment of Patients with Advanced Colorectal Cancer

Carmen J. Allegra

Colorectal cancer is the second highest cause of cancer death in the United States and represents the third most common cancer in men and women. An estimated 130,200 new cases of colorectal cancer are diagnosed annually, and this is associated with an annual mortality of approximately 56,300 individuals. Approximately 60% of all patients diagnosed with colorectal carcinoma will present with locally advanced or advanced disease. For these individuals, chemotherapy plays an important and clinically beneficial role. The mainstay of adjuvant therapy for patients with local and locally advanced disease is the combination of 5-fluorouracil (5-FU) plus leucovorin (LV) for 6 months. This therapy may be used weekly for 6 of 8 weeks or as a daily regimen for 5 days on an every-28-day schedule. Adherence to either of these schedules results in approximately a 30% decrease in mortality as compared to treatment with surgery alone. For patients with metastatic disease, the three-drug regimen of 5-FU, LV, and irinotecan (CPT-11) has recently supplanted the two-drug regimen of 5-FU plus LV (5-FU/LV) as standard therapy. Two large, prospectively randomized investigations in patients without prior therapy for metastatic colorectal cancer have demonstrated a statistically significant advantage for the three-drug regimen over 5-FU/LV in response rate (39% vs 21%), time to disease progression (7.0 vs 4.3 months), and overall survival (14.8 vs 12.6 months).[1]

In addition, CPT-11 as a single agent has been approved in the United States for use as second-line therapy in patients with metastatic colorectal cancer that is refractory to fluoropyrimidine. The use of CPT-11 in this setting has been demonstrated to prolong survival and enhance quality of life as compared to individuals treated only with the best supportive care.

Oral fluoropyrimidine analogs have also been developed, and clinical testing in large, randomized investigations involving untreated patients with advanced colorectal cancer have demonstrated that at least two of these agents, capecitabine and uracil-ftorafur-LV, have activity that appears equivalent to that of 5-FU and LV, as measured by response rate, time to disease progression, and survival.[2,3] The similar clinical activity of these agents coupled with a favorable toxicity profile and an oral route of administration make these compounds attractive clinical agents. Despite these advances in the treatment of patients with colorectal carcinoma, approximately 27% of patients with lymph node–positive disease and almost 95% of patients with metastatic disease will succumb to their disease within 5 years of diagnosis. Thus, there is an urgent need for the identification and development of new therapeutic agents for the treatment of patients with colorectal carcinoma.

Platinum compounds, including cisplatin and carboplatin, have been approved by the U.S. Food and Drug Administration since 1978 and 1989, respectively. Although these agents have been highly successful for the treatment of testicular cancer and various epithelial malignancies (including lung, head and neck, bladder, ovary, and upper gastrointestinal malignancies), they have not been found to have meaningful activity for the treatment of malignancies arising in the lower gastrointestinal tract. Oxaliplatin is a diaminocyclohexane-substituted (DACH-substituted) platinum analog that has been shown to have anticancer activity distinct from that of either cisplatin or carboplatin (Fig. 8.1). DACH-substituted platinum analogs were first synthesized and tested as anticancer agents almost 30 years ago; however, it was the work of Dr. Kidani et al[4] in the early 1980s that demonstrated the relative efficacy of the various isomers of specific DACH-substituted platinum analogs in the L1210 mouse leukemia model. These investigators found that the *trans*-l-DACH analogs with an oxalato leaving group had activity similar to that observed with cisplatin in this murine model. These same authors subsequently demonstrated that oxaliplatin and cisplatin were similarly active in a series of tumor-bearing murine models, including P388 leukemia, B16 melanoma, Lewis lung carcinoma, colon 26 and colon 38 adenocarcinomas, and M5076 fibrosarcoma. Of interest was the finding that oxaliplatin did not share cross-resistance to a highly cisplatin-resistant L1210 leukemia cell line.[5]

The mechanism of action of oxaliplatin is similar to that of other platinum compounds in that the primary lesion associated with oxaliplatin exposure is the formation of DNA intrastrand adducts, which result in the interruption of DNA

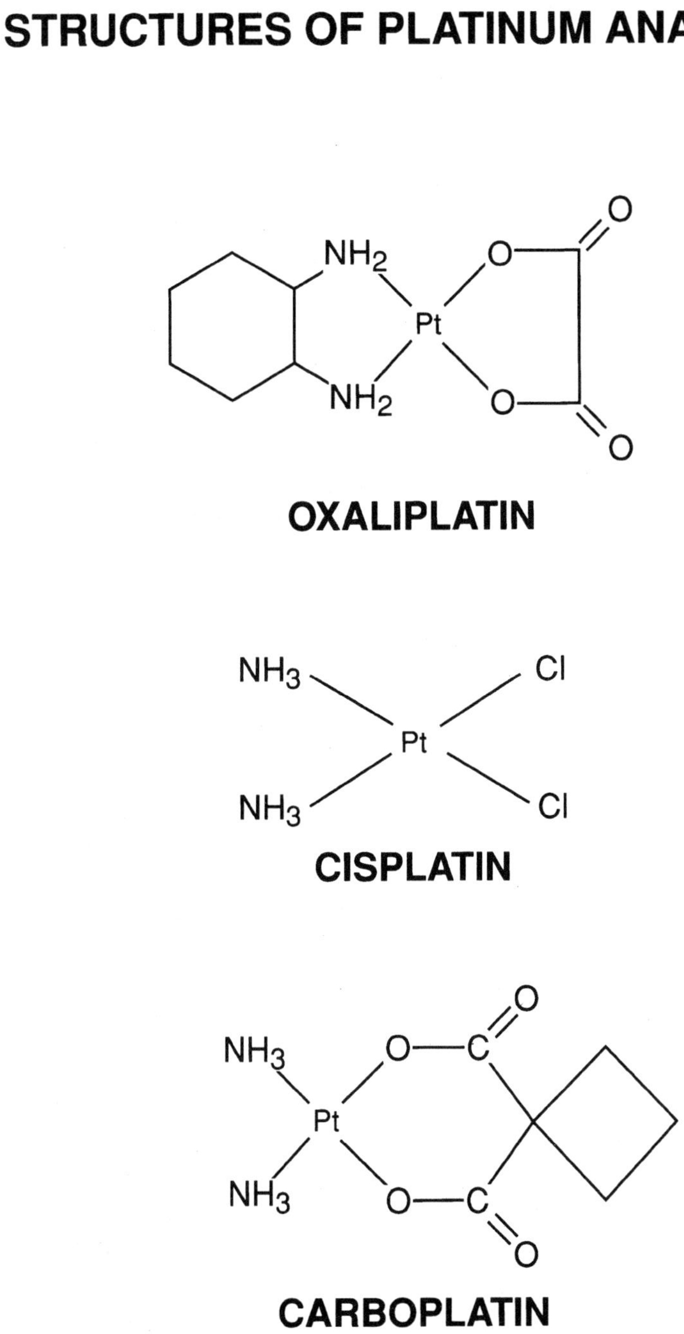

STRUCTURES OF PLATINUM ANALOGS

OXALIPLATIN

CISPLATIN

CARBOPLATIN

FIGURE 8.1 Chemical structures of platinum analogs in clinical use.

replication.[6–8] As shown in Figure 8.2, oxaliplatin requires activation to its aquated form, the active species responsible for its interaction with DNA. Displacement of the "leaving group" may occur via chloride, bicarbonate, or phosphate salts or by a sulfur-containing amino acid displacement such as methionine and cysteine.[9]

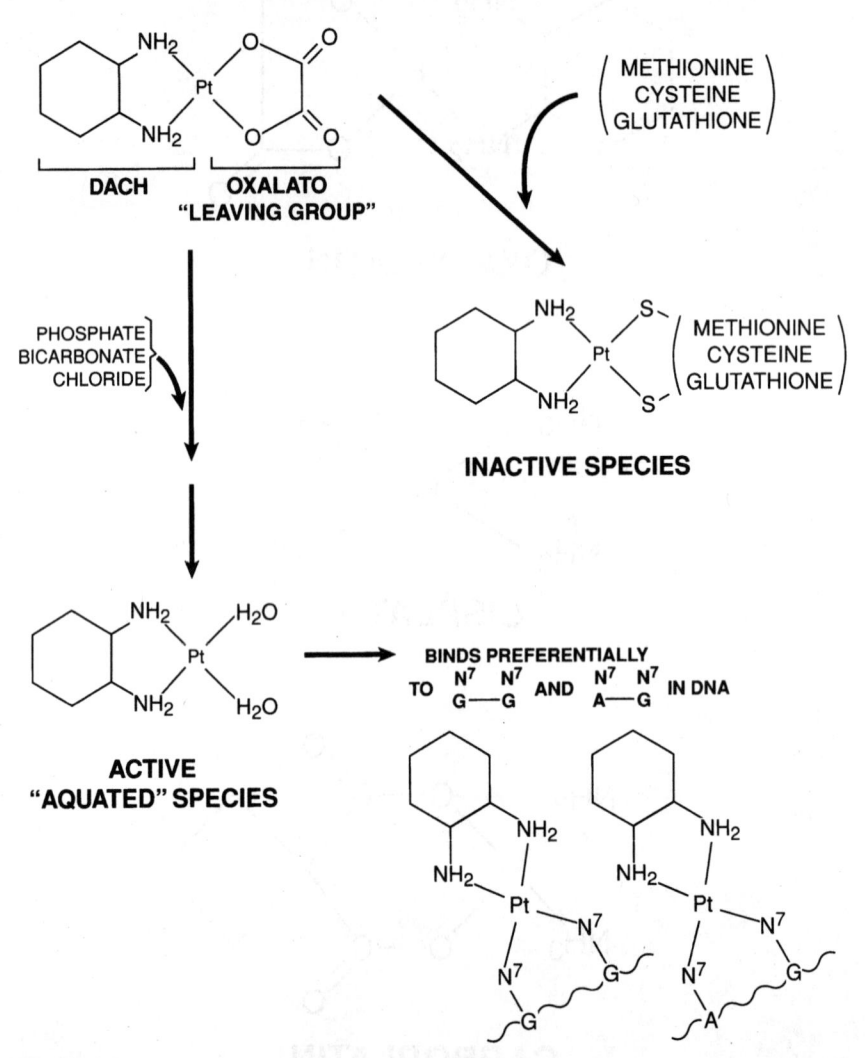

FIGURE 8.2 Proposed metabolism of oxaliplatin to its active form and its interaction with DNA.

Binding of the sulfur-containing amino acids to the DACH platinum compounds results in inactive species, whereas activation through the salts results in intermediates that may be converted to the active aquated form of the analog. Recent evidence suggests that the intracellular conversion of oxaliplatin via the chloride displacement pathway is unlikely to be a major source of activation of oxaliplatin and that alternative activation routes via displacement of the "leaving group" by either bicarbonate or phosphate may constitute the major routes of intracellular activation. Several investigations have demonstrated that platinum analogs containing a bidentate leaving group, such as oxalato and malonato, are substantially more stable than those containing chloride leaving groups, such as cisplatin. The DACH analog containing a malonate leaving group was shown to be approximately 100 times more stable in water when compared with cisplatin. The DACH analogs were found to have a half-life of approximately 9.5 hours in tissue culture media at 37°C and 21–28 minutes in L1210 mouse leukemia cells.[10]

Once activated, oxaliplatin has been shown to interact with DNA in a fashion very similar to that of cisplatin, both with regard to the types of platinum adducts formed as well as in the location of the formed adducts.[11-14] The primary platinum DNA lesions formed by oxaliplatin are GpG and ApG intrastrand diadducts, which form through the N-7 position of the purine nucleotides. While interstrand GG diadducts occur, they appear to constitute less than 1% of the total adducts and may not represent a major mechanism of cytotoxicity associated with exposure to oxaliplatin.

Despite these similarities between oxaliplatin and cisplatin, studies have demonstrated that their mechanisms of action and cellular resistance differ. The reason for these differences is not clear; however, the various forms of human DNA polymerases possess differing abilities to read past platinum DNA adducts formed by oxaliplatin as opposed to cisplatin and possess varying levels of "read-through" fidelity. The ability of repair enzymes, such as the mismatch repair enzymes, clearly distinguishes between platinum adducts formed by cisplatin and those formed by oxaliplatin. Mismatch repair–deficient cell lines have been shown to be resistant to cisplatin, though they demonstrate no significant difference in the cytotoxicity associated with exposure to oxaliplatin.[7,15,16] The oxaliplatin adducts are unrecognizable by the mismatch repair complex, thus accounting for the lack of resistance in mismatch repair–deficient cell lines as compared to their wild-type counterparts. Such differences between cisplatin and oxaliplatin in the cellular recognition and repair of formed adducts may explain the noted lack of cross-resistance between these two platinum compounds as well as the different spectrum of anticancer effects and toxicities associated with the use of each agent.

The mechanisms of resistance to the DACH platinum analogs were investigated in a series of L1210 murine leukemia cell lines resistant to either cisplatin or DACH platinum analogs and were compared with the wild-type cells in an effort to understand the critical mechanisms accounting for DACH platinum analog sensitivity. Similar studies also were conducted in matched cisplatin-resistant and wild-type human ovarian carcinoma (A2780), human KB3-1 squamous carcinoma, and human colon carcinoma cell lines (HCT8).[17-19] Although the potential mechanisms of resistance to platinum analogs are manifold, the in vitro data suggest that the major mechanism of insensitivity specifically for the DACH platinum analogs is due to differences in platinum accumulation and cellular differences in tolerance of the platinum DNA adducts. Presumably, the increased ability to tolerate the platinum DNA adducts is explainable by differences in the ability of various DNA polymerases to bypass the platinum DNA adducts in resistant cells. Whereas differences in accumulation of the DACH platinum analogs appear to play a role in several of the models, tolerance of the DACH platinum DNA adducts appears to be the most commonly observed mechanism of resistance, particularly in the human cell lines. Several other potential mechanisms of resistance were not found to be relevant as explanations of DACH platinum resistance, at least in the models investigated. These mechanisms included the efficiency of incorporation of platinum into DNA, the intracellular levels of glutathione, and the rate of repair specifically of intrastrand platinum adducts. Unfortunately, these studies did not address the importance of the formation or repair of interstrand cross-links whose role in the mechanism of action and resistance of DACH platinum analogs remains unclear.

In preclinical model systems, oxaliplatin has been shown to be remarkably less cross-resistant to a host of both human and murine cisplatin-resistant cell lines, including murine L1210 leukemia cells, human A2780 ovarian carcinoma, human KB3-1 squamous carcinoma, and human HT-29 colon carcinoma cell lines.[4,5,17-21] Oxaliplatin has also been associated with a different spectrum of preclinical activity when compared to cisplatin and carboplatin in the 60–cell line National Cancer Institute's (NCI's) Anticancer Drug Screen, consistent with the notion that oxaliplatin has different mechanisms of action, or resistance, or both, as compared to cisplatin and carboplatin.[17] Of note and in contrast to cisplatin and carboplatin, oxaliplatin was found to have remarkable activity against six of eight colorectal cancer lines contained in NCI's drug screen. Using the human tumor-cloning assay, activity was observed for oxaliplatin against colon, renal, and gastric cancers, sarcoma, and melanoma. In these studies, the activity of oxaliplatin was found to be both dose- and time-dependent.[22] In addition to its preclinical activity as a single agent, oxaliplatin has also been shown to have greater than additive activity when combined with gemcitabine (if gemcitabine administration precedes exposure to oxaliplatin),[23] topotecan,[24] cisplatin,[17] CPT-11 (particularly when oxaliplatin is used prior to CPT-11 exposure),[24,25] and in combination with 5-FU and the thymidylate synthase inhibitor AG337,[26] for which there does not appear to be a sequence dependency.

PHARMACOKINETICS

The pharmacokinetics of oxaliplatin have been studied both in murine model systems and in patients with cancer, using either relatively brief, 2- to 4-hour infusions or prolonged constant-rate or chronomodulated infusion schedules. Oxaliplatin pharmacokinetics have been investigated using two distinct methodologies, flameless atomic absorption spectrometry (FAAS) and inductively coupled plasma-mass spectrometry (ICP-MS), which has a sensitivity that is approximately tenfold greater than that of FAAS.

At the end of 2- to 4-hour infusions, approximately 37%–40% of the administered platinum rapidly crosses the red blood cell membranes and resides within the red blood cells, from which there appears to be little, if any, exchange. The oxaliplatin associated with the red blood cells has a half-life approximating that of the erythrocytes (10–48 days).[8,27,28] Ultrafilterable or free platinum accounts for only 5%–27% of the total plasma platinum. Using the FAAS methodology, the terminal half-life of free platinum has been found to be 25.2–27.3 hours,[28,29] whereas the terminal half-life of free platinum measured using the more sensitive ICP-MS assay was found to be 172 and 273 hours.[27,30] The marked difference in reported terminal half-lives most likely reflects the increased sensitivity of the ICP-MS technology. The maximum concentrations of free platinum reached at the end of 2- and 4-hour infusions has been found to be 454 ± 75 to 1210 ± 100 and 1612 ± 553 µg/L, respectively, whereas total platinum concentrations reach approximately 3100 µg/L. The area under the curve for free platinum after a dose of 130 mg/m^2 of oxaliplatin ranged from 5.21 to 20.2 µg/mL · h.

The major route of clearance for oxaliplatin appears to be the kidney, wherein approximately 54% ± 20% of the dose is eliminated; bilirubin excretion accounts for approximately 2% of the administered dose. Although no formal investigations have yet been performed in patients with impaired hepatic function, such an investigation is ongoing at the NCI.[31] The pharmacokinetics of oxaliplatin have been studied in 10 patients with moderate renal insufficiency who received 130 mg/m^2 oxaliplatin as a 2-hour infusion (mean creatinine clearance = 42 mL/min; range, 27–57 mL/min), as compared to a group of 13 individuals with normal renal function (mean creatinine clearance = 70 mL/min; range, 63–136 mL/min). Those patients with moderate renal impairment were found to have a twofold increase in the free platinum area under the curve coupled with a clearance that was almost one-half that of the normal subjects. The maximum concentrations of free and total platinum did not differ between the two groups. These investigators identified an association between the free platinum area under the curve and clearance with the calculated creatinine clearance. Although the investigation involved relatively few patients, no associations were found between the various pharmacokinetic parameters in patients with normal or moderately impaired renal function and toxicity. No pharmacokinetic or pharmacodynamic relationships have been identified yet with oxaliplatin, and no pharmacokinetic interactions between oxaliplatin and either 5-FU or CPT-11 have as yet been clearly defined.[8,32]

Oxaliplatin has also been extensively studied both in preclinical murine model systems and in patients on a circadian administration schedule. Unlike 5-FU, for which constant drug infusions result in a circadian rhythmicity of plasma concentration owing to the circadian rhythm of the critical catabolizing enzyme dihydropyrimidine dehydrogenase, oxaliplatin does not demonstrate circadian pharmacokinetics.[33] Despite the lack of circadian variation associated with oxaliplatin, investigators from France used a murine model system to demonstrate the effect of dosing time on mortality and tissue toxicity associated with oxaliplatin.[8,34,35] These investigators found that oxaliplatin was least toxic to normal tissues such as the jejunum and the blood-forming elements and was associated with the least mortality when given at 16 hours after light onset. In contrast, they found that the greatest mortality and tissue toxicity occurred when the drug was administered at 7 hours after light onset in the murine model.[8,34,35] These investigators also showed that the time of administration associated with the least toxic effects was also associated with the lowest tissue levels of platinum, thus suggesting that the reason for the diminished toxicity may well be due to diminished metabolism of oxaliplatin in the susceptible tissues. Whether this effect would be favorable or unfavorable with respect to the anticancer activity of oxaliplatin remains to be demonstrated; however, the prolonged terminal half-life associated with oxaliplatin suggests that prolonged venous infusions may be unnecessary for anticancer activity. In an attempt to address this issue, several clinical investigations have focused on the use of a circadian infusion schedule for the administration of oxaliplatin (vide infra).

CLINICAL INVESTIGATIONS

Phase I Studies

The initial phase I trials of oxaliplatin were conducted using single, brief intravenous infusions given on an every-3-to-4-week schedule. In an early trial by Mathè et al,[20] a dose of 45 mg/m^2 was proposed as a starting dose for phase II studies; however, a maximum tolerated dose was not achieved in this investigation. Although it is now appreciated that the major dose-limiting toxicity of oxaliplatin is neurotoxicity, this particular toxicity was not noted in the initial phase I trial owing to the low dose of drug administered. A subsequent investigation starting at a dose of 45 mg/m^2 and progressing up to 200 mg/m^2 given over 6 hours every 4 weeks identified 135 mg/m^2 as the recommended dose for phase II studies and found neurotoxicity to be the critical dose-limiting toxicity.[36] Gastrointestinal toxicity, primarily in the form of moderate to severe nausea and vomiting, occurred in more than 50% of patients and was not clearly dose-dependent. Hematologic toxicity, primarily in the form of thrombocytopenia, was dose-dependent and was noted at doses equal to or exceeding 135 mg/m^2. Mild to moderate thrombocytopenia occurred in 13% of patients receiving 135–150 mg/m^2 and in 28.5% of those treated at doses equal to or greater than 175 mg/m^2. Of particular note was the apparent lack of nephrotoxicity.

With regard to neurotoxicity, Extra et al[36] noted that this toxicity was predominantly sensory in nature, with an acute component of dysesthesias that was noted to be exacerbated with touching of cold surfaces or liquids and with paresthesias occurring in the fingers and toes. At a dose of 135 mg/m^2 (grade 2 + 3 = 13%), half of the individuals were noted to develop neurotoxicity during the first course of therapy. This incidence increased with increasing doses, such that all patients experienced some degree of neurotoxicity at a dose of 200 mg/m^2 (grade 2 + 3 = 30%). These investigators also noted that neurotoxicity was cumulative, with a particularly high incidence of grade II to III neurotoxicity (67%) occurring at cumulative doses in excess of 540 mg/m^2. It was noted that the duration of symptoms associated with the neurotoxicity were brief after a single course of therapy; however, the neurotoxicity tended to be slower to resolve after the fourth cycle of therapy, implying that careful neurologic follow-up should be undertaken at cumulative doses in excess of 500 mg/m^2. Electromyographic investigations conducted in six patients demonstrated an axonal sensory neuropathy with axonal degeneration and no change in motor nerve conduction velocities.

In an effort to mitigate toxicities associated with oxaliplatin, Caussanel et al[37] performed a randomized phase I investigation of continuous-infusion oxaliplatin for 5 days versus circadian-modulated infusion, with a peak administration occurring at 1600 hours for 5 days. Courses were repeated every 3 weeks. These investigators found that the circadian-modulated schedule resulted in a marked diminution of neurotoxicity and gastrointestinal toxicities when compared with the constant-infusion schedule and recommended the use of a circadian-modulation at a dose of 35 mg/m^2 daily for 5 days (175 mg/m^2 total dose). Despite the use of either constant infusion or the circadian-modulated schedule, approximately one-third of individuals suffered from moderate to severe nausea and vomiting, whereas 42% developed grade Ic, and 14% grade II, peripheral neuropathy. In all cases, peripheral neuropathy was found to resolve within a 2-month period with either discontinuation or decreased dosing of oxaliplatin. However, subsequent investigations suggest that the recovery time from neurotoxicity may be substantially longer. In a subsequent investigation using the circadian infusion schedule, electromyograms performed in three patients demonstrated decreases in conduction velocities in two individuals and suggested sensory axonal degeneration with demyelination.[38] In these phase I investigations, responses were noted in patients with breast cancer (three patients), esophageal cancer (two patients), lung cancer (two patients), urothelial cancer (one patient), and melanoma (one patient) (Table 8.1).

Phase II Studies

In early trials, patients with advanced colorectal cancer were treated with oxaliplatin as a single agent using either a 2-hour intravenous infusion given every 3 weeks or a circadian infusion schedule as described previously. Two consecutive phase II trials were reported by Machover et al[39] and represent their experience with the use of oxaliplatin as a single agent in 106 patients with refractory

TABLE 8.1 Phase I Studies with Oxaliplatin Alone

Study	No. of Patients	Dose, Schedule of Drugs	MTD (mg/m²)	Rec. Dose (mg/m²)
Mathè[20]	23	0.045–67.000 mg/m² IV q3wk	NR	45
Extra[36]	44	45–200 mg/m² IV over 6 hr q4wk	200	135
Caussanel[37]	14	125–175 mg/m² flat infusion × 5 days q3wk	150	150
	11	125–200 mg/m² CMI × 5 days (peak 1600 hr) q3wk	175	175

CMI, chronomodulated infusion; MTD, maximum tolerated dose; NR, not reached; Rec., recommended.

colorectal cancer (Table 8.2). This group identified an overall response rate of 10%, with no complete responses noted. A smaller study reported from Milan found no responses in 13 patients with refractory colorectal cancer who were treated with a dose and schedule of oxaliplatin identical to that used by the French group.[40] Using a circadian schedule of oxaliplatin given over a 5-day period every 3 weeks, starting with doses of 150 mg/m² per course and escalating, as tolerated, up to 200 mg/m² per course, Levi et al[38] identified an overall response rate of 10% in 30 individuals with advanced and refractory colorectal cancer.

Using a dose and schedule of 130 mg/m² given by 2-hour intravenous infusion every 2 weeks, oxaliplatin as a single agent was also tested in patients with advanced colorectal cancer who had no prior chemotherapeutic exposure and was found to be associated with partial response rates of 12% and 24.3% in two independent trials of 25 and 38 patients, respectively.[41,42] For both trials, the overall time to disease progression was approximately 4 months, with overall survivals of 13.2 and 14.5 months. These outcomes are similar to those using fluoropyrimidine-alone therapies. The major toxicities associated with the use of single-agent oxaliplatin are summarized in Table 8.3 and are drawn from five phase II trials (215 patients, 959 cycles) in which oxaliplatin was used as a single agent.

By far, the most common toxicity noted with the use of oxaliplatin alone in these phase II trials is neurotoxicity, primarily in the form of a peripheral sensory neuropathy highlighted by paresthesias, which can lead to functional impairment and acute dysesthesias of the hands and feet that is exacerbated by contact with cold surfaces or liquids as discussed previously. Peripheral neuropathy appears to occur to some degree in more than 90% of individuals treated with oxaliplatin; however, moderate to severe toxicity occurs in approximately 23% of treated

TABLE 8.2 Phase II with Oxaliplatin Alone in Patients with Advanced Colorectal Cancer

Study	No. of Patients	Prior Chemotherapy	Dose Schedule	Response Rate (%)	Time to Disease Progression (mo)	Survival (mo)
DeBraud[40]	13	Yes	130 mg/m^2 IV over 2 hr q3wk	0.0	2.0	NR
Machover[39]	109	Yes	130 mg/m^2 IV over 2 hr q3wk	10.0	NR	NR
Levi[38]	30	Yes	35 mg/m^2/day × 5 escalated to 40 mg/m^2/day circadian infusion (peak 1600 hr) q3wk	10.0	5.0	10.0
Diaz-Rubio[41]	25	No	130 mg/m^2 IV over 2 hr q3wk	12.0	4.0	14.5
Becouarn[42]	38	No	130 mg/m^2 IV over 2 hr q3wk	24.3	4.2+	13.2

NR, not reported.

TABLE 8.3 Grade III and IV Toxicities (%) Associated with Two Regimens Incorporating Single-Agent Oxaliplatin in Patients with Advanced Colorectal Cancer

Dose Schedule	No. of Patients	No. of Cycles	Neurotoxicity[a]	N&V	Diarrhea	Leukopenia	Thrombocytopenia	Laryngopharyngeal[b] Dysesthesia
130 mg/m² over 2 hr q3wk[39–42]	172	815	22[c]	11[c]	5[c]	2[c]	2[c]	24[c]
	51	214	15[d]	4[d]	3[d]	2[d]	2[d]	39[d]
Circadian infusion × 5 days q3wk[38]	29	105	12[d]	2[d]	6[d]	1[d]	1[d]	NR

N&V, nausea and vomiting; NR, none reported.
[a] National Cancer Institute–common toxicity criteria grades 2–4 or equivalent (i.e., mild functional impairment or greater).
[b] Any grade.
[c] Percentage of patients treated.
[d] Percentage of cycles administered.

individuals or approximately 12%–15% of administered cycles (see Table 8.3). Gastrointestinal upset in the form of nausea and vomiting or diarrhea occurs as the next most frequent toxicity, followed by a modest level of myelosuppression. The toxicities associated with the 2-hour infusion versus the circadian administration schedule appear to be similar, with the possible exception of slightly more nausea and vomiting with the 2-hour infusion and slightly more diarrhea with the circadian schedule.

As previously discussed, the neurotoxicity associated with oxaliplatin appears to depend on the cumulative drug dose, with approximately a 20% incidence of moderate to severe neuropathy at cumulative doses between 520 and 780 mg/m^2 and approximately half this incidence at doses of less than 520 mg/m^2. The cumulative effect of drug on neurotoxicity appears to be the case with either the 2-hour infusion or the chronomodulated schedule.[38–42] In general, recovery from the neurotoxicity associated with oxaliplatin is slow and appears to occur over a 6- to 12-month period after drug discontinuation. However, in many cases, only a partial regression of neurologic symptoms has been reported to occur, even after several years of follow-up.[43] Thus, the rate and completeness of recovery from the oxaliplatin-associated neurotoxicity remains to be more fully defined.

Phase II Trials in Combination with 5-FU/LV

Given the activity of oxaliplatin as a single agent for the treatment of patients with advanced colorectal cancer, several investigators combined 2-hour infusions of oxaliplatin given every 2–3 weeks with various schedules of 5-FU/LV. Principal among these regimens are those developed by de Gramont et al[44–48] and based on a bimonthly schedule of 2-day infusions of 5-FU/LV. These regimens have been designated *FOLFOX 2–7* and represent variations in the dose of 5-FU and LV or oxaliplatin with or without bolus 5-FU, coupled with a subsequent 2-day infusion of 5-FU.[44–48] As shown in Table 8.4, these regimens are associated with response rates of 20%–46% in previously treated individuals, most of whom had been treated with a similar bimonthly regimen of 5-FU/LV. The time to disease progression in patients treated on these studies averaged approximately 6 months, with overall median survivals of 10.8 to 17.0 months. These data are very interesting, considering that most of the individuals entered into these studies had progressed on prior therapy with 5-FU/LV, and suggest that oxaliplatin favorably interacts with 5-FU at the cellular level. The most frequent dose-limiting toxicities associated with the FOLFOX regimens include grade 3 to 4 neutropenia (~20%), mucositis (~10%), and neurotoxicity, manifest by at least mild functional impairment (~15%–25%).

A trial based on a compassionate use of oxaliplatin in patients with refractory advanced colorectal carcinoma was reported by Brienza et al[50] and included 111 individuals who were certified as 5-FU-refractory. Patients were treated with 2- to 6-hour infusions of oxaliplatin on an every-2-to-3-week basis using doses of

TABLE 8.4 Phase II Oxaliplatin with 5-Fluorouracil and Leucovorin in Patients with Advanced Colorectal Cancer

Study	No. of Patients	Prior Chemo-therapy	Dose Schedule	Response Rate (%)	Time to Disease Progression (mo)	Survival (mo)
Oxaliplatin given as a 2-hr infusion						
de Gramont[44]	46	Yes	5-FU, 1.5–2.0 gm/m^2/day × 2 days q2wk + LV 500 mg/m^2 on days 1 + 2 Oxaliplatin, 100 mg/m^2 over 2 hr on day 1 q2wk (FOLFOX2)	46	7	17
Andre[45]	30	Yes	5-FU, 1.5–2.0 gm/m^2/day × 2 + LV, 500 mg/m^2 + oxaliplatin, 85 mg/m^2 over 2 hr q2wk (FOLFOX3)	20	6.5	13.3
Andre[46]	40	Yes	5-FU, 1.5–2.0 gm/m^2/day × 2 + LV, 500 mg/m^2 + oxaliplatin, 85 mg/m^2 over 2 hr q2wk (FOLFOX3)	18.4	4.6	10.6
Andre[46]	57	Yes	Oxaliplatin, 85 mg/m^2 on day 1 over 2 hr + LV, 200 mg/m^2 over 2 hr, followed by bolus 5-FU, 400 mg/m^2 days 1 + 2 5-FU, 1.2 gm/m^2 over 46 hr q2wk (FOLFOX4)	23.5	5.1	11.1
Maindrault-Goebel[47]	60	Yes	Oxaliplatin, 100 mg/m^2 on day 1 over 2 hr + LV, 400 mg/m^2 over 2 hr, followed by bolus 5-FU, 400 mg/m^2 + 5-FU, 2.4–3.0 gm/m^2 over 46 hr q2wk (FOLFOX6)	27	5.3	10.8

Maindrault-Goebel[48]	38	Yes	Oxaliplatin, 130 mg/m² on day 1 over 2 hr + LV, 400 mg/m² over 2 hr + 5-FU, 400 mg/m² bolus, then 5-FU, 2.4 gm/m² over 46 hr q3wk (FOLFOX7)	44	6.2	NR
Gerard[49]	37	Yes	Oxaliplatin, 130 mg/m² q3wk over 2 hr after 5-FU, 2.6 gm/m² over 24 hr weekly, preceded by 500 mg/m² LV × 2 q3wk	17	NR	10
Janinis[52]	32	Yes	5-FU, 2.5 gm/m² over 24 hr + LV, 500 mg/m² over 2 hr + oxaliplatin, 50 mg/m² over 2 hr weekly × 6 q7wk	13	3	9
Kallen[53]	12	Yes	5-FU, 2.6 gm/m² over 24 hr + LV, 500 mg/m² + oxaliplatin, 60 mg/m² over 2 hr weekly × 4 q6wk	25	5.8	12.8
Guerin-Meyer[51]	47	Yes	5-FU, 8-hr weekly infusion with PK-guided dosing (3 mg/L) + LV, 200 mg/m² bolus at midpoint of 5-FU infusion + oxaliplatin, 130 mg/m² over 2 hr q3wk	25	5	NR
deBraud[40]	12	Yes	5-FU, 200–300 mg/m² CI (6 pts) or bolus (6 pts) + LV, 100 mg/m² daily × 5 d + oxaliplatin, 130 mg/m² over 2 hr q3wk	33	3	NR
Brienza[50]	111	Yes	5-FU/LV (various schedules) + oxaliplatin, 80–100 mg/m² q2wk or 100–135 mg/m² q3wk (2- to 6-hr infusion)	25.5	4.1	9.6

C, chronomodulated infusion; CR, complete response; F, flat infusion; 5-FU, 5-fluorouracil; LV, leucovorin; pts, patients.

TABLE 8.4 *Continued*

Oxaliplatin + 5-FU/LV given as a prolonged 4- to 5-day flat or chronomodulated schedule (peak oxaliplatin, 1600 hr; peak 5-FU/LV, 0400 hr)

Study	No. of Patients	Prior Chemo-therapy	Dose Schedule	Response Rate (%)	Time to Disease Progression (mo)	Survival (mo)
Levi[54]	52 41	No Yes	5-FU, 700 mg/m^2/day + LV, 300 mg/m^2/day + Oxaliplatin, 25 mg/m^2/day × 5 days q3wk, chronomodulated infusion	59 (11% CR) 57 (2% CR)	11 10	15 13
Garufi[66]	35	Yes	5-FU, 700 mg/m^2/day + LV, 300 mg/m^2/day + oxaliplatin, 25 mg/m^2/day × 4–5 days q2–3wk, chronomodulated infusion	23	6	11
Levi[55]	F 47 C 45	No No	5-FU, 600 mg/m^2/day + LV, 300 mg/m^2/day + Oxaliplatin, 20 mg/m^2/day × 5 days q3wk, flat vs chronomodulated infusion	F 32 C 53 ($P = 0.04$)	F 8 C 11 ($P = 0.19$)	F 14.9 C 19 ($P = 0.03$)
Levi[43]	F 93 C 93	No No	5-FU, 600 mg/m^2/d + LV, 300 mg/m^2/d + Oxaliplatin, 20 mg/m^2/day × 5 days q3wk, flat vs chronomodulated infusion	F 29 C 51 ($P = 0.003$)	F 7.9 C 9.8 ($P = 0.2$)	F 16.9 C 15.9 ($P = 0.46$)

Levi[56]	F 140 C 138	No No	5-FU, 600 mg/m²/day + LV, 300 mg/m²/day + Oxaliplatin, 20 mg/m²/day × 5 days q3wk, flat vs chronomodulated infusion	F 30 C 51 ($P < 0.001$)	F 7.5 C 10.3 ($P = 0.039$)	F 16.5 C 18.6 ($P = 0.22$)
Bertheault- Cuitkovic[57]	37 13	Yes No	5-FU, 700 mg/m²/day + LV, 300 mg/m²/day + Oxaliplatin, 25 mg/m²/day × 4 days q2wk, chronomodulated infusion	40 69	10.3 9.3	16.9 20.7
Levi[65]	90	No	5-FU, 700 mg/m²/day + LV, 300 mg/m²/day + Oxaliplatin, 25 mg/m²/day × 4 days q2wk, chronomodulated infusion	66	8.4	18.5

C, chronomodulated infusion; CR, complete response; F, flat infusion; 5-FU, 5-fluorouracil; LV, leucovorin; pts, patients.

80–135 mg/m² in addition to various schedules of 5-FU/LV. Overall, a 25.5% response rate was noted, with a median survival of 9.6 months, again supporting the activity of oxaliplatin added to 5-FU/LV regimens in 5-FU/LV failures. This trend of activity in previously treated patients is supported by various other trials that use 2-hour oxaliplatin infusions, as summarized in Table 8.4.[44–53] The median overall response rate in all 12 trials is 25% (range, 13%–46%).

The principal toxicities (grade 3 to 4) associated with 2-hour infused oxaliplatin plus various 5-FU/LV regimens in 522 individuals are summarized in Table 8.5 and include diarrhea (17%), neutropenia (20%), neuropathy with at least mild functional impairment (22%), and an interesting, and probably underreported, incidence of laryngopharyngeal dysesthesias (8%). Of interest, laryngopharyngeal dysesthesias have not been reported with the prolonged infusion schedules, although the incidence of peripheral sensory neuropathy is similar to that observed with the 2-hour oxaliplatin infusions (see Table 8.5).

Given their long-standing interest in the use of chronomodulated 5-FU/LV, Levi et al[54] combined their chronomodulated oxaliplatin regimen with 5-FU/LV (which also was given on a chronomodulated infusion schedule) using a programmable ambulatory infusion pump (see Table 8.4). These investigators developed a regimen using 5-FU, 700 mg/m²/day, plus folinic acid, 300 mg/m²/day, combined with oxaliplatin, 25 mg/m²/day for 5 consecutive days every 3 weeks. The peak infusion rate for 5-FU/LV was set at 4:00 AM, whereas that for oxaliplatin was regulated to occur at 4:00 PM based on investigations in murine models, suggesting that these times were optimal for antitumor efficacy with the least amount of normal tissue toxicity. The initial investigations using this regimen were performed in 93 patients with advanced colorectal cancer, of whom 52 patients, or 66%, had not received prior chemotherapy. Regardless of prior exposure to chemotherapy, these authors reported an overall response rate of 58%, with a 6% complete response rate and an overall median survival of 15 months.[54] Toxicities associated with this regimen were similar to those previously reported with oxaliplatin alone given by the circadian infusion schedule and included grade 3 and 4 nausea and vomiting in 8%, diarrhea in 5%, and peripheral neuropathy in 11% of 784 administered courses.

Given the interesting clinical activity of the chronomodulated three-drug regimen, two sequential, randomized trials were undertaken to evaluate the value of a chronomodulated (45 + 93 = 138 patients total) versus a fixed infusion (47 + 93 = 140 patients total) of the three-drug regimen, using doses identical to those previously reported (see Table 8.4).[43,55,56] These investigators demonstrated that the chronomodulated schedule was associated with a significantly higher response rate as compared with the flat schedule (51% vs 30%; $P < 0.001$). Although the time to disease progression was modestly improved with the chronomodulated schedule, the overall survival between the two groups (18.6 vs 16.5 months) was not statistically different.

Of interest are the differences in toxicity profiles reported in the two sequential investigations using identical treatment regimens. Whereas the rate of grade 3 to

TABLE 8.5 Grade 3 to 4 Toxicities Associated with 5-Fluorouracil and Leucovorin Plus Oxaliplatin

	No. of Patients	Stoma-titis (%)	Diarrhea (%)	N&V (%)	Neuro-pathy[a] (%)	Thrombo-cytopenia (%)	Neutro-penia (%)	H/F (%)	LPD (%)
Prolonged infusion schedules									
Flat 3-drug infusion × 5 days q3wk[54-56]	138	79	29	19	23	NR	8[b]	8[b]	NR
Chronomodulated 3-drug infusion × 5 days q3wk[54-56]	138	15	29	24	19	NR	3[b]	3[b]	NR
Chronomodulated 5-FU/LV plus 6-hr infusion oxaliplatin (data from phase III trial)[58]	100	10	43	25	13	1	2	0	NR
Chronomodulated 3-drug infusion × 4 days q2wk[57,65]	140	29	41	34	26	3	8	10	NR
2-Hr infusion schedules									
Oxaliplatin over 2 hr q2–3wk plus 5-FU/LV (various schedules)[44-51]	522	6	15	9	24	7	21	1	5
Oxaliplatin over 2 hr plus 5-FU/LV bimonthly (data from phase III trial)[59]	209	6	12	6	18	3	42	0	23

5-FU, 5-fluorouracil; H/F, palmar/plantar erythrodysesthesia (hand-foot syndrome); LPD, laryngopharyngeal dysesthesias; LV, leucovorin; NR, not reported; N&V, nausea and vomiting.
[a]National Cancer Institute–common toxicity criteria grades 2 to 4 or equivalent (i.e., mild functional impairment or greater).
[b]Combined neutropenia and H/F.

4 stomatitis was consistent between the two studies in demonstrating that the flat infusion was associated with this toxicity in five times more patients, the degree of neuropathy associated with each regimen as reported in these two trials was strikingly different.[55,56] In the first trial, the chronomodulated schedule was associated with a fourfold higher incidence of grade 2 neuropathy, whereas in the second trial, the incidence of grade 2 neuropathy in the flat infusion rate group was twofold higher as compared with the chronomodulated group. The reasons for this discrepancy are not clear given that identical regimens were explored with each study. However, combining the toxicities from both trials suggests little difference in toxicities between the flat and chronomodulated schedules. Furthermore, the toxicities associated with the infusion schedules may be compared with those associated with 2-hour oxaliplatin infusion regimens (see Table 8.5). Of note, the incidence of grade 3 to 4 gastrointestinal toxicities and hand-foot syndrome appears somewhat higher with the prolonged infusion schedules. Whether the toxicity and cumbersome logistics associated with chronomodulated or flat prolonged infusions of oxaliplatin plus 5-FU/LV can be justified by enhanced efficacy when compared with the 2-hour oxaliplatin regimens remains to be determined by prospective randomized investigations. However, the outcomes associated with treatment of chemotherapy-naive patients having advanced colorectal cancer using a chronomodulated three-drug regimen suggest the clinical benefit may be similar to that achieved with the shorter infusion schedules.

In an effort to enhance the efficacy of the chronomodulated three-drug regimen (see Table 8.4), a more dose-intense schedule was developed using a 4-day, every-2-week regimen. An initial investigation of 13 patients with colorectal cancer who had not received prior therapy yielded a 69% response rate and an overall median survival in excess of 20 months.[57] Of note, peripheral neuropathy requiring patient withdrawal from the study occurred in 30% of the 50 patients treated with this regimen. A subsequent investigation using an identical dose-intensified regimen in 90 patients confirmed a high response rate of 66%, with a progression-free survival (8.4 months) and median overall survival (18.5 months) similar to that previously reported using the every-3-week chronomodulated schedule.[65] Of note, the dose-intensified schedule was associated with a 40% rate of grade 3 to 4 nausea, vomiting, and diarrhea, as well as a 25.6% rate of grade 2 peripheral neuropathy, which resulted in withdrawal from the study for 19% of treated patients. The added value of the more dose-intense chronomodulated schedule as compared to either the every-3-week flat or chronomodulated schedule requires further investigation.

Phase III Studies

Two multiinstitutional, prospectively randomized trials have been reported this year.[58,59] Both trials were designed to address the value of adding oxaliplatin to

5-FU/LV. The first of these investigations explored the addition of a 6-hour infusion of oxaliplatin (125 mg/m^2/day) preceding a 5-day course of chronomodulated 5-FU (700 mg/m^2/day) and LV (300 mg/m^2/day), with a peak delivery rate occurring at 0400 hours and repeated every 21 days.[58] The 6-hour infusion was designed to avoid the occurrence of laryngopharyngeal dysesthesias associated with the shorter infusion schedules. One hundred previously untreated patients with measurable advanced colorectal cancer were randomized to each of the two arms of the study (200 patients total). The demographics associated with patients on each of the two arms was balanced with the exception of twice as many patients having carcinoembryonic antigen levels $\leq$ 10 ng/mL on the oxaliplatin-containing arm and twofold more individuals having received prior adjuvant chemotherapy on the control arm. These two imbalances tend to favor the experimental arm.

The reported overall response rates for individuals on the control versus experimental arms were 16% and 53%, respectively; however, only a portion of these responses were confirmed by subsequent scans performed at 9 weeks.[58] Thus, the response rates confirmed by repeat scanning and documented by external review were 12% and 34%, which, although lower than the investigator-reviewed responses, maintained a difference that was highly statistically significant ($P < 0.001$). Of note, three complete responses were observed in the oxaliplatin-containing arm. The median progression-free survival was 2.5 months longer for the experimental group, and this difference was also statistically significant ($P = 0.048$). Overall median survival for each of the groups was nearly identical at 19.9 and 19.4 months for the control and experimental arms, respectively. Although the chronomodulated regimen of 5-FU/LV was well tolerated, the toxicities associated with the addition of oxaliplatin included a marked increase (two- to eightfold) in the incidence of severe gastrointestinal toxicities, including diarrhea, nausea and vomiting, and mucositis. In addition, a 45% incidence of sensory neuropathy was noted. Neurotoxicity included paresthesias lasting for longer than 14 days (32%) or functional impairment in the activities of daily living (13%), which ultimately led to the withdrawal from treatment for 77% of these individuals (10 patients total). The median cumulative dose of oxaliplatin that led to functional impairment was 1.1 gm/m^2, whereas that leading to paresthesias lasting for more than 14 days was 716 mg/m^2.

A second randomized multicenter trial assessed the value of oxaliplatin given as a 2-hour infusion at 85 mg/m^2 every 2 weeks when added to a bimonthly regimen of LV given by a 2-hour infusion followed by bolus 5-FU, then infusional 5-FU for 2 days.[59] Four hundred twenty previously untreated individuals with advanced and measurable colorectal carcinoma were entered into this study. The patient demographics were equally balanced on the two arms. The investigators found an overall response rate of 50.7% in the experimental arm containing oxaliplatin, as compared with 22.3% in the control group ($P = 0.0001$). The progression-free survival, as measured by external review, was 6.0 months in the control arm and 8.2 months in the experimental arm ($P = 0.0003$), and the overall survival was not different between the two groups (14.7 months vs 16.2 months). As was the case for the chronomodulated schedule, the addition of oxaliplatin to the bimonthly regimen resulted in remarkably greater incidence of toxicity in the form of grade 3 and 4 neutropenia (eightfold) and gastrointestinal toxicities (two- to threefold). In particular, grade 3 peripheral neurosensory toxicity associated with functional impairment occurred in 18% of patients treated on the oxaliplatin-containing arm. Eight patients (4%) were withdrawn from the study owing to neurotoxicity. The occurrence of neuropathy was clearly cumulative, with estimates for the occurrence of grade 3 neuropathy of 10% after 9 cycles and 50% after 14 cycles of therapy. The median time to recovery from grade 3 neurotoxicity was approximately 3 months.

A quality-of-life assessment associated with this trial demonstrated comparability between the two arms; however, the time to deterioration of global health status to 20% or 40% was significantly longer for patients on the oxaliplatin-containing arm.[59] The toxicities associated with the oxaliplatin-containing arm in this randomized trial were very similar to those previously reported in 12 separate phase II trials (as summarized in Table 8.5), with the exception of neutropenia, which appears to have occurred at twice the frequency as compared with prior regimens using 2-hour infusional oxaliplatin with 5-FU/LV. However, the level of neuropathy is similar and the incidence of gastrointestinal disturbance is substantially less than that reported on the various chronomodulated schedules. Of interest is the reported 23% incidence of laryngopharyngeal dysesthesias associated with patients treated on the oxaliplatin-containing arm. Given that prior reports have probably underreported this particular toxicity, the 23% occurrence appears to be a realistic estimate.

These two randomized studies comparing 5-FU/LV therapy with and without oxaliplatin are consistent in that they both show highly statistically significant increases in overall response rates and time to disease progression in the oxaliplatin-containing arms (Table 8.6).[58,59] However, neither study demonstrates an overall survival advantage, and both studies are associated with substantial additional toxicity attributable to oxaliplatin, particularly neurosensory toxicity requiring treatment modification or termination for a substantial minority of individuals. One possible reason for the lack of a survival advantage is the availability of active agents for 5-FU/LV failures, including oxaliplatin (for those who did not receive oxaliplatin in the original treatment assignment) and CPT-11 (which clearly has demonstrated clinical benefit as second-line therapy in patients with recalcitrant disease). Given the incremental clinical benefit associated with the addition of oxaliplatin, it may be a reasonable expectation that the use of second-line agents would confound the interpretation of overall survival. Thus, the clinical value of the addition of oxaliplatin to 5-FU/LV and its role in the clinical armamentarium remains to be defined.

TABLE 8.6 Phase III 5-Fluorouracil (5-FU) and Leucovorin (LV) With or Without Oxaliplatin in Patients with Advanced Colorectal Cancer

Study	No. of Patients	Dose Schedule	Response Rate (%)	Time to Disease Progression (mo)	Median Survival (mo)
de Gramont[59]	420	LV 200 mg/m^2/day followed by 5-FU bolus, 400 mg/m^2/day and 22-hr infusion 600 mg/m^2/day × 2 days q2wk, alone or with oxaliplatin, 85 mg/m^2 over 2 hr (FOLFOX4)	22.3 vs 50.7 ($P = 0.0001$)	6.0 vs 8.2 ($P = 0.0003$)	14.7 vs 16.2 ($P = 0.12$)
Giacchetti[58]	200	Chronomodulated 5-FU/LV, 700/300 mg/m^2/day (peak 0400 hr) × 5 days, alone or with oxaliplatin, 125 mg/m^2 IV over 6 hr on day 1 q21d	16 vs 53 ($P < 0.0001$)	6.1 vs 8.7 ($P = 0.048$)	19.9 vs 19.4

A three-arm randomized trial sponsored by NCI should provide additional insight. This trial is designed to compare a weekly regimen of CPT-11 plus 5-FU/LV, which has previously been shown to significantly improve overall survival compared with 5-FU/LV alone, a bimonthly 48-hour 5-FU/LV regimen coupled with a brief infusion of oxaliplatin and, finally, a non-fluoropyrimidine-containing combination of oxaliplatin plus CPT-11 given on an every-3-week basis.

Phase I and II Trials Using Oxaliplatin in Non-5-FU-Containing Combination Regimens

Clinical trials have been initiated combining oxaliplatin with other agents with known activity in the treatment of patients with colorectal carcinoma, including CPT-11 and raltitrexed. Three phase II trials involving a total of 160 patients with advanced colorectal carcinoma who had not received prior chemotherapy combined raltitrexed, 3 mg/m² intravenously over 15 minutes, and oxaliplatin, 130 mg/m² over 2 hours given 45 minutes after the raltitrexed dose, and called for dosing every 3 weeks.[60-62] Encouraging response rates between 40% and 62% coupled with a convenient administration schedule and acceptable toxicity should encourage further development of this particular combination.

An interesting non–thymidylate synthase–directed combination of oxaliplatin and CPT-11 has been developed and tested in preliminary studies by two groups. Using oxaliplatin, 85 mg/m² on days 1 and 15, coupled with CPT-11, 80 mg/m² on days 1, 8, and 15 of an every-4-week cycle, investigators from Austria identified a 42% overall response rate in 36 previously treated individuals with advanced colorectal carcinoma.[63] Similar encouraging preliminary data in patients with previously treated disease comes from a phase I investigation conducted at the Memorial Sloan-Kettering Cancer Center and calling for a 2-hour oxaliplatin infusion followed by weekly CPT-11 for 4 weeks, administered on an every-6-week schedule.[64] The investigators in these trials identified a 26% overall response rate in 23 patients treated at the recommended dose of oxaliplatin (60 mg/m²) and CPT-11 (65 mg/m²). Both of these investigations identified neutropenia and diarrhea as dose-limiting,[63,64] and peripheral sensory neuropathy as a common toxicity (grade 2 to 3 = 22%) in the Austrian schedule.[63] The combination of oxaliplatin and CPT-11 is of particular interest given the absence of a thymidylate synthase–directed agent. This combination may have especially interesting activity in those patients whose cancers contain high levels of thymidylate synthase and thus are relatively insensitive to regimens containing thymidylate synthase–directed agents such as 5-FU.

FUTURE DIRECTIONS

From the current literature, it is clear that oxaliplatin has notable clinical activity in patients with colorectal carcinoma. As a single agent, oxaliplatin clearly has activity both in chemotherapy-naive patients and in individuals whose disease is refractory to standard agents. When combined with various schedules of 5-FU/LV, oxaliplatin is associated with approximately a 25% response in previously treated individuals whose colorectal cancer is advanced and a 50% response in chemotherapy-naive patients. The use of the three-drug regimen in this population is reproducibly associated with a time–to–disease progression of 8–9 months and an overall survival of 15–19 months.

Although no direct comparisons have been explored, the clinical outcomes associated with prolonged infusions, whether chronomodulated or flat, versus the relatively brief 2- to 6-hour infusions, appear similar. Hence, it is unclear whether the use of infusional therapy, with its attendant logistic issues and somewhat greater degree of gastrointestinal toxicities, can be justified. Ongoing randomized investigations will provide direct comparisons of clinical efficacy and toxicity of fluoropyrimidine-based regimens in combination with either oxaliplatin or CPT-11. The clinical outcomes associated with the oxaliplatin-containing regimens and those regimens combining CPT-11 and 5-FU/LV might emerge as being very similar in terms of response rates, time to tumor progression, and overall survival, given the recently reported results of CPT-11 and 5-FU/LV combinations.[1] A central and prevalent toxicity that makes oxaliplatin less attractive is peripheral sensory neuropathy, which is cumulative and only slowly reversible. Quality-of-life assessments associated with ongoing randomized trials should help to balance this particular toxicity with other measures of clinical benefit.

How and where oxaliplatin ultimately will fit into the clinical armamentarium for the treatment of patients with colorectal carcinoma remains to be defined. Although it is unlikely that oxaliplatin as a single agent will have clinical utility, its use with fluoropyrimidine-based regimens appears highly likely as either first-line or second-line therapy for the treatment of advanced colorectal disease. It also is likely that a three-drug combination using oxaliplatin will prove to be efficacious in the adjuvant setting as either sole therapy or, potentially, as part of a sequential regimen. Finally, given the recent evidence that high levels of thymidylate synthase expression are associated with nonresponse to fluoropyrimidine-containing regimens, it is likely that a CPT-11 and oxaliplatin combination would prove highly useful in the subset of patients whose cancer overexpresses thymidylate synthase. Clinical investigations designed to address many of the aforementioned issues are ongoing. The outcome of these clinical investigations should provide clarity for the role of oxaliplatin in the treatment of advanced disease and as adjuvant therapy for patients with colorectal carcinoma.

ACKNOWLEDGMENTS

I would like to thank Ms. Janet Edds for her careful editing of this manuscript and Dr. William Dahut for his review and suggestions concerning the clinical science surrounding the development of oxaliplatin.

REFERENCES

1. Saltz LB, Cox JV, Blanke C et al. Irinotecan plus fluorouracil and leucovorin for metastatic colorectal cancer. Irinotecan Study Group. N Engl J Med 2000;343:905–914.
2. Pazdur R, Douillard J-Y, Skillings JR et al. Multicenter phase III study of 5-fluorouracil (5-FU) or UFT in combination with leucovorin (LV) in patients with metastatic colorectal cancer. Proc Am Soc Clin Oncol 1999;18:1009.
3. Twelves C, Harper P, Van Cutsem E et al. A Phase III trial (S014796) of Xeloda (capecitabine) in previously untreated advanced/metastatic colorectal cancer. Proc Am Soc Clin Oncol 1999;18:1010.
4. Kidani Y, Noji M, Tashiro T. Antitumor activity of platinum(II) complexes of 1,2-diamino-cyclohexane isomers. Japan J Cancer Res (Gann) 1980;71:637–643.
5. Tashiro T, Kawada Y, Sakurai Y et al. Antitumor activity of a new platinum complex, oxalato (trans-L-1,2-diaminocycohexane)platinum (II): new experimental data. Biomed Pharmacother 1989;43:251–260.
6. Luo FR, Wyrick SD, Chaney SG. Cytotoxicity, cellular uptake, and cellular biotransformation of oxaliplatin in human colon carcinoma cells. Oncol Res 1998;10:595–603.
7. Vaisman A, Masutani C, Hanaoka F et al. Efficient translesion replication past oxaliplatin and cisplatin GpG adducts by human DNA polymerease η. Biochemistry 2000;39:4575–4580.
8. Levi F, Metzger G, Massari C et al. Oxaliplatin: pharmacokinetics and chronopharmacological aspects. Clin Pharmacokinet 2000;38:1–21.
9. Mauldin SK, Plescia M, Richards FA et al. Displacement of the bidentate malonate ligand from (D,L-trans-1,2-diaminocyclohexane) malonatoplatinum(II) by physiologically important compounds in vitro. Biochem Pharmacol 1988;37:3321–3333.
10. Mauldin SK, Gibbons G, Wyrick SD et al. Intracellular biotransformation of platinum compounds with the 1,2-diaminocyclohexane carrier ligand in the L1210 cell line. Cancer Res 1988;48:5136–5144.
11. Page JD, Husain I, Sancar A et al. Effect of the diaminocyclohexane carrier ligand on platinum adduct formation, repair, and lethality. Biochemistry 1990;29:1016–1024.
12. Boudny V, Vrana O, Gaucheron F et al. Biophysical analysis of DNA modified by 1,2-diaminocyclohexane platinum(II) complexes. Nucleic Acids Res 1991;20:267–272.
13. Saris CP, van de Vaart PJM, Rietbrock RC et al. In vitro formation of DNA adducts by cisplatin, lobaplatin, and oxaliplatin in calf thymus DNA in solution and in cultured human cells. Carcinogenesis 1996;17:2763–2769.
14. Woynarowski JM, Chapman WG, Napier C et al. Sequence- and region-specificity of oxaliplatin adducts in naked and cellular DNA. Mol Pharmacol 1998;54:770–777.
15. Vaisman A, Varchenko M, Umar A et al. The role of hMLH1, hMSH3, and hMSH6 defects in cisplatin and oxaliplatin resistance: correlation with replicative bypass of platinum-DNA adducts. Cancer Res 1998;58:3579–3585.
16. Nehme A, Baskaran R, Nebe S et al. Induction of JNK and c-Abl signaling by cisplatin and oxaliplatin in mismatch repair-proficient and -deficient cells. Br J Cancer 1999;79:1104–1110.
17. Rixe O, Ortuzar W, Alvarez M et al. Oxaliplatin, tetraplatin, cisplatin, and carboplatin: spectrum of activity in drug-resistant cell lines and in the cell lines of the National Cancer Institute's Anticancer Drug Screen panel. Biochem Pharmacol 1996;52:1855–1865.
18. Schmidt W, Chaney SG. Role of carrier ligand in platinum resistance of human carcinoma cell lines. Cancer Res 1993;53:799–803.
19. Gibbons GR, Page JD, Mauldin SK et al. Role of carrier ligand in platinum resistance in L1210 cells. Cancer Res 1990;50:6497–6501.

20. Mathè G, Kidani Y, Segiguchi M et al. Oxalato-platinum or L-OHP, a third-generation platinum complex: an experimental and clinical appraisal and preliminary comparison with cis-platinum and carboplatinum. Biomed Pharmacother 1989;43:237–250.
21. Pendyala L, Creaven PJ. In vitro cytotoxicity, protein binding, red blood cell partitioning, and biotransformation of oxaliplatin. Cancer Res 1993;53:5970–5976.
22. Raymond E, Lawrence R, Izbicka E et al. Activity of oxaliplatin against human tumor colony-forming units. Clin Cancer Res 1998;4:1021–1029.
23. Faivre S, Raymond E, Woynarowski JM et al. Supraadditive effect of 2′,2′-diflourodeoxycytidine (gemcitabine) in combination with oxaliplatin in human cancer cell lines. Cancer Chemother Pharmacol 1999;44:117–123.
24. Plasencia C, Taron M, Abad A et al. Synergism of oxaliplatin (OXA) with either 5-fluorouracil (5FU) or topoisomerase I inhibitor in sensitive and 5FU-resistant colorectal cell lines is independent of DNA-mismatch repair and p53 status. Proc Am Soc Clin Oncol 2000;19:793.
25. Zeghari-Squalli N, Raymond E, Cvitkovic E et al. Cellular pharmacology of the combination of the DNA topoisomerase I inhibitor SN-38 and the diaminocyclohex and platinum derivative oxaliplatin. Clin Cancer Res 1999;5:1189–1196.
26. Raymond E, Buquet-Fagot C, Djelloul S et al. Antitumor activity of oxaliplatin in combination with 5-fluorouracil and the thymidylate synthase inhibitor AG337 in human colon, breast, and ovarian cancers. Anticancer Drugs 1997;8:876–885.
27. Gamelin E, Bouil AL, Boisdron-Celle M et al. Cumulative pharmacokinetic study of oxaliplatin, administered every three weeks, combined with 5-fluorouracil in colorectal cancer patients. Clin Cancer Res 1997;3:891–899.
28. Kern W, Braess J, Bottger B et al. Oxaliplatin pharmacokinetics during a four-hour infusion. Clin Cancer Res 1999;5:761–765.
29. Massari C, Brienza S, Rotarski M et al. Pharmacokinetics of oxaliplatin in patients with normal versus impaired renal function. Cancer Chemother Pharmacol 2000;45:157–164.
30. Graham MA, Gamelin E, Misset JL et al. Clinical pharmacokinetics of oxaliplatin. Proc Am Assoc Cancer Res 1998;39:1088.
31. CancerNet, National Cancer Institute, NIH. Phase I Study of Oxaliplatin in Patients with Advanced Malignancies and Varying Degrees of Liver Dysfunction. Clinical Study 00-C-0172. Bethesda, MD: National Institutes of Health, National Cancer Institute, 2001. http://cancernet.nci.nih.gov.
32. Joel SP, Richards F, Seymour M et al. Oxaliplatin (L-OHP) does not influence the pharmacokinetics of 5-fluorouracil (5FU). Proc Am Soc Clin Oncol 2000;19:748.
33. Metzger G, Massari C, Etienne M-C et al. Spontaneous or imposed circadian changes in plasma concentrations of 5-fluorouracil coadministered with folinic acid and oxaliplatin: relationship with mucosal toxicity in patients with cancer. Clin Pharmacol Ther 1994;56:190–201.
34. Boughattas NA, Levi F, Fournier C et al. Circadian rhythm in toxicities and tissue uptake of 1,2-diammino-cyclohexane(*trans*-L) oxalatoplatinum(II) in mice. Cancer Res 1989;49:3362–3368.
35. Boughattas NA, Hecquet B, Fournier C et al. Comparative pharmacokinetics of oxaliplatin (L-OHP) and carboplatin (CBDCA) in mice with reference to circadian dosing time. Biopharm Drug Dispos 1994;15:1–13.
36. Extra JM, Espie M, Calvo F et al. Phase I study of oxaliplatin in patients with advanced cancer. Cancer Chemother Pharmacol 1990;25:299–303.
37. Caussanel J-P, Levi F, Brienza S et al. Phase I trial of 5-day continuous venous infusion of oxaliplatin at circadian rhythm-modulated rate compared with constant rate. J Natl Cancer Inst 1990;82:1046–1050.

38. Levi F, Perpoint B, Garufi C et al. Oxaliplatin activity against metastatic colorectal cancer. A phase II study of 5-day continuous venous infusion at circadian rhythm modulated rate. Eur J Cancer 1993;294:1280–1284.
39. Machover D, Diaz-Rubio E, de Gramont A et al. Two consecutive phase II studies of oxaliplatin (L-OHP) for treatment of patients with advanced colorectal carcinoma who were resistant to previous treatment with fluoropyrimidines. Ann Oncol 1996;7:95–98.
40. DeBraud F, Munzone E, Nole F et al. Synergistic activity of oxaliplatin and 5-fluorouracil in patients with metastatic colorectal cancer with progressive disease while on or after 5-fluorouracil. Am J Clin Oncol 1998;21:279–283.
41. Diaz-Rubio E, Sastre J, Zaniboni A et al. Oxaliplatin as single agent in previously untreated colorectal carcinoma patients: a phase II multicentric study. Ann Oncol 1998;9:105–108.
42. Becouarn Y, Ychou M, Ducreux M et al. Phase II trial of oxaliplatin as first-line chemotherapy in metastatic colorectal cancer patients. J Clin Oncol 1998;16:2739–2744.
43. Levi F, Zidani R, Misset J-L. Randomized multicentre trial of chronotherapy with oxaliplatin, fluorouracil, and folinic acid in metastatic colorectal cancer. Lancet 1997;350:681–686.
44. de Gramont A, Vignoud J, Tournigand C et al. Oxaliplatin with high-dose leucovorin and 5-fluorouracil 48-hour continuous infusion in pretreated metastatic colorectal cancer. Eur J Cancer 1997;33:214–219.
45. Andre T, Louvet C, Raymond E et al. Bimonthly high dose leucovorin, 5-fluorouracil infusion and oxaliplatin (FOLFOX3) for metastatic colorectal cancer resistant to the same leucovorin and 5-fluorouracil regimen. Ann Oncol 1998;9:1251–1253.
46. Andre T, Bensmaine A, Louvet C et al. Multicenter phase II study of bimonthly high-dose leucovorin, fluorouracil infusion, and oxaliplatin for metastatic colorectal cancer resistant to the same leucovorin and fluorouracil regimen. J Clin Oncol 1999;17:3560–3568.
47. Maindrault-Goebel F, Louvet C, Andre T et al. Oxaliplatin added to the simplified bimonthly leucovorin and 5-fluorouracil regimen as second-line therapy for metastatic colorectal cancer (FOLFOX6). Eur J Cancer 1999;35:1338–1342.
48. Maindrault-Goebel F, De Gramont A, Louvet C et al. High-dose oxaliplatin with the simplified 48h bimonthly leucovorin (LV) and 5-fluorouracil (5FU) regimen in pretreated metastatic colorectal cancer (FOLFOX). Proc Am Soc Clin Oncol 2000;19:1017.
49. Gerard B, Bleiberg H, Van Daele D et al. Oxaliplatin combined to 5-fluorouracil and folinic acid: an effective therapy in patients with advanced colorectal cancer. Anticancer Drugs 1998;9:301–305.
50. Brienza S, Bensmaine A, Soulie P et al. Oxaliplatin added to 5-fluorouracil-based therapy (5-FU ± FA) in the treatment of 5-FU-pretreated patients with advanced colorectal carcinoma (ACRC): results from the European compassionate-use program. Ann Oncol 1999;10:1311–1316.
51. Guerin-Meyer V, Delva R, Lortholary A et al. Combination of oxaliplatin (OXA/5-FU/FA) in 5-FU refractory advanced colorectal cancer (RACRC) patients (pts) treated with 5-FU/FA weekly PK guided regimen. Proc Am Soc Clin Oncol 2000;19:1001.
52. Janinis J, Papakostas P, Samelis G et al. Second-line chemotherapy with weekly oxaliplatin and high-dose 5-fluorouracil with folinic acid in metastatic colorectal carcinoma: a Hellenic Cooperative Oncology Group (HeCOG) phase II feasibility study. Ann Oncol 2000;11:163–167.
53. Kallen K-J, Hofmann MAK, Timm A, et al. Weekly oxaliplatin, high-dose infusional 5-fluorouracil and folinic acid as palliative third-line therapy of advanced colorectal carcinoma. Z Gastroenterol 2000;38:153–157.
54. Levi F, Misset J-L, Brienza S et al. A chronopharmacologic phase II clinical trial with 5-fluorouracil, folinic acid, and oxaliplatin using an ambulatory multichannel programmable pump. Cancer 1992;69:893–900.

55. Levi F, Zidani R, Vannetzel J-M et al. Chronomodulated versus fixed-infusion-rate delivery of ambulatory chemotherapy with oxaliplatin, fluorouracil, and folinic acid (leucovorin) in patients with colorectal cancer metastases: a randomized multi-institutional trial. J Natl Cancer Inst 1994; 86:1608–1617.
56. Levi FA, Zidani R, Llory J et al. Final efficacy update at 7 years of flat vs chronomodulated infusion (chrono) of oxaliplatin, 5-fluorouracil and leucovorin as first line treatment of metastatic colorectal cancer. Proc Am Soc Clin Oncol 2000;19:936.
57. Bertheault-Cvitkovic F, Jami A, Ithzaki M et al. Biweekly intensified ambulatory chronomodulated chemotherapy with oxaliplatin, 5-fluorouracil and folinic acid in patients with metastatic colorectal cancer. J Clin Oncol 1996;14:2950–2958.
58. Giacchetti S, Perpoint B, Zidani R et al. Phase III multicenter randomized trial of oxaliplatin added to chronomodulated fluorouracil-leucovorin as first-line treatment of metastatic colorectal cancer. J Clin Oncol 2000;18:136–147.
59. de Gramont A, Figer A, Seymour M et al. Leucovorin and fluorouracil with or without oxaliplatin as first-line treatment in advanced colorectal cancer. J Clin Oncol 2000;18:2938–2947.
60. Seitz FJ, Douillard JY, Paillot B et al. Tomudex (raltitrexed) plus oxaliplatin as first-line chemotherapy in metastatic colorectal cancer (MCRC) patients: a promising combination. Proc Am Soc Clin Oncol 1999;18:986.
61. Scheithauer W, Kornek GV, Ulrich-Pur H et al. Promising therapeutic potential of oxaliplatin + raltitrexed in patients with advanced colorectal cancer (ACC): results of a Phase I/II trial. Proc Am Soc Clin Oncol 2000;19:997.
62. Douillard JY, Michel P, Gamelin E et al. Raltitrexed ('Tomudex') plus oxaliplatin: an active combination for first-line chemotherapy in patients with metastatic colorectal cancer. Proc Am Soc Clin Oncol 2000;19:971.
63. Scheithauer W, Kornek GV, Raderer M et al. Combined irinotecan and oxaliplatin plus granulocyte colony-stimulating factor in patients with advanced fluoropyrimidine/leucovorin-pretreated colorectal cancer. J Clin Oncol 1999;17:902–906.
64. Kemeny N, Tong W, Stockman J et al. Phase I trial of weekly oxaliplatin and irinotecan in previously treated patients with metastatic colorectal cancer. Proc Am Soc Clin Oncol 2000;19: 948.
65. Levi F, Zidani R, Brienza S et al. A multicenter evaluation of intensified, ambulatory, chronomodulated chemotherapy with oxaliplatin, 5-fluorouracil, and leucovorin as initial treatment of patients with metastatic colorectal carcinoma. Cancer 1999;85:2532–2540.
66. Garufi C, Brienza S, Pugliese P et al. Overcoming resistance to chronomodulated 5-fluorouracil and folinic acid by the addition of chronomodulated oxaliplatin in advanced colorectal cancer patients. Anticancer Drugs 2000;11:495–501.

Chapter 9

Chemoradiation for Patients with Cervical Cancer

Franco Muggia

Silvia Formenti

John Curtin

Recently completed clinical trials in locally advanced cancers of the uterine cervix have put under intense focus current therapeutic practices in the management of this disease. The finding from five prospective randomized trials that cisplatin-based chemotherapy provides an advantage in both progression-free survival and overall survival over radiation alone or radiation with other radiosensitizers across five trials prompted a clinical alert by the National Cancer Institute (NCI) in February 1999.[1] The salient findings of these trials are summarized in Table 9.1.[2-6] The relative risk reductions for death from cervical cancer in these series vary between 0.5 and 0.71.[7]

Rather than representing a prescription for the current treatment of cervical cancer, these trials are best considered a stepping stone for the more rational integration of locally directed modalities (surgery, irradiation) with systemic therapy. In this chapter, we begin with a historical perspective on how the focus on chemoradiation arose and follow with a review of systemic therapy and its implications when combined with radiation and a discussion of the rational exploration of such therapies in the light of state-of-the-art roles of radiation and

TABLE 9.1 Chemoradiation Versus Radiation Trials: National Cancer Institute Clinical Alert

Study	Study Population	Irradiation Arm	Chemotherapy	Chemoradiation Arm
Peters (SWOG, GOG)	IA2, IB, IIA after surgery, positive PLNs	$N = 127$; 3-yr survival, 77%	5-FU $1000/m^2 \times 4$ days + cis, $70/m^2$ q3wk	$N = 116$; 3-yr survival, 87%
Keys (GOG123)	Bulky IB (tumor ≥ 4 cm)	$N = 186$; 3-yr survival, 74%	Cis, $40/m^2$ weekly	$N = 183$; 3-yr survival, 83%
Morris (RTOG)	IB, IIA with $N+$ or $T \geq 5$ cm; IIB–IV	$N = 195$; 5-yr survival, 58%; DFS, 40%	5-FU $1000/m^2 \times 4$ days + cis, $75/m^2$ q3wk	$N = 193$; 5-yr survival, 73%; DFS, 67%
Rose (GOG120)	IIB, IIIA, B, IVA; negative paraLNs	$N = 176$ (+HU); 3-yr PFS, 47%	Cis, $40/m^2$/wk, or cis/5-FU/HU, q4wk	$N = 177$; 3-yr survival, 67%; $N = 173$; 3-yr survival, 64%
Whitney (GOG85)	IIB, III, IVA; negative paraLNs	$N = 191$ (+HU); 5-yr PFS, 49%	5-FU, $1000/m^2 \times 4$ days + cis, $50/m^2$ q3wk	$N = 177$; 5-yr PFS, 67%

5-FU, 5-fluorouracil; cis, cisplatin; DFS, disease-free survival; GOG, Gynecologic Oncology Group; HU, hydroxyurea; paraLN, paraortic lymph node; PFS, progression-free survival; PLN, pelvic lymph nodes; RTOG, Radiation Therapy Oncology Group; SWOG, Southwest Oncology Group.

surgery. We conclude (rather than begin) with a stage-by-stage description of current treatment of women with cancer of the uterine cervix, so that the full impact of chemoradiation can be discussed. Except where specifically noted, no distinction is made between squamous and nonsquamous cancers as regards response to chemotherapy.

These issues must be placed in the perspective of the known epidemiology and outcome of this disease.[8-11] Worldwide, cancer of the uterine cervix is second only to breast cancer as the most common malignancy in women with respect to both incidence and mortality.[12] Close to half a million cases of cervical cancer are diagnosed annually. In both underdeveloped and industrialized nations, the majority of women who develop the disease are most often economically disadvantaged and have poor access to medical care and screening programs.

In the United States, there has been a sharp decline in the incidence and mortality from cervical cancer over the last 50 years.[13] The decline of the total number of cases and a shift to an earlier stage at diagnosis is directly related to cervical cytology screening. Mass use of the Papanicolaou (Pap) smear for cervical cancer screening here and in other countries has consistently proven to be one of the most effective tools applied for the control of a disease. However, there are still approximately 13,000 cases per year diagnosed in this country with approximately 5,000 deaths attributed annually to this disease.[9] In the majority of patients with a diagnosis of invasive cancer of the cervix, inadequate screening remains a common problem, especially among older women. The peak age of cervical cancer is 47 years, with only some 22% of cases diagnosed in women older than 65. However, older women typically present with more advanced stage of disease and account for more than 50% of the fatal cases in the United States.

Until the NCI clinical alert, standard treatment included surgery or radiation (or both) for nearly all localized stages—treatments that were known to be fairly inadequate for the 25% of these patients presenting with bulky primary cancers (stage IB2) or those extending to parametria and vagina (stages IIB, IIIB, and IVA). For these locally advanced, bulky stages, the local control rate from radiation varied from 80% to 87% in stage IB2 to only 25% in stage IVA. The 5-year survival rate varied from 63% to 75% in stage IB2 to 18% to 34% in stage IVA. Any impact from chemoradiation on these measures of outcome would have notable repercussions on disease mortality in both the United States and in developing countries, although implementation of these strategies is difficult without upgrading medical facilities.

HISTORICAL PERSPECTIVE

During the first 50 years of the twentieth century, cervical cancer became characterized as a disease afflicting young women and, in at least 70% of instances, presenting in locally advanced stages. The pioneering work of Papanicolaou established the value of routine screening programs that identified a stage of the disease in a preinvasive form that was 100% curable by limited surgery. In the United States, such programs coupled with an awareness of the role of sexual transmission as a risk factor led to a gradual decrease in the death rate from cervical cancer. Nevertheless, the treatment of locally advanced stages by radiation therapy was progressively refined by major centers that have continued to care for women discovered with such late cancers. Observations from recurrence patterns after treatment of advanced stages with radiation have provided the foundations for subsequent combined modality approaches.

Importance of Local Control

Absence of local control or pelvic failure is defined as persistent or recurrent disease after potentially curative treatment to the original tumor site in the pelvis. Kim et al[14] have reviewed the incidence of pelvic failures by Federation International de Gynecologie et Obstetrique (FIGO) stage (Table 9.2)[15] in 569 patients treated with radiation therapy alone. Stage IA patients had 4.6% pelvic failures, IB patients had 11.2% failures, and IIA patients had 8.4% failures. In the more advanced stages, the incidence of pelvic failures (with or without distant metastases) increases remarkably: 30.1% in stage IIB, 52.3% in stage III, and 69.2% in stage IVA. Most pelvic failures appeared within 36 months with approximately 80% appearing within 24 months of the initial therapy. Not surprisingly, in this and in other series,[16–18] patients with pelvic tumor control have 5-year survival rates higher than those in patients with pelvic failures, emphasizing the point that the quality of local treatment is a crucial condition for cure. Table 9.3 illustrates in one series the comparison of the 5-year survival rates for different stages of cervical cancer when the disease is controlled in the pelvis versus when the disease in persistent or recurrent (or both). These data convey the guiding principle that treatment combinations should not compromise local control rates and require adherence to radiation protocols with adequate dose and appropriate schedule. Some of the key variables in the successful treatment with radiation are treatment duration and oxygenation.

Effect of Treatment Duration on Outcome

The continuity of treatment has been shown to be a crucial factor in the outcome of cervical cancer treated with radiation alone. Excessive interruptions are presumably associated with increased tumor regeneration and consequently loss of local tumor control. Maciejewski et al[19] studied the effect of tumor cell repopulation in various clinical tumors and found an increased recurrence rate with protracted treatment at every level in a series of increasing total doses. Two large clinical studies reported findings compatible with such tumor repopulation as a cause of decreased local control and survival in cervical cancer. The first study, by the Patterns-of-Care group, analyzed the effect of total treatment time on pelvic control and survival using a database dating from 1973 to 1978.[20] The results

TABLE 9.2 International Federation of Gynecology and Obstetrics Staging of Carcinoma of the Cervix Uteri

	Definition
I	Carcinoma strictly confined to the cervix (extension to the corpus should be disregarded).
IA	Invasive carcinoma diagnosed only by microscopy. All macroscopically visible lesions, even with superficial invasion, are stage IB. Stromal invasion with a maximal depth of 5.0 mm measured from the base of the epithelium and a horizontal spread of 7.0 mm or less. Vascular space involvement, venous or lymphatic, does not affect classification.
IA1	Measured stromal invasion 3.0 mm or less in depth and 7.0 mm or less in horizontal spread.
IA2	Measured stromal invasion more than 3.0 mm and not more than 5.0 mm with a horizontal spread 7.0 mm or less.
IB	Clinically visible lesion confined to the cervix or microscopic lesion greater than IA2.
IB_1	Clinically visible lesion 4cm or less in greatest dimension.
IB_2	Clinically visible lesion more than 4cm in greatest dimension.
II	Cervical carcinoma invades beyond the cervix but not to the pelvic wall or to the lower third of the vagina.
IIA	Tumor without parametrial invasion.
IIB	Tumor with parametrial invasion.
III	Tumor extends to the pelvic wall and/or involves the lower third of the vagina and/or causes hydronephrosis or a nonfunctioning kidney.
IIIA	Tumor involves the lower third of the vagina, no extension to the pelvic wall.
IIIB	Tumor extends to the pelvic wall and/or causes hydronephrosis or a nonfunctioning kidney.
IV	Carcinoma has extended beyond the true pelvis or has clinically involved the mucosa of the bladder or rectum.
IVA	Tumor invades mucosa of the bladder or rectum, and/or extends beyond the true pelvis.

TABLE 9.3 Relationship Between Local Control and Five-Year Survival

	Five-Year Survival	
Disease Stage	Pelvic Control (%)	Pelvic Failure (%)
IB	92	19
IIA	88	15
IIB	87	20
III	70	5

of this study demonstrate a highly significant decrease in survival ($P = 0.0001$) and pelvic control ($P = 0.0001$) as treatment time was increased from fewer than 6 to 6–7.9 to 8–8.9 and 10 or more weeks (Table 9.4). Noticeably, the incidence of major complications was not significantly increased with the less protracted treatment. Multivariate analysis revealed three independent prognostic factors for in-field recurrence: stage of disease (stage I vs stage III), total treatment time (at each one of the time intervals), and age (> 50 vs < 50 years).

The second study reviewed 830 cervical cancer patients treated at the Princess Margaret Hospital, Toronto.[21] Three different statistical methods were used to analyze the data, and all yielded an approximate 1% loss of pelvic control per day beyond 30 days required to complete the radiation. As in the preceding study, this study identified stage, age, and treatment time as independent variables. In quantitative terms, a 20-day extension beyond 30 days in completing radiation would result in a 20% decrease in the expected local control rate for a given age and stage.

Role of Oxygenation

Again, a prospective experience from the Princess Margaret Hospital provided a clear demonstration of the role of hemoglobin levels in predicting pelvic recurrences from cervical cancer: transfusion over 12 gm/dl decreased the local recurrence rate in stage IIB and stage III patients receiving radiation.[22] This study, emanating from principles of radiation cytotoxicity in relation to oxygenation, pointed to the likely relationship of hypoxia and failure to achieve local control in cancer of the cervix. Hypoxic radiosensitizers, such as misonidazole, were, therefore, studied in phase III clinical trials.[23–25] However, the therapeutic index of this drug proved inadequate, and it required more than a decade to rekindle interest in such an approach. A retrospective study of seven centers across Canada indicated that the average weekly nadir hemoglobin was highly predictive of outcome.[26] Recent trials using chemoradiation, and increasing the likelihood of anemia, also bring attention to such an issue. In fact, discussion of a trial testing chemoradiation versus radiation alone by the National Cancer Institute of Canada[27] raised the issue of anemia as one possible explanation for a lack of significant differences between the two arms (G. Thomas and D. Pearcey, personal communication at the American Society of Clinical Oncology meeting, May 2000). There-

TABLE 9.4 Four-Year Actuarial Outcome by Total Treatment Time

4-Year Actuarial	< 6 Wk	6 to < Wk	8 to < 10 Wk	> 10 Wk	P
Pelvic recurrence	6%	12%	16%	20%	.0001
Survival	81%	74%	73%	66%	.0001
Major complications	15%	11%	12%	17%	NS

fore, renewed interest in this area is expected, particularly with the availability of recombinant erythropoietin formulations.

Optimal Sequencing of Combined Modalities

Early trials emanating from Roswell Park used hydroxyurea during radiation and formed the basis for subsequent Gynecologic Oncology Group (GOG) phase III trials.[28,29] Such trials provided the rationale for additional studies of radiosensitization, culminating in the chemoradiation studies indicated in Table 9.1. The modest effects of hydroxyurea in improving results and the failure of such hypoxic sensitizers as misonidazole[23–25] emphasized the importance of trying newer approaches. The success of conventional chemotherapeutic drugs in enhancing the effects of radiation in carcinoma of the anal canal[30] encouraged the exploration of such drugs as 5-fluorouracil (5-FU), mitomycin C, and cisplatin for better control of local and distant recurrences from cervical cancer.

After this experience with concomitant hydroxyurea and the recognition that approaches for advanced cervical cancer require improvements in both local-regional control and control of distant metastases fueled interest in adding chemotherapy to local modalities. Though simultaneous chemoradiation became the subject of randomized clinical trials, medical oncologists reported striking effects of chemotherapy[31,32]—and occasionally such agents as interferon-α and 13-cis retinoic acid[33]—on primary tumors when given prior to irradiation or surgery. In several instances, these encouraging pilot studies gave rise to phase III studies (Table 9.5).[34–39] No improved outcome was documented in fully accruing studies and detailed published reports[34–39]; in fact, two studies actually reported inferior results for neoadjuvant chemotherapy.[36,38] The rarity of complete pathologic responses from preoperative chemotherapy does cast doubt on the potential for such sequential therapy to match the current accomplishments of simultaneous chemoradiation in unresectable cervical cancer.

The role of preoperative chemotherapy or chemoradiation, however, deserves further study. A recently published series used chemoradiation followed by surgical resection for patients with FIGO stage IIB–IIIA, with 13 of 24 (54.2%) of surgical specimens demonstrating no residual tumor.[40] Among patients with stage IB subjected to surgery, one randomized study claimed superiority of neoadjuvant chemotherapy with vincristine, bleomycin, and cisplatin prior to surgery and irradiation as opposed to surgery and irradiation alone.[41] After this lead, the GOG sponsored a phase II study of neoadjuvant chemotherapy followed by radical hysterectomy for women with stage IB2 cancers of the cervix.[42] On the basis of the encouraging results of this study, an ongoing trial by the GOG (GOG 141) is exploring whether preoperative vincristine plus cisplatin will yield improved results as compared to surgery for "bulky" stage IB (J. Blessing, GOG, personal communication). Interpretation of this trial, however, will be complicated by the frequent use of postoperative irradiation in both arms. Such use is in accordance

TABLE 9.5 Prospective Randomized Trials of Sequential Chemotherapy Prior to Radiation Versus Radiation

Study	No. of Patients	Stage	Chemotherapy Arm	Outcome vs. RT Alone
Sundfor et al[34]	94	IIB–IVA	Cis/FU × 3 cycles → RT	5-yr PFS vs NS RT alone
Tattersall et al[35]	71	IB–IIA (pN+*)	Cis/VLB/Bleo × 3 cycles → RT	NS vs RT alone
Souhami et al[36]	107	IIIB	Cis/VLB/Bleo/MTC × 3 cycles → RT	Worse 5-yr survival for chemo + RT arm: 23% vs 39% (0.02)
Kumar et al[37]	184	IIB-IV	Bleo/IFX-mesna/Cis × 2 cycles → RT	NS vs RT alone
Tattersall et al[38]	260	IIIB–IVA	Cis + epirubicin × 3 cycles → RT	Worse 3-yr DFS for chemo + RT arm: 40% vs 50% (0.02)
Herod et al[39]	172	IB–IVA	Bleo/IFX/Cis × 2/3 cycles → RT	NS vs RT alone Projected 5-yr survival, 32%

Bleo, bleomycin; Cis, cisplatin; DFS, disease-free survival; FU, 5-fluorouracil; IFX, ifosfamide; MTC, mitomycin C; NS, not significant; PFS, progression-free survival; RT, radiation therapy; VLB, vinblastine.

with the demonstration that postoperative pelvic irradiation is associated with a reduction in pelvic and distant metastases as compared to observation in "high-risk" (lymphovascular space involvement), lymph node–negative patients after radical hysterectomy.[43] For patients subjected to radical hysterectomy and positive lymph nodes, chemoradiation including cisplatin plus 5-FU was shown to improve survival over irradiation alone.[3] Therefore, a number of questions arise as to the use of irradiation, chemotherapy, or both in accordance with the findings at radical hysterectomy. Three small randomized studies[44–46] already explored the role of chemotherapy alone in these patients, but the most appropriate comparator—chemoradiation—was used only in one.[46] Further studies in this area are needed.

SYSTEMIC CHEMOTHERAPY

The choice of cisplatin or cisplatin plus 5-FU as the preferred regimen accompanying irradiation was based on (1) the effect of these drugs against metastatic cervical cancer and (2) the favorable experience of combining these drugs with irradiation in a number of different primary cancer sites, including non–small cell lung and head and neck cancers (cisplatin) and esophageal and head and neck cancers (cisplatin + 5-FU). However, the contribution of cisplatin or cisplatin-based regimens to the systemic chemotherapy of metastatic cervical cancer is not clearly superior to that of other agents. The results of single-agent or combination chemotherapy in metastatic cervical cancer are consistently fairly modest. In fact, over the years, the enthusiasm has dampened in conducting comparative phase III trials (in the United States mostly by the GOG), as opposed to piloting new regimens or exploring the activity of new drugs. With the current interest in chemoradiation, we first review drugs of interest because of their antitumor activity and their potential as radiosensitizers and then comment on combination chemotherapy regimens, whether used for treatment of advanced disease or as part of a neoadjuvant strategy. Finally, we mention the emerging interest in new cytotoxic oral agents to combine with irradiation, drugs acting as biochemical modulators, and other noncytotoxic, biological approaches.

Cytotoxic Drugs

Platinums Cisplatin's activity in cervical cancer was identified by the GOG in publications dating to 1979.[47,48] The drug was capable of inducing objective responses in 20%–30% of patients, but emesis and renal toxicity complicated its use. A subsequent GOG study (GOG 43) failed to demonstrate a dose-response beyond from 50 to 100 mg/m^2 per cycle,[49] and the platinum analogs carboplatin or iproplatin were disappointing in phase II studies.[50] However, in the absence of comparative data, other experience suggests that carboplatin may have equivalent activity and better tolerance.[51] Oxaliplatin and new platinum compounds under development have not been adequately tested in cervical cancer; a GOG study is ongoing in previously treated patients (P. Fracasso, personal communication). Cisplatin has been part of many combinations studied in the neoadjuvant setting and in other phase III studies. Interest in radiosensitization by cisplatin dates to the 1970s,[52] but its delivery is problematic because of the need for hydration and control of vomiting. A daily schedule was the superior arm in combination with radiation for non–small cell lung cancer.[53] Carboplatin, with its slower intracellular kinetics of platinum-DNA adduct formation,[54] may provide analogous chemotherapy-irradiation interactions on a twice-weekly schedule that has been tested clinically with encouraging results.[55] Moreover, experimental evidence suggests that the cellular uptake of carboplatin is enhanced by irradiation.[56]

Fluoropyrimidines The activity of 5-FU against cervical cancer was demonstrated several decades ago in various studies using inaccurate assessments of response.[57] Studies by the GOG (GOG 26II) during the last decade have shown activity with this drug when modulated by high weekly doses of leucovorin.[58,59] In addition, encouraging activity was demonstrated in combination with cisplatin as first-line therapy.[60] As noted, this combination, particularly with 5-FU given as continuous infusion for 4–5 days, has frequently been used together with irradiation in cancers of gastrointestinal and upper aerodigestive origin. Protracted infusion schedules of 5-FU alone have been used as radiosensitization for cervical cancer in randomized trials,[61] including one recently completed and reported by Pearcey at the American Society of Clinical Oncology meeting in May 2000.[27] Only a trend favoring combined treatment has been shown in these studies. Therefore, in spite of this drug capturing considerable attention, questions remain as to its role, optimal schedule, and use of modulators.

Gemcitabine (difluorodeoxycytidine) has antitumor activity against cervical cancer when given alone[62] and in combination with cisplatin.[63] It is also a potent radiosensitizer,[64] and interest in its use in combined modality trials in cervical cancer is mounting.[65]

Taxanes Paclitaxel in advanced cervical cancer was first studied by the GOG (with the 24-hour and then 3-hour schedules) and was found by this group and others to have some activity (but not exceeding 20%) in advanced or recurrent squamous cancer.[66,67] Activity was also shown by the group in nonsquamous cancer of the cervix.[68] Plans to study docetaxel similarly are under way in the GOG. In the meantime, paclitaxel, 135 mg/m² by 24-hour infusion, in combination with cisplatin, 50 mg/m², has shown promising activity.[69] This regimen has been compared with cisplatin as a single agent in a phase III study (J. Blessing, GOG 169, personal communication). Regardless of whether they add to the activity of cisplatin in metastatic disease, taxanes hold interest as radiosensitizers.[70,71] Accordingly, several pilot studies using paclitaxel in weekly or twice-weekly schedules in combination with irradiation and platinums have either been published[72] or are planned by the GOG and by studies at New York University and the University of Southern California.

Ifosfamide and Conventional Alkylating Drugs Of the bischloroethyl alkylating agents, ifosfamide (always given with Mesna bladder protection) has been part of combination chemotherapy for cervical cancer during the last decade, primarily on the basis of its single-agent activity[73,74] and its incorporation into an active combination with bleomycin and cisplatin.[75] Comparative studies in the GOG indicated that cisplatin plus ifosfamide had improved activity and time-to-failure relative to cisplatin alone or to cisplatin plus the alkylating epoxide dibromodulcitol, but cisplatin alone was eventually retained as the control arm for a subsequent randomized study (GOG 110) because of toxicity considerations.[76] Chlorambucil has been used in some of the European studies because of its subjective tolerance by the oral route.[77] In general, this class of drugs is not considered to radiosensitize tumors independent of their antitumor activity.

Topoisomerase 1 Inhibitors Both topotecan and irinotecan, camptothecin derivatives, have shown activity against untreated cervical cancer (GOG 76U) and previously treated cervical cancer (GOG 127F).[78,79] GOG studies have completed accrual in a study combining irinotecan with cisplatin (J. Blessing, GOG 76BB, personal communication), whereas cisplatin plus topotecan is an arm of a currently active phase III study (vs cisplatin alone and MVAC in GOG 179; J. Blessing, personal communication). As topoisomerase 1 may be involved in DNA repair after use of DNA-damaging agents, a sequence-dependent enhancing effect on toxicity and efficacy has been noted in combination with irradiation.[80,81] Similarly, enhanced efficacy and toxicity were documented when cisplatin preceded the topotecan.[82] Analogous mechanisms may lead to radiosensitization, which is being exploited in a number of disease sites.[83] Irinotecan is a prodrug of SN-38 and shows less schedule dependence, presumably because of the potent and persistent inhibition of topoisomerase 1 by SN-38.[84]

Anthracyclines Activity of doxorubicin and epirubicin used as single agents was documented more than two decades ago; in the recent past, their use has been in combination, mostly as part of phase III studies (described later). Only slight activity has been documented in GOG trials with other topoisomerase 2 inhibitors that are DNA-intercalating agents, such as menogaril[85] and amonafide.[86] The enhancement of irradiation in normal tissues renders their use as selective radiosensitizers unpredictable. Nevertheless, one randomized clinical trial using epirubicin in combination with cisplatin and irradiation versus irradiation alone with negative results has been reported.[38] Recently, liposomally encapsulated doxorubicin that preferentially localizes in tumors rekindled interest in such formulation in combination with irradiation.

Vinca Alkaloids Vincristine was among one of the first chemotherapeutic drugs to be used in the treatment of advanced cervical cancer, and it has been used in several combinations (discussed later), primarily because it triggered little if any myelosuppression. Studies by the GOG documented the activity of vinblastine,[87] and, more recently, the group has been studying the use of vinorelbine alone[88] (J. Blessing, GOG127L and 128E, personal communication) and in combination with cisplatin[89] (J. Blessing GOG 76Z, personal communication). Presumably, because these drugs induce mitotic arrest, they sensitize cells to irradiation. Synergy against animal tumors and clinical benefit have also been reported when these drugs have been combined with taxanes.[90]

Mitomycin C Mitomycin C and its analog porfiromycin were widely used in treating cervical cancer during the 1970s (often in combination with bleomycin), primarily on the basis of Japanese data. However, the GOG documented only modest activity in untreated patients.[91] Nevertheless, the drug is a hypoxic radiosensitizer, as it undergoes bioreductive activation in a hypoxic environment,[92] and interest in combination with irradiation persists.

Miscellaneous Drugs Among commercially available drugs, methotrexate and bleomycin have been frequently used in the treatment of advanced cancer of the cervix, and trials demonstrating activity have been published for either drug.[57] Insufficient activity coupled with problematic toxicity has curtailed their use except in combinations such as bleomycin, ifosfamide, and cisplatin (Platinol)[39] or methotrexate, vinblastine, doxorubicin (Adriamycin), and cisplatin[93] (J. Blessing, GOG 179, personal communication). Oral drugs that have been considered for evaluation include etoposide[94]; the folate thymidylate synthase inhibitor raltitrexed; the oral platinum derivative JM216; oral topotecan; and altretamine.[95] Etoposide deserves special mention because of its established role in small-cell cancers arising in the cervix.

Cytotoxic Drug Combinations

As noted for each drug class, most of the agents deemed promising have proceeded to combinations with cisplatin. However, how they perform relative to cisplatin alone must await results from the few randomized studies that are ongoing. To date, no persuasive evidence that has appeared substantiates that these combinations will emerge as superior to cisplatin for advanced disease. Nevertheless, combinations have usually been the choice to be used simultaneously with irradiation in comparison to irradiation alone (as in some of the recent randomized trials shown in Table 9.1) and have been the choice, rather than single agents, for neoadjuvant randomized trials.

In fact, drug combinations became established in the treatment of advanced cervical cancer primarily because of activity when given prior to surgery. The Southwest Oncology Group performed one of the first randomized studies investigating the role of chemotherapy in cervical cancer. However, slow accrual led to dropping the cisplatin control arm while completing the study with the combination of mitomycin C, bleomycin, and vincristine that proved disappointing.[96]

Other randomized studies have been done by the European Organization for Research and Treatment of Cancer and by the GOG. These studies have generally failed to show a survival advantage for the combination, although some improvement in response rates or in time-to-failure was documented for cisplatin plus ifosfamide relative to cisplatin.[76] Because of toxicity considerations, some randomized phase III trials by the GOG in advanced or recurrent cervical cancer have reverted to using cisplatin alone as the control arm.

Radiosensitizers and Modulators

Misonidazole as a hypoxic radiosensitizer in the GOG phase III trial proved inferior to hydroxyurea.[25] The clinical trials within the GOG establishing a role for intermittent hydroxyurea during the course of irradiation were not convincingly accepted outside this group. After the trial showing that cisplatin plus 5-FU plus hydroxyurea yielded results superior to irradiation and hydroxyurea[5] (see Table 9.1), radiosensitization with this last agent ceased to be the standard in any group. Also, an ongoing pilot study evaluating intravenous hydroxyurea as a radiosensitizer by the New York GOG will likely not complete study without some modification. More recently, other hypoxic radiosensitizers with improved therapeutic indices, such as tirapazamine, have been undergoing clinical study. This drug has added interest because of its ability to enhance the effect of such cytotoxic drugs as cisplatin and cyclophosphamide.[97] As noted, many of the chemotherapeutic agents also have the potential to be radiosensitizers. Currently, the focus has been on cisplatin and, to a lesser extent, on 5-FU. However, taxanes, topoisomerase I inhibitors, and gemcitabine have generated considerable interest in combination with irradiation in cancers of various origins, including the uterine cervix.

Among noncytotoxic drugs, retinoids represent another drug class that has the potential for radio- and chemosensitization and represent potentially attractive agents for future trials.[98,99] Combinations with interferon-α were reported to be active, but this observation has subsequently not been confirmed.[100] Inhibitors of the epidermal growth factor receptor are receiving wide testing in cancers of lung and head and neck origin. These will undoubtedly receive testing in cervical cancer. Laboratory studies suggest that expression of epidermal growth factor receptor varies inversely with sensitivity to cisplatin.[101] Antiangiogenic strategies also hold some promise and await clinical study, whether as consolidation for patients in remission or in combination with other modalities.

Treatment Modalities According to Stage

Stage IA The exact definition of early-stage cervical cancer has been debated for several decades.[102] The widely accepted staging criteria has been published by FIGO and is presented in Table 9.2. The confusion regarding the ongoing debate over classifying early-stage disease can be inferred from the fact that FIGO has changed the definition of stage IA disease five times between 1960 and 1995. In 1973, the Society of Gynecologic Oncologists suggested a definition for microinvasive carcinoma of the cervix: microscopic invasive cancer with a maximum depth of invasion of 3 mm. This definition gained many advocates as it was thought that it could be used as a guide for therapy. Those patients with microinvasive cancers could be treated conservatively, possibly with a conization, whereas those who had more than 3 mm but less than 5 mm of invasion or vascular-lymphatic involvement might be considered for more radical therapy. Owing to estimates of nodal involvement of 4%–10%, the recommended treatment for patients with stage IA2 disease continues to be radical hysterectomy with bilateral pelvic lymphadenectomy or radiation therapy. In the rare patient who is considered a candidate for primary radiation therapy for stage IA cervical cancer, addition of chemotherapy is not indicated.

Stage IB Surgery has the advantages of shorter treatment time, removal of the primary tumor, more limited tissue injury, and the potential to preserve ovarian and, in select cases, reproductive function. The standard approach has been radical hysterectomy with pelvic lymphadenectomy and aortic lymph node sampling. Several large series have reported on the outcome after radical hysterectomy. One single-institution study reported a primarily surgical approach to the management of stage IB and stage IIA cervical carcinoma.[103] In addition to that of reporting on the long-term survival rates, the intention of the review was to correlate pathologic characteristics of the primary tumor with the incidence of recurrence after surgery so that consideration could be given to the development of adjunctive trials for high-risk patients.

The study included 431 patients who underwent radical hysterectomy as primary therapy from 1959 to 1977. Two hundred ninety-five patients had stage IB disease, and the other 136 patients had stage IIA disease. Complete pelvic lymphadenectomy was performed in 410 patients, and 8 patients had partial node dissections that were abbreviated because of the presence of extensive nodal disease or intraoperative complications. The 5-year survival rate for the entire group of 431 patients was 81.7%. Of the 418 patients who had complete or partial node dissections, 71 (17%) had lymph node metastases. Five-year survival in patients with negative nodes was 85% as compared to 50% for those with positive lymph nodes.

After stratification for nodal metastases, other histopathologic factors associated with an increased risk of recurrence and decreased survival were (1) nonsquamous histology, (2) primary tumor size of 4 cm or greater, (3) deep invasion into the outer one-third of the cervical stroma, and (4) grade 3 cancers. In a prospective study of the GOG, reported by Delgado et al[104] in 1990, additional risk factors were identified for patients treated by radical hysterectomy without obvious involvement of the pelvic lymph nodes. A subset of high-risk features (Table 9.6) derived from this prospective study was used to define the study population for GOG trial 92, which compared adjuvant pelvic radiation therapy versus no treatment.[43] Analysis of this study indicated a statistically significant (47%) reduction in risk of recurrence (relative risk, 0.53; $P = 0.008$, one-tail) among the radiation therapy group, with recurrence-free rates at 2 years of 88% for the radiation therapy group versus 79% for the group of patients who received no further treatment after radical hysterectomy. One important finding in this study was that radiation therapy not only had an impact on the reduction of local recurrences but was associated with a decrease in distant metastases.

One group of patients who would appear to benefit from the information derived from GOG 92 consists of the patients who present with stage IB2 disease. However, the "best practice" management of these patients is controversial. In part, this controversy persists owing to the competing protocols open to patients with locally advanced cervical cancer; the definition of *locally advanced* is also debated. During the same time that the GOG was conducting protocol 92, with a key eligibility factor being cervical lesion greater than 5 cm in diameter, patients were alternatively eligible for GOG protocol 123. This study was also recently reported and was included among the studies announced in the NCI clinical alert. Protocol 123[105] was a randomized study; all women with stage IB2 cervical cancer were treated with external radiation therapy, intracavitary irradiation, and extrafascial hysterectomy. The experimental arm of this randomized study was the addition of weekly *cis*-diamminedichloroplatinum during the external radiation therapy at a dose of 40 mg/M^2. The results of this study suggest that for patients with large cervical cancers without evidence of regional metastases, the optimal treatment may be external radiation therapy combined with weekly *cis*-diamminedichloroplatinum and one intracavitary implant followed by extrafascial hysterectomy. Some authors have suggested that patients may not need the hysterectomy; however, until that is proven in a prospective study, our opinion is that this is the preferred method of management for patients with stage IB2 cervical cancer.

Advanced-Stage Disease Many of the GOG studies of combined chemotherapy and irradiation required surgical staging prior to enrollment to exclude aortic

TABLE 9.6 Risk Factors for Determining Need for Postoperative Pelvic Radiation Therapy After Radical Hysterectomy with Negative Pelvic Lymph Nodes

Lymph-vascular space involvement
  Deep one-third invasion
  Middle third invasion and tumor >2 cm in diameter
  Superficial cervical stromal invasion and tumor >5 cm in diameter
No lymph-vascular space involvement
  Middle or deep one-third involvement and tumor >4 cm

Reprinted with permission from reference 37.

lymph node metastases and to exclude intraperitoneal extension of the primary cervical cancer. Many authors have questioned the routine value of surgical staging prior to pelvic radiation therapy in patients with negative aortic lymph nodes on either computed tomography scan or magnetic resonance imaging studies, whereas others have reported that information obtained from surgical staging has a significant impact on treatment planning and prognosis.[106,107] If surgical staging is performed, the preferred approach is an extraperitoneal technique to minimize adhesions and bowel toxicity during the subsequent irradiation. More recently, laparoscopic approaches have been used, and preliminary results suggest comparable sensitivity in detecting lymph node metastases without an increase in toxicity. The advantage of the laparoscopic approach includes the decrease in recovery time, which allows for initiation of treatment sooner as compared to the extraperitoneal approach.

As discussed, the GOG has published data from a randomized trial of chemotherapy plus radiation therapy followed by surgical resection of the cervical primary in large stage IB2 cervical cancer but, in the United States, this approach has not been used in the management of advanced-stage disease. Various other centers have reported on either neoadjuvant chemotherapy or combination chemotherapy plus radiation therapy followed by radical hysterectomy for stage IIB-III cervical cancers.[46,108] Although such treatment is feasible, there appears to be a significant increase in toxicity associated with the combination of chemotherapy and irradiation followed by radical surgery but without striking improvement in outcome. With the exception of biopsy-proven recurrences, we do not recommend radical surgery after chemotherapy and curative-intent radiation therapy for patients with stage IIB-IVA cervical cancer.

UNRESOLVED ISSUES AND FUTURE DIRECTIONS

The value of randomized clinical trials in resolving issues about the proper integration of therapeutic modalities is well illustrated by the five recently published trials included in Table 9.1. The trials address questions including different patient populations and use somewhat different regimens of cisplatin plus 5-fluorouracil; in two instances, they use a weekly schedule of cisplatin. One question that arises is whether cisplatin as a single agent in a chemoradiation regimen should be the building block for subsequent chemoradiation regimens. An obvious lead to follow is whether carboplatin can substitute for cisplatin in the combined treatment. This will not only facilitate the logistics of treatment but the twice-weekly administration of carboplatin has the potential to approach more closely the schedule considered optimal for radiosensitization—constant exposure to platinum adducts during irradiation.

The integration of such other drugs as a taxane, gemcitabine, a topoisomerase I inhibitor, or a vinca alkaloid with a platinum is another direction that might be considered to improve the systemic effects of the combination. In these explorations, however, it is imperative that the principles of optimal irradiation be observed (i.e., adequate dose, shortest duration of treatment, adequate oxygenation). Moreover, proponents of building systemic therapy at the expense of irradiation need to be reminded of the negative neoadjuvant trials and the relatively poor results of chemotherapy in advanced cervical cancer, regardless of response rates. Questions concerning chemotherapy, therefore, should not obscure the need to adhere to a standard irradiation protocol and to avoid such problems as treatment interruptions and emerging anemia that might be fostered by more aggressive chemotherapy regimens.

This new focus on chemoradiation certainly should not preclude inquiry into new treatment modalities, such as those targeting angiogenesis and signal transduction inhibitors. This review, in fact, identifies several areas that are controversial, and participation in clinical trials should further stimulate systematic testing of new agents and concepts. Improvements in imaging may facilitate characterizing the effects of certain interventions being considered for subsequent phase III studies.

Finally, one might reflect on reasons for the superiority of chemoradiation over the sequential use of the modalities. One hypothesis to advance is that the achievement of profound tumor destruction associated with pathologic complete remissions could perhaps trigger an immunologic response against the tumor. Some preliminary data by our group in locally advanced breast cancer support this hypothesis.[109]

REFERENCES

1. National Cancer Institute. Concurrent Chemoradiation for Cervical Cancer. Clinical Announcement. Washington, DC: National Cancer Institute, 1999.
2. Keys HM, Bundy BN, Stehman FB et al. Cisplatin, radiation and adjuvant hysterectomy compared with radiation and adjuvant hysterectomy for bulky stage IB cervical carcinoma. N Engl J Med 1999;340:1154–1161.
3. Peters WA III, Liu PY, Barrett RJ et al. Concurrent chemotherapy and pelvic radiation therapy compared to radiation therapy alone as adjuvant therapy after radical surgery in high-risk early stage carcinoma of the cervix. J Clin Oncol 2000;18:1606–1613.
4. Rose PG, Bundy BN, Watkins EB et al. Concurrent cisplatin-based radiotherapy and chemotherapy for locally advanced cervical cancer. N Engl J Med 1999;340:1144–1153.
5. Whitney CW, Sause W, Bundy BN et al. Randomized comparison of fluorouracil plus cisplatin versus hydroxyurea as an adjunct to radiation therapy in stage IIB-IVA carcinoma of the cervix with negative para-aortic lymph nodes: a Gynecologic Oncology Group and Southwest Oncology Group Study. J Clin Oncol 1999;17:1330–1348.
6. Morris M, Eifel PJ, Lu J et al. Pelvic radiation with concurrent chemotherapy compared with para-aortic radiation for high-risk cervical cancer. N Engl J Med 1999;340:1137–1143.
7. Thomas GM. Improved treatment for cervical cancer—concurrent chemotherapy and radiotherapy [editorial]. N Engl J Med 1999;340:1198–1199.
8. Whelan SL, Parkin DM, Masuyer E. Patterns of cancer in five continents. IARC Monogr Eval Carcinog Risks Hum, 1990.

9. Landis SH, Murray T, Bolden S, Wingo PA. Cancer statistics, 1999. CA Cancer J Clin 1999;49: 8–31.
10. Reeves WC, Brinton LA, Garcia M et al. Human papillomavirus infection and cervical cancer in Latin America. N Engl J Med 1989;320:1437–41.
11. Zur Hausen HH. Viruses and human cancers. Eur J Cancer 1999;35:1878–1885.
12. Bosch FX, Manos MM, Munoz N et al. Prevalence of human papillomavirus in cervical cancer: a worldwide perspective. J Natl Cancer Inst 1995;87:796–802.
13. National Institutes of Health. Cervical cancer. NIH Consensus Statement 1996;14:1–38.
14. Kim RY, Trotti A, Wu CJ et al. Radiation alone in the treatment of cancer of the uterine cervix: analysis of pelvic failure and dose response relationship. Int J Radiat Oncol Biol Phys 1989;17: 973–978.
15. International Federation of Gynecology and Obstetrics. Staging announcement: FIGO staging of gynecologic cancers: cervical and vulva. Int J Gynecol Cancer 1995;5:319.
16. Coia L, Won M, Lanciano R et al. The Patterns of Care Outcome Study for cancer of the uterine cervix. Results of the Second National Practice Survey. Cancer 1990;66:2451–2456.
17. Perez CA, Breaux S, Madoc-Jones H et al. Radiation therapy alone in the treatment of carcinoma of uterine cervix: I. Analysis of tumor recurrence. Cancer 1983;51:1393–1402.
18. Perez CA, Kuske RR, Camel HM et al. Analysis of pelvic tumor control and impact on survival in carcinoma of the uterine cervix treated with radiation therapy alone. Int J Radiat Oncol Biol Phys 1988;14:613–621.
19. Maciejewski B, Withers HR, Taylor JM, Hliniak A. Dose fractionation and regeneration in radiotherapy for cancer of the oral cavity and oropharynx: tumor dose-response and repopulation. Int J Radiat Oncol Biol Phys 1989;16:831–843.
20. Lanciano RM, Pajak TF, Martz K, Hanks GE. The influence of treatment time on outcome for squamous cell cancer of the uterine cervix treated with radiation: a patterns-of-care study. Int J Radiat Oncol Biol Phys 1993;25:391–397.
21. Fyles A, Keane TJ, Barton M, Simm J. The effect of treatment duration in the local control of cervix cancer. Radiother Oncol 1992;25:273–279.
22. Bush RS, Jenkin RP, Allt WE et al. Definitive evidence for hypoxic cells influencing cure in cancer therapy. Br J Cancer 1978;37:302–306.
23. Leibel S, Bauer M, Wasserman T et al. Radiotherapy with or without misonidazole for patients with stage IIIB or IVA squamous cell carcinoma of the uterine cervix. Preliminary report of a Radiation Therapy Oncology Group randomized trial. Int J Radiat Oncol Biol Phys 1987;13: 541–549.
24. Stehman FB, Bundy BN, Keys H et al. A randomized trial of hydroxyurea vs misonidazole adjunct to radiation therapy in carcinoma of the cervix: a preliminary report of a Gynecologic Oncology Group study. Am J Obstet Gynecol 1988;159:87–94.
25. Stehman FB, Bundy BN, Thomas G et al. Hydroxyurea versus misonidazole with radiation in cervical carcinoma: long-term follow-up of a Gynecologic Oncology Group trial. J Clin Oncol 1993;11:1523–1528.
26. Grogan M, Thomas GM, Melamed I et al. The importance of hemoglobin levels during radiotherapy for carcinoma of the cervix. Cancer 1999;86:1528–1536.
27. Pearcey RG, Brundage MD, Drouin P et al. A clinical trial comparing concurrent cisplatin and radiation therapy versus radiation alone for locally advanced squamous cell carcinoma of the cervix carried out by the National Cancer Institute of Canada Clinical Trial Group [abst 1497]. Proc Am Soc Clin Oncol 2000;19:378a.

28. Hreshchyshyn MM, Aron BS, Boronow RC et al. Hydroxyurea or placebo combined with radiation to treat stages IIIB and IV cervical cancer confined to the pelvis. Int J Radiat Oncol Biol Phys 1979;5:317–322.
29. Piver MS, Barlow JJ, Vongstma V et al. Hydroxyurea: a radiation potentiator in carcinoma of the uterine cervix—a randomized double-blind study. Am J Obstet Gynecol 1983;147:803–808.
30. Cummings BJ, Keane TJ, O'Sullivan B et al. Epidermoid anal cancer: treatment by radiation alone or by radiation and 5-fluorouracil with and without mitomycin C. Int J Radiat Oncol Biol Phys 1992;21:1115–1125.
31. Friedlander M, Kaye S, Sullivan A et al. Cervical carcinoma: a drug-responsive tumour experience with combined cisplatin, vinblastine, and bleomycin therapy. Gynaecol Oncol 1983;16:275–281.
32. Tobias J, Buxton EJ, Blackledge G et al. Neoadjuvant bleomycin, ifosfamide and cisplatin in cervical cancer. Cancer Chemother Pharmacol 1990;26[suppl]:S59–62.
33. Lippman SM, Kavanagh JJ, Paredes-Espinosa M et al. 13-*cis* retinoic acid plus interferon alpha 2a in locally advanced squamous cell carcinoma of the cervix. J Natl Cancer Inst 1993;85:499–500.
34. Sundfor K, Trope CG, Hogberg T et al. Radiotherapy and neoadjuvant chemotherapy in cervical carcinoma: a randomized multicenter study of sequential cisplatin and 5-fluorouracil and radiotherapy in advanced cervical carcinoa stage IIB and IVA. Cancer 1996;77:2371–2378.
35. Tattersall MHN, Ramirez C, Coppleson M. A randomized trial of adjuvant chemotherapy and radical hysterectomy in stage Ib-IIA cervical cancer patients with pelvic nodes metastases. Gynecol Oncol 1992;46:176–181.
36. Souhami L, Gil RA, Allan SE et al. Randomized trial of chemotherapy followed by pelvic radiation therapy in stage IIIB carcinoma of the cervix. J Clin Oncol 1991;9:970–977.
37. Kumar L, Kaushal R, Nandy M. Chemotherapy followed by radiotherapy vs radiotherapy in locally advanced cervical cancer: a randomized study. Gynecol Oncol 1994;54:307–315.
38. Tattersall MHN, Lorvidhaya S, Vootiprux V et al. Randomized trial of epirubicin and cisplatin chemotherapy followed by pelvic radiation in locally advanced cervical cancer. J Clin Oncol 1195;13:444–451.
39. Herod J, Burton A, Buxton J et al. A randomized, prospective, phase III clinical trial of primary bleomycin, ifosfamide and cisplatin (BIP) chemotherapy followed by radiotherapy versus radiotherapy alone in inoperable cancer of the cervix. Ann Oncol 2000;11:1175–1181.
40. Mancuso S, Smaniotto D, Benedetti Panici P et al. Phase I-II trial of preoperative chemoradiation in locally advanced cervical carcinoma. Gynecol Oncol 2000;78:324–328.
41. Sardi JE, Giaroli A, Sananes C et al. Long-term follow-up of the first randomized trial using neoadjuvant chemotherapy in stage Ib squamous carcinoma of the cervix. The final results. Gynaecol Oncol 1997;67:61–69.
42. Eddy GL, Manetta A, Alvarez RD et al. Neoadjuvant chemotherapy with vincristine and cisplatin followed by radical hysterectomy and pelvic lymphadenectomy for FIGO stage IB bulky cervical cancer: a Gynecologic Oncology Group pilot study. Gynecol Oncol 1995;57:412–416.
43. Sedlis A, Bundy BN, Rotman MZ et al. A randomized trial of pelvic radiation therapy versus no further therapy in selected patients with stage IB carcinoma of the cervix after radical hysterectomy and pelvic lymphadenectomy: a Gynecologic Oncology Group study. Gynecol Oncol 1999;73:177–183.
44. Iwasaka T, Kamura T, Yokoyama M et al. Adjuvant chemotherapy after radical hysterectomy for cervical carcinoma: a comparison with effects of adjuvant radiotherapy. Obstet Gynecol 1998;91:977–981.

45. Lahousen M, Haas J, Pickel H et al. Chemotherapy versus radiotherapy versus observation for high-risk cervical carcinoma after radical hysterectomy: a randomized, prospective, multicenter trial. Gynecol Oncol 1999;73:196–201.
46. Curtin JP, Hoskins WJ, Venkatraman ES et al. Adjuvant chemotherapy versus chemotherapy plus pelvic irradiation for high-risk cervical cancer patients after radical hysterectomy and pelvic lymphadenectomy (RH-PLND): a randomized phase III trial. Gynecol Oncol 1996;61:3–10.
47. Thigpen T. Cisplatin for the treatment of cervical and ovarian cancers: experience of the Gynecologic Oncology Group. Cancer Treat Rep 1979;63:1549–1555.
48. Thigpen T, Shingleton H, Homesley H et al. Cis-platinum in treatment of advanced or recurrent squamous cell carcinoma of the cervix: a phase II study of the Gynecologic Oncology Group. Cancer 1981;48:899–903.
49. Bonomi P, Blessing JA, Stehman FB et al. Randomized trial of three cisplatin dose schedules in squamous cell carcinoma of the cervix: a Gynecologic Oncology Group study. J Clin Oncol 1985; 3:1079–1085.
50. McGuire WP, Arseneau J, Blessing JA et al. A randomized comparative trial of carboplatin and iproplatin in squamous carcinoma of the uterine cervix: a Gynecologic Oncology Group study. J Clin Oncol 1989;7:1462–1468.
51. Lira-Puerto V, Silva A, Morris M et al. Phase II trial of carboplatin or iproplatin in cervical cancer. Cancer Chemother Pharmacol 1991;28:391–396.
52. Muggia FM and Glatstein E. Summary of investigations on platinum compounds and radiation interactions. Int J Rad Oncol Biol Phys 1979;5:1407–1409.
53. Schaake-Koning C, van den Bogaert W, Dalessio O et al. Effects of concomitant cisplatin and radiotherapy on inoperable non–small cell lung cancer. N Engl J Med 1992;326:524–530.
54. Knox RJ, Friedlos F, Lydall DA, Roberts JJ. Mechanism of cytotoxicity of anticancer platinum drugs: evidence that cisdiamminedichloroplatinum (II) and cis-diammine-(1,1-cyclobutane) dichloroplatinum(II) differ in the kinetics of their interactions with DNA. Cancer Res 1986;46: 1972–1979.
55. Muderspach LI, Curtin JP, Roman LD et al. Carboplatin as a radiation sensitizer in locally advanced cervical cancer: a pilot study. Gynecol Oncol 1997;65:336–342.
56. Yang LX, Douple EB, Wang HJ. Irradiation enhances cellular uptake of carboplatin. Int J Radiat Oncol Biol Phys 1995;33:641–646.
57. Wasserman T, Comis R, Goldsmith M et al. Tabular analysis of the clinical therapy of solid tumors. Cancer Treat Rep 1975;6:399–419.
58. Look KY, Muss HB. A phase II trial of 5-fluorouracil and high-dose leucovorin in advanced or recurrent cancer squamous cell carcinoma of the cervix. Am J Clin Oncol 1996;19:439–441.
59. Look KY, Muss HB. A phase II trial of 5-fluorouracil and high-dose leucovorin in advanced or recurrent nonsquamous cancer of the cervix. Gynecol Oncol 1997;67:255–258.
60. Bonomi P, Blessing J, Ball H et al. A phase II evaluation of cisplatin and 5-fluorouracil in patients with advanced squamous cell carcinoma of the cervix: a Gynecologic Oncology Group Study. Gynecol Oncol 1989;34:357–359.
61. Thomas G, Dembo A, Ackerman I et at. A randomized trial of standard vs partially hyperfractionated radiation with or without concurrent 5-fluorouracil in locally advanced cervical cancer. Gynecol Oncol 1998;69:52–58.
62. Schilder R, Blessing JA, Morgan M et al. Evaluation of gemcitabine in patients with squamous cell carcinoma of the cervix. A phase III study of the Gynecologic Oncology Group. Gynecol Oncol 2000;76:204–207.

63. Bouzid K, Mahlouf H. A study with gemcitabine (G) and cisplatin (C) in locally advanced, recurrent or metastatic squamous cell carcinoma of the cervix [abst 1549]. Proc Am Soc Clin Oncol 2000;19:391a.
64. Shewach DS, Lawrence TR. Radiosensitization of human solid tumor cell lines with gemcitabine. Semin Oncol 1996;23[suppl 10]:65–71.
65. Pattaranutaporn P, Thirapakawong C, Chansilpa Y et al. Study of concurrent gemcitabine and radiotherapy in locally advanced stage of cervical carcinoma [abst 1545]. Proc Am Soc Clin Oncol 2000;19:390a.
66. McGuire WP, Blessing JA, Moore D et al. Paclitaxel has moderate activity in squamous cervix cancer: a Gynecologic Oncology Group study. J Clin Oncol 1996;14:792–795.
67. Kudelka AP, Winn R, Edwards CL et al. An update of a phase II study of paclitaxel in advanced or recurrent squamous cell cancer of the cervix. Anti-Cancer Drugs 1997;8:657–661.
68. Curtin JP, Blessing JA, Webster KD et al. Paclitaxel in persistent or recurrent nonsquamous cancer of the cervix. J Clin Oncol 2001;19:1275–1278.
69. Rose PG, Blessing JA, Gershenson DM, McGehee R. Paclitaxel and cisplatin as first-line therapy in recurrent or advanced squamous cell carcinoma of the cervix: a Gynecologic Oncology Group study. J Clin Oncol 1999;73:196–201.
70. Tishler RB, Schiff PB, Geard CR, Hall EJ. Taxol: a novel radiation sensitizer. Int J Radiat Oncol Biol Phys 1992;22:613–617.
71. Britten RA, Perdue S, Opoku J, Craighead P. Paclitaxel is preferentially cytotoxic to human cervical tumor cells with low Raf-1 kinase activity: implications for paclitaxel-based chemoradiation regimens. Radiother Oncol 1998;43:329–334.
72. Chen MD, Paley PJ, Potish RA, Twiggs LB. Phase I trial of taxol as a radiation sensitizer with cisplatin in advanced cervical cancer. Gynecol Oncol 1997;67:131–136.
73. Meanwell C, Mould J, Blackledge G et al. Phase II study of ifosfamide in cervical cancer. Cancer Treat Rep 1986;70:727–730.
74. Sutton GP, Blessing JA, McGuire WP et al. Phase II trial of ifosfamide and Mesna in patients with advanced or recurrent squamous carcinoma of the cervix who had received chemotherapy: a Gynecologic Oncology Group study. Am J Obstet Gynecol 1993;168:805–807.
75. Buxton EJ, Meanwell CA, Hilton CA et al. Combination bleomycin, ifosfamide and cisplatin chemotherapy in cervical cancer. J Natl Cancer Inst 1989;81:359–361.
76. Omura GA, Blessing JA, Vaccarello L et al. Randomized trial of cisplatin versus cisplatin plus mitolactol versus cisplatin plus ifosfamide in advanced squamous carcinoma of the cervix: a Gynecologic Oncology Group study. J Clin Oncol 1997;15:165–171.
77. Chauvergne J, Robart J, Heron J et al. Randomized phase III trial of neoadjuvant chemotherapy (CT) + radiotherapy (RT) vs RT in stage IIB, III carcinoma of the cervix: a cooperative study of the French Oncology Centers. Proc Am Soc Clin Oncol 1988;7:136.
78. Muderspach L, Blessing JA, Levenbach C, Moore DL Jr. A phase II study of topotecan in patients with advanced squamous cell carcinoma of the cervix. Gynecol Oncol (in press).
79. Bookman MA, Blessing JA, Hanjani P et al. Topotecan in squamous cell carcinoma of the cervix. Gynecol Oncol 2000;77:446–449.
80. Lamond JP, Wang M, Kinsella TJ et al. Concentration and timing dependence of lethality enhancement between topotecan, a topoisomerase I inhibitor, and ionizing radiation. Int J Radiat Oncol Biol Phys 1996;36:361–368.
81. Rich TA, Kirichenko AV. Camptothecin radiation sensitization: mechanisms, schedules, and timing. Oncology 1998;12[suppl 6]:114–120.

82. Rowinsky EK, Kaufman SH, Baker SD et al. Sequences of topotecan and cisplatin: phase I, pharmacologic and in vitro studies to examine schedule dependence. J Clin Oncol 1996;14: 1074–1084.
83. Muggia FM, Dimery I, Arbuck S. The camptothecins: from discovery to the patient. NY Acad Sci 1997;803:213–223.
84. Jaxel C, Kohn KW, Wani MC et al. Structure activity study of the actions of camptothecin derivatives on mammalian topoisomerase I: evidence for a specific receptor site and a relation to antitumor activity. Cancer Res 1989;49:5077–5082.
85. Sutton GP, Blessing JA, Barrett RJ, Gallup DG. Phase II trial of menogaril in patients with squamous carcinoma of the cervix: a Gynecologic Oncology Group study. Gynecol Oncol 1994; 52:229–231.
86. Asbury RF, Blessing JA, Soper JT. A Gynecologic Oncology Group phase II study of amonafide (NSC 308847) in squamous cell carcinoma of the cervix. Am J Clin Oncol 1994;17:125–128.
87. Sutton GP, Blessing JA, Barnes W, Ball H. Phase II study of vinblastine in previously treated squamous carcinoma of the cervix. A Gynecologic Oncology Group study. Am J Clin Oncol 1990;13:470–471.
88. Lhomme C, Vermorken JB, Mickiewicz E et al. Phase II trial of vinorelbine in patients with advanced and/or recurrent cervical carcinoma: an EORTC Gynaecological Cancer Cooperative Group Study. Eur J Cancer 2000;36:194–199.
89. Pignata S, Silvestro G, Ferrari E et al. Phase II study of cisplatin and vinorelbine as first-line chemotherapy in patients with carcinoma of the uterine cervix. J Clin Oncol 1999;17:756–760.
90. Miller VA, Krug LM, Ng KK et al. Phase II trial of docetaxel and vinorelbine in patients with advanced non-small-cell lung cancer. J Clin Oncol 2000;18:1346–1350.
91. Thigpen T, Blessing JA, Gallup DG et al. Phase II trial of mitomycin-C in squamous cell carcinoma of the uterine cervix: a Gynecologic Oncology Group study. Gynecol Oncol 1995;57:376–379.
92. Sartorelli AC. Role of hypoxic cells in the therapeutic response of solid tumors [presidential address]. Proc Am Assoc Cancer Res 1987;28:461.
93. Long HJ 3rd, Cross WG, Wieand HS et al. Phase II trial of methotrexate, vinblastine, doxorubicin, and cisplatin in advanced/recurrent carcinoma of the uterine cervix and vagina. Gynecol Oncol 1995;57:235–239.
94. Rose PG, Blessing JA, Van Le L, Waggoner S. Prolonged oral etoposide in recurrent or advanced squamous cell carcinoma of the cervix: a Gynecologic Oncology Group study. Gynecol Oncol 1998;70:263–266.
95. Rose PG, Blessing JA, Arseneau J. Phase II evaluation of altretamine for advanced or recurrent squamous cell carcinoma of the cervix: a Gynecologic Oncology Group Study. Gynecol Oncol 1996;62:100–102.
96. Alberts DS, Masson-Liddil N. The role of cisplatin in the management of advanced squamous cell cancer of the cervix. Semin Oncol 1989;16[suppl 6]:66–78.
97. Dorie MJ, Brown JM. Modification of the antitumor activity of chemotherapeutic drugs by the hypoxic cytotoxic agent tirapazamine. Cancer Chemother Pharmacol 1997;39:361–366.
98. Benbrook DM, Shen-Gunther J, Nunez ER, Dynlacht JR. Differential retinoic acid radiosensitization of cervical carcinoma cell lines. Clin Cancer Res 1997;3:939–945.
99. Oridate N, Lotan D, Mitchell MF et al. Inhibition of proliferation and induction of apoptosis in cervical carcinoma cells by retinoids. Implications for chemoprevention. J Cell Biochem 1995; 23S:80–86.
100. Look KY, Blessing JA, Nelson BE et al. A Phase II trial of isotretinoin and alpha interferon in patients with recurrent squamous cell carcinoma of the cervix: a Gynecologic Oncology Group study. Am J Clin Oncol 1998;21:591–594.

101. Donato DJ, Perez M, Kang H et al. EGF receptor and p21WAF1 expression are reciprocally altered as ME-180 cervical carcinoma cells progress from high to low cisplatin sensitivity. Clin Cancer Res 2000;6:193–202.
102. Morrow CP, Curtin JP. Surgery for cervical neoplasia. In Morrow CP, Curtin JP, eds. Gynecologic Cancer Surgery. New York: Churchill Livingstone, 1996:381–392.
103. Fuller AF, Elliot N, Kosloff C et al. Determinants of increased risk for recurrence in patients undergoing radical hysterectomy for stage IB and IIA carcinoma of the cervix. Gynecol Oncol 1989;33:34–39.
104. Delgado G, Bundy B, Zaino R et al. Prospective surgical-pathological study of disease-free interval in patients with stage IB squamous cell carcinoma of the cervix: a Gynecologic Oncology Group study. Gynecol Oncol 1990;38:352–357.
105. Keys H, Gibbons SK. Optimal management of locally advanced cervical carcinoma. J Natl Cancer Inst Monogr 1996;21:89–92.
106. Goff BA, Muntz HG, Paley PJ et al. Impact of surgical staging in women with locally advanced cervical cancer. Gynecol Oncol 1999;74:436–442.
107. Potish RA, Downey GO, Adcock LL et al. The role of surgical debulking in cancer of the uterine cervix. Int J Radiat Oncol Biol Phys 1989;17:979–984.
108. Jurado M, Martinez-Monge R, Garcia-Foncillas J et al. Pilot study of concurrent cisplatin, 5-fluorouracil, and external beam radiotherapy prior to radical surgery ± intraoperative electron beam radiotherapy in locally advanced cervical cancer. Gynecol Oncol 1999;74:30–37.
109. Demaria S, Volm MD, Shapiro RL et al. Development of tumor infiltrating lymphocytes in breast cancer after neoadjuvant paclitaxel chemotherapy. Cancer (submitted).

Tyrosine Kinase Inhibitors in the Treatment of Chronic Myelogenous Leukemia

Brian J. Druker

Chronic myelogenous leukemia (CML) is a clonal hematopoietic stem cell disorder with an annual incidence of one to two cases per 100,000 population per year. The chronic or stable phase of the disease is characterized by excess numbers of myeloid cells that differentiate normally. Within an average of 4–6 years, the disease transforms through an "accelerated phase" to an invariably fatal acute leukemia, also known as *blast crisis*, as the leukemic clone progressively loses the capacity for terminal differentiation.[1,2]

Current treatment choices for CML include stem cell transplantation, hydroxyurea, or interferon-α-based regimens, with allogeneic stem cell transplantation being the only proven curative therapy for CML.[3] As the average age of onset of CML is greater than 50 years of age, this factor, plus the inability to identify a suitably matched donor, limits this option to a minority of patients. Thus, fewer than 20% of CML patients are cured with current treatment options.[1,2]

CHRONIC MYELOGENOUS LEUKEMIA

Molecular Pathogenesis

Four decades of scientific discovery have contributed to our knowledge of the molecular etiology of CML, beginning with the identification of the Philadelphia chromosome.[4] This subsequently was shown to result from a reciprocal translocation between the long arms of chromosomes 9 and 22.[5] The molecular consequence of this translocation is the juxtaposition of Bcr-encoded sequences on chromosome 22 with c-Abl sequences translocated from chromosome 9.[6,7] The *Bcr-Abl* fusion gene is transcribed and translated into a 210-kd chimeric protein in which the first exon of c-Abl is replaced by Bcr sequences.[8,9] The fusion protein p210Bcr-Abl, which is present in virtually all patients with CML, has increased protein tyrosine kinase activity as compared to c-Abl.[10] This same 210-kd fusion protein is present in approximately one-half of adult acute lymphoblastic leukemia (ALL) patients whose disease is positive for the Philadelphia chromosome (Ph). The remainder of the Ph-positive adult ALL patients and the majority of pediatric Ph-positive ALL patients express a 185-kd Bcr-Abl fusion protein (Fig. 10.1).[11,12]

Bcr-Abl Kinase Activity as a Molecular Target for CML Therapy

As noted, the Bcr-Abl tyrosine kinase is present in virtually all patients with CML. In a variety of animal models, Bcr-Abl, as the sole oncogenic event, has been conclusively established as a leukemic oncogene.[13–16] Although numerous signaling pathways have been demonstrated to be activated by the expression of Bcr-Abl, all transforming functions of the Bcr-Abl protein are dependent on the tyrosine kinase activity of the Abl portion of this protein.[11,17] Thus, an inhibitor of the Abl protein tyrosine kinase would be predicted to be an effective and

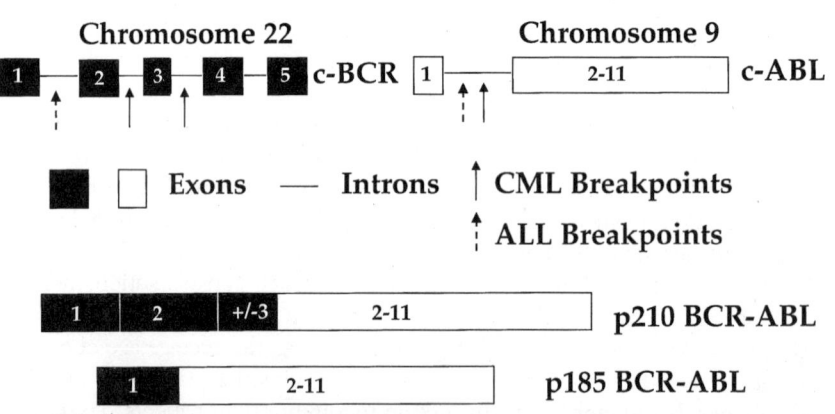

FIGURE 10.1 Common breakpoints in chronic myelogenous leukemia (CML) and Philadelphia chromosome–positive (Ph+) acute lymphoblastic leukemia (ALL) and the molecular consequences of these rearrangements. In CML and Ph+ ALL, a break occurs between the first and second exon of c-abl. Thus, virtually all the c-abl locus is translocated to chromosome 22, into the *bcr* gene. In CML, the breakpoints in *Bcr* occur after what was historically called the second or third exon, resulting in a chimeric mRNA and protein of 210 kd. In some cases of Ph+ ALL, the breakpoints in the *Bcr* gene occur after the first exon, creating a smaller fusion mRNA and protein, termed *p185Bcr-Abl*.

selective therapeutic agent for CML and other Bcr-Abl–positive leukemias. (Fig. 10.2)

DESIGNING A TYROSINE KINASE INHIBITOR

Given the prominent role of tyrosine kinases in regulating cellular proliferation, considerable effort has been directed toward the development of inhibitors of this enzyme activity as potential antineoplastic agents.[18,19] Compounds that possess inhibitory activity for protein tyrosine kinases were initially isolated from natural sources in the early to mid-1980s and include the flavinoid quercetin, the isoflavinoid genistein, the antibiotic herbimycin A, and erbstatin.[20–22] These compounds are relatively nonspecific tyrosine kinase inhibitors and may have activities independent of their tyrosine kinase inhibitory activity that contribute to cellular cytotoxicity.[21]

In 1988, Yaish et al[23] reported a series of synthetic compounds, called *tyrphostins*, that displayed specificity for individual tyrosine kinases. Working independently, scientists at Novartis identified a lead kinase inhibitor by the time-consuming process of random screening (i.e., testing large compound libraries for inhibition of protein kinases in vitro). In this case, the initial lead compound was a relatively weak inhibitor of protein kinase Cα and the platelet-derived

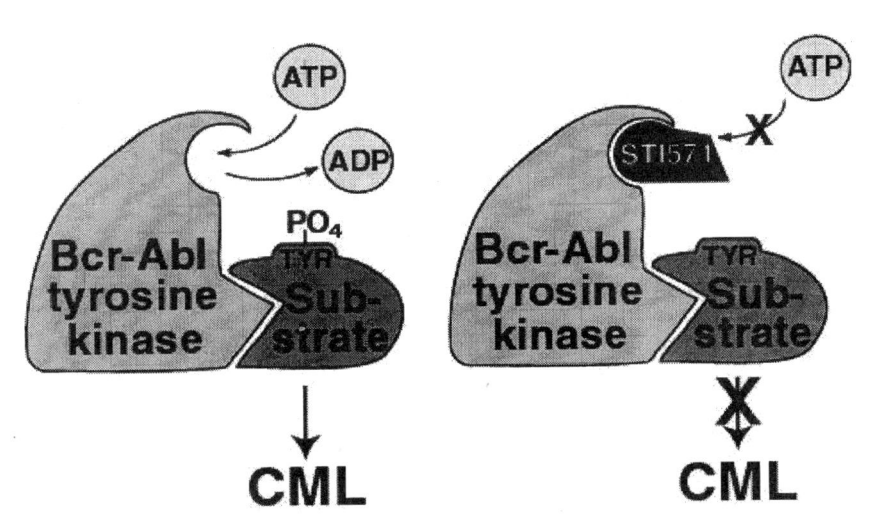

FIGURE 10.2 The Bcr-Abl tyrosine kinase is a constitutively active kinase that functions by binding adenosine triphosphate (ATP) and transferring phosphate from ATP to tyrosine residues on various substrates. This activity causes the excess proliferation of myeloid cells characteristic of chronic myelogenous leukemia (CML). STI571 functions by blocking the binding of ATP to the Bcr-Abl tyrosine kinase, thus inhibiting the activity of the kinase. In the absence of tyrosine kinase activity, substrates required for Bcr-Abl function cannot be phosphorylated. ADP, adenosine diphosphate.

growth factor receptor.[24] The specificity and potency for target kinase was improved by synthesizing a series of chemically related compounds and analyzing the relationship between structure and activity for each compound. From this program, dual inhibitors of the v-Abl and the platelet-derived growth factor receptor kinases were generated.[25,26] STI571 (formerly CGP 57148B) emerged from these efforts as the lead compound for preclinical development (Fig. 10.3).

STI571

Preclinical Testing

STI571 has been tested in a number of preclinical models, including in vitro assays of enzyme inhibition, cellular assays of proliferation, and in vivo assays of tumor formation. These studies demonstrate that STI571 inhibits all Abl kinases at submicromolar concentrations, including p210Bcr-Abl, p185Bcr-Abl, v-Abl, and the c-Abl tyrosine kinase.[27] Numerous tyrosine and serine–threonine protein kinases have been tested for inhibition by STI571 and, except for the platelet-derived growth factor receptor and the c-Kit tyrosine kinases, no others are inhibited.[27]

In a pivotal set of preclinical experiments, STI571 was shown to suppress the proliferation of Bcr-Abl-expressing cells in vitro and in vivo.[28] In this and subsequent studies, STI571, at concentrations of 1 and 10 μM, has been shown to kill or inhibit the proliferation of all Bcr-Abl-expressing cell lines tested.[27,29–32] In contrast, a variety of immortalized or transformed cell lines that do not express Bcr-Abl are not sensitive to STI571. In colony-forming assays using CML bone marrow or peripheral blood samples, treatment with STI571 decreases the number

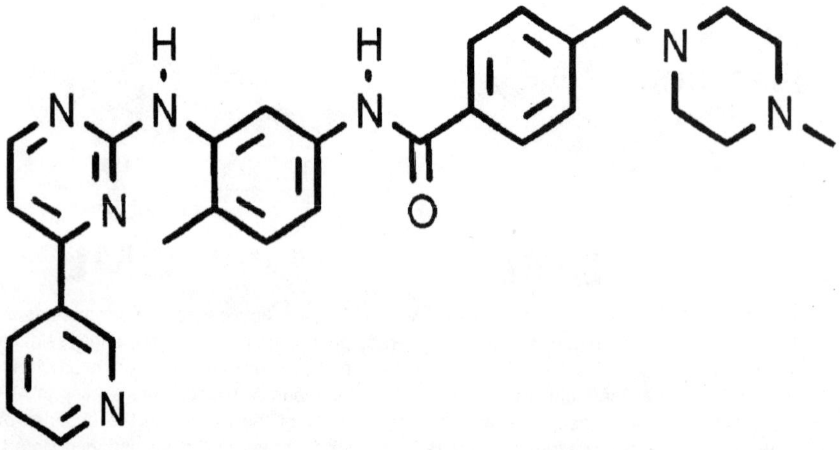

FIGURE 10.3 Structure of STI571.

of colonies formed and may select for the growth of Bcr-Abl-negative progenitor cells.[28,30,33] Minimal inhibition of the colony-forming potential of normal bone marrow has been observed. Similar results, showing selective depletion of Bcr-Abl-positive cells, have been observed in long-term marrow cultures.[34] Thus, STI571 appears to be selectively toxic to cells expressing the constitutively active Bcr-Abl protein tyrosine kinase (Fig. 10.3).

Early pharmacokinetic studies in rats and dogs demonstrated that bioactive concentrations are readily achieved in the circulation with an oral formulation of STI571 with a half-life of 4–6 hours. Studies in mice showed that STI571 had in vivo activity against Bcr-Abl-expressing tumor cells. Initial experiments, using a once-daily injection schedule of STI571, showed inhibition of tumor proliferation but failed to eradicate Bcr-Abl-expressing tumors.[28] However, administration of STI571 thrice daily over an 11-day period cured 87%–100% of treated mice, whereas once- or twice-daily administration did not.[35] This data suggested that continuous exposure to STI571 would be important for optimal antileukemic effects.

Toxicity testing by daily oral administration to rats for 13 weeks showed occasional renal calcifications and mild bladder mucosal hyperplasia at the lowest dose of 6 mg/kg. In dogs, a no-effect level was seen at 3 mg/kg, but progressive liver toxicity was seen at the highest dose of 100 mg/kg. At the highest dose levels, some vomiting, diarrhea, mild anemia, and neutropenia were observed.

Phase I Trials of STI571 in Chronic-Phase CML Patients

On the basis of the efficacy of STI571 in a variety of preclinical models and an acceptable animal toxicology profile, phase I clinical trials with STI571 were begun in June 1998. The initial study was a dose escalation study designed to establish the maximum tolerated dose with a secondary endpoint of clinical efficacy. Patients were eligible if they were in the chronic phase of CML and had failed therapy with interferon-α. STI571 was administered as once-daily oral therapy, and no other cytoreductive agents were allowed. Eighty-three patients have been enrolled in 14 dose levels, ranging from 25 to 1000 mg. The median duration of disease at study entry was 3.8 years, and one-third of patients had signs of disease acceleration with increased blasts or basophils in peripheral blood or marrow.

Once doses of 300 mg or greater were reached, 53 of 54 patients (98%) achieved a complete hematologic response.[36] Responses were typically seen within the first 3 weeks of therapy and have been maintained in 51 of 53 patients, with a median follow-up duration of 310 days. At STI571 doses of 300 mg or greater, cytogenetic responses were seen within 5 months in 17 of 31 patients (53%), with 10% achieving a complete cytogenetic response. Although the follow-up on this group of patients is relatively short, these data indicate that an Abl-specific, tyrosine kinase inhibitor has significant activity in CML, even in interferon-refractory patients.

Side effects of STI571 have been minimal, with no dose-limiting toxicities encountered. The most common side effects have been nausea, muscle cramps, periorbital edema, peripheral edema, and diarrhea, with most of these being grade 1 toxicities. Grade 2–4 myelosuppression was observed at a dose of at least 300 mg in up to 26% of patients.[36] The myelosuppression might be consistent with a therapeutic effect, as the Ph-positive clone contributes the majority of hematopoiesis in these patients. Although hepatotoxicity was a concern from preclinical toxicology studies, elevations in transaminases have been uncommon.

Pharmacokinetics of STI571

Pharmacokinetic studies showed that the half-life of STI571 is 13–16 hours, which is sufficiently long to permit once-daily dosing.[37] At doses of 300 mg or greater, at which significant clinical responses were observed, plasma levels equivalent to the predicted, effective, in vitro level of 1 μM were achieved. STI571 is metabolized primarily by the CYP3A4 P450 enzyme system. This suggests that STI571 levels would be lower in patients being treated with such medications as phenytoin, which are known inducers of this enzyme system. This also suggests that increased STI571 levels might be observed if STI571 were given concomitantly with drugs known to interfere with the activity of the CYP3A4 enzyme, potentially resulting in toxicity.

Phase I Trials in CML Blast Crisis and Other Bcr-Abl-Positive Acute Leukemias

Given the effectiveness of STI571 in chronic-phase patients in whom interferon therapy had failed, the phase I studies were expanded to include CML patients in myeloid and lymphoid blast crisis and patients with relapsed or refractory Ph chromosome–positive ALL. Patients have been treated with daily doses of 300–1000 mg of STI571; 21 of 38 patients (55%) with myeloid blast crisis responded to therapy, defined by a decrease in percentage of marrow blasts to less than 15%; and 17 of 38 (45%) cleared their marrow of blasts (< 5%), with four of these patients (11%) meeting criteria for a complete remission with full recovery of peripheral blood counts. Seven myeloid blast crisis patients remain on therapy, with fewer than 5% marrow blasts, with or without recovery of peripheral blood counts and with follow-up of between 101 and 349 days.[38]

Among patients with lymphoid phenotype, Ph-positive ALL, and lymphoid blast crisis of CML, 14 of 20 (70%) responded, 11 of 20 (55%) completely clearing their marrow of blasts and 4 patients (20%) meeting criteria for a complete hematologic response. However, all but one of the lymphoid phenotype patients have relapsed between days 45 and 117.[38] Thus, STI571 has significant single-agent activity in Bcr-Abl-positive acute leukemias, but resistance to STI571 can occur, at least in more advanced stages. However, these studies demonstrate that in the majority of cases, the leukemic clone in Bcr-Abl-positive acute leukemias, including CML blast crisis, remains at least partially dependent on Bcr-Abl kinase activity for survival.

As the outcome of stem cell transplantation is improved for patients who are returned to a second chronic phase as compared to transplantation while in blast crisis,[39] the clearance of blasts from the marrow of the majority of blast crisis patients could render STI571 useful as a bridge to transplantation. Similarly, improved therapeutic outcomes might be possible by combining STI571 with standard antileukemic agents.

Phase II Trials

The phase I data have been confirmed in rapidly accruing, multiinstitutional, international phase II studies. These studies have included 532 CML patients in whom interferon therapy has failed, 233 accelerated-phase patients, and 260 myeloid blast crisis patients. Remarkably, in the 532 chronic-phase patients in whom interferon therapy has failed, the complete cytogenetic response rate was 28% within 3–9 months of beginning therapy. Only 3% of patients have been resistant to therapy or relapsed in the first year of treatment, and 2% of patients discontinued therapy owing to side effects, with skin rashes being the most frequent severe side effect causing discontinuation.[40]

In the phase II studies, accelerated phase was defined as blasts of greater than or equal to 15% but less than 30%; blasts plus promyelocytes equal to or greater than 30% in peripheral blood or marrow; more than 20% basophils in peripheral blood; or platelets less than 100×10^9 per liter unrelated to therapy. In this strictly defined population, 44% achieved a complete hematologic response, and 21% of patients had major cytogenetic responses, with a complete cytogenetic response rate of 14%. The median survival has not been reached with 73% of patients alive at 1 year.[41] In myeloid blast crisis patients, an overall response rate of 62% was achieved, and the median survival of this patient population was between 6 and 9 months.[42]

Dose

Unlike most anticancer therapies, a maximum tolerated dose for STI571 was not identified. However, there are several endpoints that could be used in place of the maximum tolerated dose to choose a biologically relevant dose for future trials. The first is an analysis of the pharmacokinetic profile. Preclinical studies suggested that maintenance of STI571 levels exceeding 1 μM would be necessary for optimal therapeutic benefits, and this correlated well with serum drug levels in patients treated with a dose of 300 mg or greater. In the dose escalation studies of chronic and blast crisis patients, there was little evidence for improved responses at doses in excess of 300 mg. However, at doses of 800 and 1000 mg, there was a greater incidence of grade 1 and 2 toxicities, particularly nausea, fluid retention, and diarrhea. Further, there was a greater incidence of serious adverse events in patients treated with 800 and 1000 mg. Thus, for phase II studies, doses of 400 and 600 mg have been chosen, as these appear to be safe doses and are at or above the plateau in the dose-response curve. The dose-response curve represents a second parameter that could be used for dose selection. In the phase II study of 233 accelerated-phase patients, approximately equal numbers of patients were treated with 400 mg and 600 mg. Analysis of this data is ongoing and could be fairly useful in determining whether a dose-response relationship exists. At present, patients in chronic phase are being treated with 400 mg, and those in accelerated and blast phases are started at 600 mg/day.

For a Bcr-Abl tyrosine kinase inhibitor, it would seem that the optimal dose would be one that resulted in maximal inhibition of the kinase. Thus far, we have been able to demonstrate that phosphorylation of Crkl, a substrate of Bcr-Abl, is decreased in patients undergoing treatment with STI571. Additional reagents to analyze the endpoint of kinase inhibition are currently being developed.[43]

WHY DO CYTOGENETIC RESPONSES OCCUR?

The success of STI571 as a therapeutic agent for CML answers several questions about CML biology but leaves many more to be addressed. The most important issue that this clinical trial has demonstrated is that the Bcr-Abl tyrosine kinase, as predicted from animal models, is critical to the development of CML. However, it has not yet been possible to determine the primary mechanism of action of Bcr-Abl or the kinase inhibitor (i.e., whether Bcr-Abl induces proliferation or protects cells from apoptotic cell death). In the former case, it is possible that STI571 would simply prevent proliferation of the leukemic clone without eliminating it. Even in this scenario, it is possible that cytogenetic responses would be observed. Presumably, with the inhibition of Bcr-Abl kinase activity, the leukemic clone would be subjected to normal marrow regulatory influences and would be eliminated at the end of the progenitor cell's natural life span. It is also likely that normal hematopoietic progenitors might regain a proliferative advantage or that progression to blast crisis could be delayed or avoided. If Bcr-Abl protects from apoptotic cell death, it is possible that treatment with a kinase inhibitor could eliminate the leukemic clone.

MECHANISMS OF RESISTANCE

The activity in blast crisis patients demonstrates that the leukemic clone remains at least partially dependent on Bcr-Abl kinase activity for survival. However, these trials also point out that resistance to STI571 as a single agent is a reality. Several publications examining cells lines that express Bcr-Abl have shown that the most common mechanism of STI571 resistance was *Bcr-Abl* gene amplification.[44-46] However, other resistant cell lines did not have detectable *Bcr-Abl* gene amplification, and at least one resistant cell line showed overexpression of the multidrug resistant P-glycoprotein.[45] Interestingly, an examination of samples from patients resistant to STI571 shows that in the majority, the Bcr-Abl kinase remains active.[47] This suggests that such mechanisms as *Bcr-Abl* amplification or reduction in uptake of STI571 may be operative in vivo. Another possibility consistent with these data would be mutations in the kinase domain of Abl that render the kinase insensitive to STI571. Last, there has been a suggestion from animal studies that protein binding of STI571 could be responsible for relapse.[48] However, samples from relapsed patients have decreased cellular sensitivity to STI571, suggesting that resistance is a cell-intrinsic phenotype and not due to protein binding.

COMBINATIONS OF STI571 WITH OTHER ANTILEUKEMIC AGENTS

Bcr-Abl is known to render cells resistant to chemotherapeutic agents, although the mechanism of resistance remains unclear.[49,50] In vitro evidence demonstrates that treatment of cells expressing Bcr-Abl with STI571 reverses this chemotherapy resistance.[51] Further, additive or even synergistic antiproliferative effects between STI571 and other antileukemic agents, including interferon-α, daunorubicin, and cytarabine, were observed.[51] Similar results were seen with etoposide plus cytarabine.[52] Such studies provide a strong rationale for combining STI571 with other active agents, both in advanced disease patients and in chronic-phase patients.

ONGOING AND ANTICIPATED USES OF STI571

The optimal use of STI571 has yet to be defined. The phase II studies using STI571 as a single agent in CML patients refractory to, or intolerant of, interferon-α and in patients in the accelerated phase or blast crisis are ongoing. These studies will provide valuable information regarding the effectiveness and safety profile of STI571 in a larger cohort of patients. Most critical will be a determination of the durability of responses. A phase III randomized study, comparing STI571 to interferon plus Ara-C, in patients with newly diagnosed disease is currently in progress. Whether even better and more durable responses will be observed in patients in early chronic phase remains to be determined. As Bcr-Abl may be the sole molecular abnormality in the early chronic phase, it is conceivable that STI571 alone could eradicate the malignant clone in this subgroup of patients. Future studies will be designed to determine whether the addition of interferon or cytarabine to STI571 will improve the outcome for chronic-phase patients. As more patients are obtaining complete cytogenetic remissions, it will become increasing important to analyze these patients for molecular responses as the level of Bcr-Abl transcripts may be useful in predicting relapses.[53]

In accelerated and blast crisis patients, STI571 will be tried in combination with a variety of antileukemic agents. For blast crisis or Ph-positive ALL, using STI571 similarly to all-*trans*-retinoic acid in acute promyelocytic leukemia would seem a reasonable paradigm. Other uses for STI571 might include treatment of patients relapsing after stem cell transplantation as an alternative to donor lymphocyte infusions, as an adjunct to autologous stem cell transplantation, and possibly as an in vitro purging agent for autologous stem cell transplantation. Additional tasks for the future will be studies aimed at predicting response to this molecularly targeted agent and ultimately combining STI571 with agents directed against pathways mediating resistance to STI571.

INTEGRATION OF STI571 INTO CML TREATMENT ALGORITHMS

The rapid success of STI571 has already rendered many CML treatment algorithms obsolete. As the duration of follow-up is relatively short, predictions regarding the potential use of STI571 range widely. However, at present, allogeneic stem cell transplant remains the only treatment known to cure CML. As is it unknown whether initial treatment with STI571 will compromise the outcome of transplant, it is difficult to know whether delaying transplant for a trial of STI571 in a younger patient is advisable. In the absence of firm data, individual decisions regarding the choice and timing of transplantation will continue to depend on such factors as patient age, availability of a well-matched donor, individual prognostic factors and, of course, patient preference. For patients who are not candidates for transplantation, STI571—at least from results of the early studies—is an attractive alternative.

CONCLUSION

The clinical trials with STI571 are a dramatic demonstration of the potential of targeting molecular pathogenetic events in a malignancy. As this paradigm is applied to other malignancies, it is worth remembering that Bcr-Abl and CML have several features that were critical to the success of this agent. One of these is that Bcr-Abl tyrosine kinase activity has clearly been demonstrated to be critical to the pathogenesis of CML. Thus, not only was the target of STI571 known, but it was directed against a critical event in the development of CML. Another important feature is that the results demonstrate, as with most malignancies, that treatment earlier in the course of the disease yields better results. Thus, identification of the crucial, early events in malignant progression is the first step in reproducing the success with STI571 in other malignancies.

ACKNOWLEDGMENT

This study was funded by grants from the National Cancer Institute, by a Translational Research Award from the Leukemia and Lymphoma Society, and by a Clinical Scientist Award from the Burroughs Wellcome Fund.

REFERENCES

1. Faderl S, Talpaz M, Estrov Z, Kantarjian HM. Chronic myelogenous leukemia: biology and therapy. Ann Intern Med 1999;131:207–219.
2. Sawyers CL. Chronic myeloid leukemia. N Engl J Med 1999;340:1330–1340.
3. Kolibaba KS, Druker BJ. Current status of treatment for chronic myelogenous leukemia. Medscape Oncol 2000;3(2). http://oncology.medscape.com/medscape/oncology/journal/public/onc.journal.html
4. Nowell PC, Hungerford DA. A minute chromosome in human chronic granulocytic leukemia. Science 1960;132:1497–1501.
5. Rowley JD. A new consistent abnormality in chronic myelogenous leukaemia identified by quinacrine fluorescence and giemsa staining. Nature 1973;243:290–293.
6. Heisterkamp N, Stephenson JR, Groffen J et al. Localization of the c-abl oncogene adjacent to a translocation break point in chronic myelocytic leukemia. Nature 1983;306:239–242.
7. Bartram CR, de Klein A, Hagemeijer A et al. Translocation of c-abl correlates with the presence of a Philadelphia chromosome in chronic myelocytic leukemia. Nature 1983;306:277–280.
8. Ben-Neriah Y, Daley GQ, Mes-Masson A-M et al. The chronic myelogenous leukemia-specific P210 protein is the product of the bcr/abl hybrid gene. Science 1986;233:212–214.
9. Shtivelman E, Lifshitz B, Gale RP, Canaani E. Fused transcript of abl and bcr genes in chronic myelogenous leukaemia. Nature 1985;315:550–554.
10. Davis RL, Konopka JB, Witte ON. Activation of the c-abl oncogene by viral transduction or chromosomal translocation generates altered c-abl proteins with similar in vitro kinase properties. Mol Cell Biol 1985;5:204–213.
11. Deininger MW, Goldman JM, Melo JV. The molecular biology of chronic myeloid leukemia. Blood 2000;96:3343–3356.
12. Clark SS, McLaughlin J, Timmons M et al. Expression of a distinctive BCR-ABL oncogene in Ph1-positive acute lymphocytic leukemia (ALL). Science 1988;239:775–777.
13. Daley GQ, Van Etten RA, Baltimore D. Induction of chronic myelogenous leukemia in mice by the P210bcr/abl gene of the Philadelphia chromosome. Science 1990;247:824–830.
14. Heisterkamp N, Jenster G, ten Hoeve J et al. Acute leukaemia in bcr/abl transgenic mice. Nature 1990;344:251–253.
15. Kelliher MA, McLaughlin J, Witte ON, Rosenberg N. Induction of a chronic myelogenous leukemia-like syndrome in mice with v-abl and BCR/ABL. Proc Natl Acad Sci USA 1990;87:6649–6653.
16. Huettner CS, Zhang P, Van Etten RA, Tenen DG. Reversibility of acute B-cell leukaemia induced by BCR-ABL1. Nat Genet 2000;24:57–60.
17. Lugo TG, Pendergast AM, Muller AJ, Witte ON. Tyrosine kinase activity and transformation potency of bcr-abl oncogene products. Science 1990;247:1079–1082.
18. Levitzki A, Gazit A. Tyrosine kinase inhibition: an approach to drug development. Science 1995;267:1782–1788.
19. Kolibaba KS, Druker BJ. Protein tyrosine kinases and cancer. Biochim Biophys Acta 1997;1333:F217–248.
20. Chang C-J, Geahlen RL. Protein-tyrosine kinase inhibition: mechanism-based discovery of antitumor agents. J Nat Prod 1992;55:1529–1560.
21. Casnellie JE. Protein kinase inhibitors: probes for the functions of protein phosphorylation. Adv Pharmacol 1991;22:167–205.

22. Boutin JA. Tyrosine protein kinase inhibition and cancer. Int J Biochem 1994;26:1203–1226.
23. Yaish P, Gazit A, Gilon C, Levitzki A. Blocking of EGF-dependent cell proliferation by EGF receptor kinase inhibitors. Science 1988;242:933–935.
24. Zimmermann J, Caravatti G, Mett H et al. Phenylamino-pyrimidine (PAP) derivatives: a new class of potent and selective inhibitors of protein kinase C (PKC). Arch Pharm (Weinheim) 1996;329: 371–376.
25. Buchdunger E, Zimmermann J, Mett H et al. Selective inhibition of the platelet-derived growth factor signal transduction pathway by a protein-tyrosine kinase inhibitor of the 2-phenylaminopyrimidine class. Proc Natl Acad Sci USA 1995;92:2558–2562.
26. Buchdunger E, Zimmermann J, Mett H et al. Inhibition of the Abl protein-tyrosine kinase in vitro and in vivo by a 2-phenylaminopyrimidine derivative. Cancer Res 1996;56:100–104.
27. Druker BJ, Lydon NB. Lessons learned from the development of an abl tyrosine kinase inhibitor for chronic myelogenous leukemia. J Clin Invest 2000;105:3–7.
28. Druker BJ, Tamura S, Buchdunger E et al. Effects of a selective inhibitor of the ABL tyrosine kinase on the growth of BCR-ABL positive cells. Nat Med 1996;2:561–566.
29. Carroll M, Ohno-Jones S, Tamura S et al. CGP 57148, a tyrosine kinase inhibitor, inhibits the growth of cells expressing BCR-ABL, TEL-ABL and TEL-PDGFR fusion proteins. Blood 1997;90: 4947–4952.
30. Deininger MW, Goldman JM, Lydon N, Melo JV. The tyrosine kinase inhibitor CGP57148B selectively inhibits the growth of BCR-ABL-positive cells. Blood 1997;90:3691–3698.
31. Beran M, Cao X, Estrov Z et al. Selective inhibition of cell proliferation and BCR-ABL phosphorylation in acute lymphoblastic leukemia cells expressing Mr 190,000 BCR-ABL protein by a tyrosine kinase inhibitor (CGP-57148). Clin Cancer Res 1998;4:1661–1672.
32. Gambacorti-Passerini C, le Coutre P, Mologni L et al. Inhibition of the ABL kinase activity blocks the proliferation of BCR/ABL+ leukemic cells and induces apoptosis. Blood Cells Mol Dis 1997; 23:380–394.
33. Marley SB, Deininger MW, Davidson RJ et al. The tyrosine kinase inhibitor STI571, like interferon-alpha, preferentially reduces the capacity for amplification of granulocyte-macrophage progenitors from patients with chronic myeloid leukemia. Exp Hematol 2000;28:551–557.
34. Kasper B, Fruehauf S, Schiedlmeier B et al. Favorable therapeutic index of a p210(BCR-ABL)-specific tyrosine kinase inhibitor; activity on lineage-committed and primitive chronic myelogenous leukemia progenitors. Cancer Chemother Pharmacol 1999;44:433–438.
35. le Coutre P, Mologni L, Cleris L et al. In vivo eradication of human BCR/ABL-positive leukemia cells with an ABL kinase inhibitor. J Natl Cancer Inst 1999;91:163–168.
36. Druker BJ, Talpaz M, Resta D et al. Efficacy and safety of a specific inhibitor of the Bcr-Abl tyrosine kinase in chronic myeloid leukemia. N Engl J Med (in press).
37. Peng B, Hayes M, Druker B et al. Clinical pharmacokinetics and pharmacodynamics of STI571 in a phase 1 trial in chronic myelogenous leukemia (CML) patients. Proc Am Assoc Cancer Res 2000;41:256a.
38. Druker BJ, Sawyers CL, Kantarjian H et al. Activity of a specific inhibitor of the Bcr-Abl tyrosine kinase in the blast crisis of chronic myeloid leukemia and acute lymphoblastic leukemia with the Philadelphia chromosome. N Engl J Med (in press).
39. Spencer A, O'Brien SG, Goldman JM. Options for therapy in chronic myeloid leukaemia. Br J Haematol 1995;91:2–7.
40. Kantarjian H, Sawyers C, Hochhaus A et al. Phase II study of STI571, a tyrosine kinase inhibitor, in patients with resistant or refractory Philadelphia chromosome positive chronic myeloid leukemia. Blood 2000;96:470a.

41. Talpaz M, Silver RT, Druker BJ et al. A Phase II study of STI571 in adult patients with Philadelphia chromosome positive chronic myeloid leukemia in accelerated phase. Blood 2000;96:469a.
42. Sawyers CL, Hochhaus A, Feldman E et al. A Phase II study to determine the safety and anti-leukemic effects of STI571 in patients with Philadelphia chromosome positive chronic myeloid leukemia in myeloid blast crisis. Blood 2000;96:503a.
43. Karamlou K, Lucas L, Druker B. Identification of molecular endpoints as a guide for clinical decision making in STI571-treated chronic myelogenous leukemia patients. Blood 2000;96:98a.
44. Weisberg E, Griffin JD. Mechanism of resistance to the ABL tyrosine kinase inhibitor STI571 in BCR/ABL-transformed hematopoietic cell lines. Blood 2000;95:3498–3505.
45. Mahon FX, Deininger MW, Schultheis B et al. Selection and characterization of BCR-ABL positive cell lines with differential sensitivity to the tyrosine kinase inhibitor STI571: diverse mechanisms of resistance. Blood 2000;96:1070–1079.
46. le Coutre P, Tassi E, Varella-Garcia M et al. Induction of resistance to the Abelson inhibitor STI571 in human leukemic cells through gene amplification. Blood 2000;95:1758–1766.
47. Gorre M, Banks K, Hsu NC et al. Relapse in Ph+ leukemia patients treated with an Abl-specific kinase inhibitor is associated with reactivation of Bcr-Abl. Blood 2000;96:470a.
48. Gambacorti-Passerini C, Barni R, le Coutre P et al. Role of alpha1 acid glycoprotein in the in vivo resistance of human BCR-ABL(+) leukemic cells to the abl inhibitor STI571. J Natl Cancer Inst 2000;92:1641–1650.
49. Bedi A, Zehnbauer BA, Barber JP et al. Inhibition of apoptosis by BCR-ABL in chronic myeloid leukemia. Blood 1994;83:2038–2044.
50. Nishii K, Kabarowski JH, Gibbons DL et al. ts BCR-ABL kinase activation confers increased resistance to genotoxic damage via cell cycle block. Oncogene 1996;13:2225–2234.
51. Thiesing JT, Ohno-Jones S, Kolibaba KS, Druker BJ. Efficacy of an Abl tyrosine kinase inhibitor in conjunction with other anti-leukemic agents against Bcr-Abl positive cells. Blood 2000;96:3195–3199.
52. Fang G, Kim CN, Perkins CL et al. CGP57148B (STI-571) induces differentiation and apoptosis and sensitizes Bcr-Abl-positive human leukemia cells to apoptosis due to antileukemic drugs. Blood 2000;96:2246–2253.
53. Hochhaus A, Reiter A, Saussele S et al. Molecular heterogeneity in complete cytogenetic responders after interferon-alpha therapy for chronic myelogenous leukemia: low levels of minimal residual disease are associated with continuing remission. German CML Study Group and the UK MRC CML Study Group. Blood 2000;95:62–66.

Rituximab for the Treatment of Patients with B-Cell Non-Hodgkin's Lymphoma

David G. Maloney

Peter McLaughlin

Antibody therapy has emerged from early clinical studies into daily oncology practice over the past 2 to 3 years. In B-cell non-Hodgkin's lymphoma (NHL), this new technology has been led by the introduction of rituximab, a chimeric anti-CD20 monoclonal antibody (mAb). Phase I and II clinical trials found that the use of the antibody in single or multiple doses had anti-tumor activity and that relatively few serious adverse events were associated with the therapy. Now, more than 3 years since rituximab was approved for use by the United States Food and Drug Administration and was introduced into the clinical practice of oncology, the uses of this agent have increased from the single-agent treatment for low-grade NHL to exploration into treatments for other B-cell NHL histologies and combinations with or after chemotherapy. Recent data presented in abstract form suggest that the addition of rituximab to standard-dose CHOP (cyclophosphamide, hydroxydaunomycin, Oncovin, prednisone) chemotherapy improves the outcome of elderly patients with aggressive-histology NHL, a finding that, if confirmed, will institute a new standard for aggressive NHL therapy.[1]

Despite these clinical observations, the mechanism of tumor cell kill that is dominant in patients treated with rituximab remains poorly understood. It is likely that there are both immune-mediated effects (complement-dependent cytotoxicity [CDC] and antibody-dependent cell-mediated cytotoxicity [ADCC]), as well as direct antiproliferative effects of the antibody. These observations are from the analysis of cell lines and tumor samples in vitro; however, in patients, it is not clear which of these mechanisms is the most important. A better understanding of the process of tumor cell inhibition will allow rational combinations of the antibody therapy with or after the administration of conventional anti-tumor agents. The hope is that these combinations and/or sequences of therapy will allow additive effects or synergy of tumor cell kill without impeding immune clearance mechanisms and will ultimately eliminate the minimal residual disease that presumably causes patients to relapse after an apparent complete response (CR) after standard chemotherapy.

This chapter explores the use of rituximab for the treatment of B-cell NHL and discusses issues ranging from the mechanism of action of this agent to the newer combination studies with chemotherapy. However, because of the explosion of studies using rituximab, limitations of space preclude a detailed discussion of all ongoing trials but instead focus on selected studies that highlight the different approaches.

CD20 ANTIGEN

The success of rituximab therapy can be traced in part to the characteristics of the target antigen CD20 (Table 11.1). The CD20 antigen is a B-cell lineage cell surface glycoprotein that is expressed from the late pre–B-cell stage of B-cell differentiation through mature B cells and is usually lost on differentiation into plasma cells.[2] The protein is tightly held in the cell surface membrane because

TABLE 11.1 CD20 Antigen Characteristics

Nonglycosylated phosphoprotein, molecular weight, 33–35 kd
Tetraspan family with sequence homology to IgE Fc receptor
Tightly held in membrane with low rate of modulation
Not secreted or shed
Function unknown, possibly involved in Ca^{2+} flux
Noncovalently associated with Src family kinases
Contains multiple intracellular serine/threonine phosphorylation sites
Expression pattern:
    Mature B cells from the pre–B-cell stage
    Minimal expression on mature plasma cells (20%)
    Most B-cell malignancies have high levels
    Low levels in CLL
Normal tissue expression
    Mature B cells
    Not on stem cells or other critical tissues

CLL, chronic lymphocytic leukemia; IgE, immunoglobulin E.

of four transmembrane domains.[3] Both the amino and the carboxyl terminal regions of the molecule are within the cytoplasm. Only a small portion of the molecule is exposed on the outer cell membrane, and most anti-CD20 mAbs bind to this small region. The function of the molecule is not known; however, it is structurally similar to proteins that may aggregate and form or control ionic channels or membrane pores.[4] It may be involved in controlling progression through the cell cycle.[5] Transfection of CD20 into T cells has been associated with increased calcium flux into the cell.[6] After anti-CD20 antibody binding, the antigen has a low rate of internalization or modulation from the cell surface, resulting in the stable expression of the antigen/antibody complex. This has been an advantage for treatments with unlabeled antibodies and with radioisotope-labeled antibodies.[7] Additional important properties of CD20 include the high-level expression on most B-cell NHL histologies (excluding chronic lymphocytic leukemia [CLL]), the absence of expression on critical host cells, and the lack of known sequence mutations. The restricted expression of CD20 to mature B cells and the lack of expression on other host hematopoietic cells limit the expected toxicity of targeting CD20 with unlabeled mAbs to the depletion of B cells. The lack of significant antigen mutation limits tumor escape due to antigen loss or the expression of antigen variants. These issues have limited antibody therapy directed against other antigens, such as the immunoglobulin (Ig) idiotype. These characteristics of the CD20 antigen appear to be an advantage for unlabeled antibody therapy and are likely in large part responsible for the success of CD20-directed antibody therapy.

RITUXIMAB

Rituximab (Rituxan, MabThera, IDEC-C2B8) is a chimeric antibody made from genetically splicing the murine variable regions of the IgG1(κ) anti-CD20 antibody IDEC-2B8 and human IgG1(κ) constant regions.[8] Characteristics of the mAb are shown in Table 11.2. The human IgG1 constant regions allows a more prolonged half-life and decreased immunogenicity (decreased human anti-mouse antibody response) and augments the ability of the antibody to kill CD20-expressing cells through interaction with the human immune effector functions of CDC and ADCC. Rituximab binds to the cell surface–exposed portion of the CD20 molecule, and preclinical studies demonstrated expected binding and clearance of B cells from the blood, spleen, and lymph nodes of macaques.[8]

IMMUNE-MEDIATED ANTI-TUMOR EFFECTS
Antibody-Dependent Cell-Mediated Cytotoxicity

The chimeric mAb is more efficient and effective than the murine parent antibody in killing cells via CDC and ADCC.[8] This has been shown in the in vitro analysis

TABLE 11.2 Rituximab Chimeric anti-CD20 Antibody Characteristics

Chimeric, mouse/human monoclonal antibody
Specific for human CD20
Containing human IgG1 heavy and κ constant regions
Containing murine CD20 binding sequences from IgG1, κ, mAb IDEC-2B8
Mediates ADCC using human effector cells
Mediates complement lysis using human complement
Serum half-life:
   76 hours after first 375-mg/m² dose in relapsed low-grade NHL
   206 hours after fourth 375-mg/m² dose in relapsed low-grade NHL
Low immunogenicity in B-cell NHL trials
Retreatment possible

ADCC, antibody-dependent all-mediated cytotoxicity; IgG1, immunoglobulin G1; NHL, non-Hodgkin's lymphoma.

of tumor cells incubated with sources of human immune effector cells or human complement and the mAb. However, it remains controversial whether these immune mechanisms are the only mechanisms responsible for the clearance of tumor cells from the blood, bone marrow, or lymph nodes/tumor masses in vivo. Studies suggest that the ability of the antibody to bind to Fc receptors is required for the mAb to be active in a murine xenograft model and that the type of Fc binding is critical to the ability to induce an anti-tumor effect.[9] These observations imply that ADCC is the most important mechanism in clearing tumor cells from tumor masses or lymph nodes. In clinical trials with rituximab, the level of immune effector cells (as measured by the natural killer cell count in the peripheral blood) has correlated with anti-tumor effect.[10] However, poor immune function is also correlated with increasing amount of prior therapy, and a decreased response rate has been observed in these patients.[11] It is not clear whether the lessened effect is due to increased tumor resistance or to a lack of immune effector cells in these patients. Augmentation of immune effector cells may be possible through the use of cytokines. Combination studies with rituximab and growth factors or cytokines, such as interferon (IFN)-α, interleukin (IL)-2, and G-CSF or granulocyte macrophage colony stimulating factor, are ongoing and are discussed in detail later in this chapter.

Complement-Mediated Lysis

The contribution of complement binding to the anti-tumor effect remains more difficult to elucidate. It is clear that the human IgG1 Fc portion of the mAb can bind and activate complement through the c1q.[8] In vitro, some cell lines are sensitive to complement-mediated lysis using human complement.[12] Sensitivity or resistance to the direct effects of mAb and complement may be determined by the expression of complement resistance proteins, such as CD55 and CD59, on the tumor cell surface.[13] These proteins can interfere with the progression and/or amplification of the complement cascade necessary for tumor cell lysis. Several studies have suggested that the sensitivity or resistance to rituximab therapy may be partly due to the variable expression of these resistance proteins.[14] This has been observed in the in vitro analysis of some tumor cell lines. In vivo, however, this remains uncertain because most nucleated cells express these complement resistance proteins. Some patients have complement consumption after rituximab therapy. This has been more common in patients with large numbers of circulating tumor cells in the peripheral blood and may be more common in patients with a brighter expression of CD20. Taken together, these data suggest that complement may be involved in the clearing of CD20-expressing cells from the blood and possibly in releasing factors responsible for the first infusion symptoms observed in some patients.[15] However, it is unclear whether complement fixation is necessary or involved in the elimination of tumor cells in lymph nodes or large masses. Experience with the CAMPATH series of anti-CD52 mAbs demonstrated that the IgM isotype was very effective in fixing complement and lysing tumor cells in vitro but was relatively ineffective in depleting tumor cells in the peripheral blood in clinical trials.[16] In contrast, the IgG1 antibody (CAMPATH1-H), which has Fc receptor binding, induced rapid clearance of tumor cells from the blood, bone marrow, and, to a lesser extent, lymph nodes. This suggests that Fc receptor binding and ADCC are more important than complement binding and raises the question that if complement binding were abolished from rituximab, would the anti-tumor effects be similar, but with decreased infusion-related toxicity?[17]

DIRECT ANTI-TUMOR EFFECTS

In addition to immune-based tumor cell clearance, there is evidence that mAbs binding to the CD20 surface protein may induce cellular changes that may result in a decrease of the tumor cell growth rate and, in some cell lines, induce apoptosis.[18,19] Although the exact function of the CD20 molecule remains poorly defined, many cellular changes have been observed in the analysis of tumor cell lines in vitro after the binding or cross-linking of anti-CD20 mAbs. These changes include induction of tyrosine protein phosphorylation, decreases in proliferation, growth arrest, increases in calcium flux, redistribution of a variety of cell surface proteins within the outer cell membrane, and apoptosis.[20-24] Numerous groups have demonstrated both early and late apoptotic changes, such as phosphatidyl serene redistribution into the outer cellular membrane and activation of programmed cell death that appears to be mediated through a mitochondrial/caspase 9 cascade. This can result in PARP cleavage and DNA fragmentation. These changes seem to require clustering of CD20 and associated molecules with involvement of src family kinase activity.[20,21,25] The induction of these changes appears to be cell line dependent and may be augmented by additional cross-linking—possibly through antibody binding to Fc receptor–expressing cells.[24]

In vivo, the importance of these "direct" effects remains unknown; however, there are several observations that suggest that the presence or absence of these direct effects may contribute to sensitivity or resistance to rituximab therapy. The first observation is that not all patients respond to rituximab. It is possible that there are either differences in ADCC or complement-mediated effector function in these patients or that the tumor cells differ in their intrinsic resistance to these immune-based effector mechanisms. However, measurement of these differences, if they exist, remains elusive. Additionally, only 40% of patients responding to a first course of rituximab respond to retreatment with rituximab at the time of progression.[26] In most of these cases it is unlikely that the patient's immune system is less functional than it was at the time of their prior treatment, implying that if ADCC were the key effector function, it should be more effective, not worse, on retreatment. The mechanism of acquired resistance to rituximab remains unknown, but it is possible that the loss of these direct effects may play a role. Last, there is increasing evidence that tumor cell kill in vivo (in CLL tumor cells) may involve the induction of apoptosis and/or growth arrest; however, it is still uncertain whether these terminal events are due to direct effects, immune-mediated effects, or a combination of effects.

RITUXIMAB AND CHEMOTHERAPY: EVIDENCE FOR SYNERGY?

As discussed later in this chapter, rituximab's minimal toxicity profile and, significantly, the lack of hematologic toxicity allow combination trials with conventional anti-tumor chemotherapeutic agents. In vitro, combining exposure of cells to rituximab and agents, such as etoposide, cyclophosphamide, doxorubicin, cisplatin, or fludarabine, leads to augmented tumor cell kill, as measured by a variety of assays.[27-29] However, detailed analysis has not yet been reported, and although the data suggest at least additivity of tumor cell kill, there has not been proof of true synergy. A better understanding of the mechanisms of tumor cell kill and interaction with conventional agents is needed.

In addition to evaluating the effects of the combination of antibody with chemotherapy on the tumor cells, consideration of the effects of the chemotherapy treatment on immune-based tumor clearance mechanisms needs to be undertaken. Clinical trials suggest a higher response rate to rituximab for patients with less prior chemotherapy.[11] Untreated patients with follicular NHL have been reported to have overall response rates of 75%, whereas patients refractory to chemotherapy have overall response rates to rituximab alone of approximately 30%. There has been a correlation with the number of natural killer cells in the peripheral blood and the overall response, suggesting that ADCC may play an important role in in vivo tumor cell kill.[30] Because courses of conventional chemotherapy may clearly affect the immune system, the effects of rituximab combined with or after conventional therapy are not easy to predict.

Combination trials may be considered, based on administration of the antibody before or simultaneously with the chemotherapy or in a sequence following completion of the chemotherapy courses. Simultaneous administration allows true synergy, whereas sequential administration may allow recovery of the immune system from the effects of the chemotherapy before the antibody treatments as well as allowing substantial tumor reduction from the chemotherapy. The optimal schedule for combining rituximab simultaneously with chemotherapy is not known; however, the prolonged half-life of the antibody likely ensures that treatments with the antibody given with or before each chemotherapy cycle achieve saturating levels of the antibody throughout the treatment course.[30]

Clinical trials are now evaluating each of these approaches. For the treatment of low-grade follicular NHL, the Southwest Oncology Group trial #9800 treated 104 patients with newly diagnosed advanced-stage disease with six cycles of CHOP followed by adjuvant rituximab. An analysis of this trial is ongoing. In a smaller trial, Czuczman et al[31] reported on the simultaneous combination of rituximab with six cycles of CHOP. Although both approaches appear promising, neither has yet been tested against or proved to be superior to CHOP alone. Multiple randomized trials evaluating the integration of rituximab and conventional therapy are ongoing. In contrast to these trials in low-grade NHL, definitive phase III comparative combination trials of rituximab and chemotherapy for elderly patients with aggressive lymphoma have now been performed. These preliminary data from the French Groupe d'Etudes des Lymphomes de l'Adulte (GELA) group suggest that simultaneous treatment with rituximab and CHOP is superior to that with CHOP alone.[1] It is hoped that the preliminary data from the GELA trial will result in sustained improvement and will be confirmed in the ongoing United States–based trials.

PHARMACOLOGY OF RITUXIMAB

After rituximab infusion, CD20 sites on cells in the blood are rapidly saturated, followed by the spleen, bone marrow, and lymph nodes. The initial clearance of the first dose of mAb represents distribution into the plasma volume and clearance by CD20 sites. Subsequent doses generally demonstrate a longer half-life once antibody excess has been obtained.[30] The initial clinical trial of single-dose rituximab evaluated doses from 10 to 500 mg/m^2 administered as a single slow intravenous infusion.[32] Dose-limiting toxicity was not observed; however, prolonged infusion times were required for the higher dose levels because of starting and stopping of the infusion as a result of infusion-related symptoms. However, the results of this single dose trial demonstrated detection of antibody on tumor biopsy specimens taken from most patients 2 weeks after treatment at dose levels of more than 100 mg/m². Subsequent trials have generally evaluated treatment with multiple doses from 125 to 500 mg/m² for four to eight doses. The dose of 375 mg/m² for four doses (one infusion each week) was approved by the US Food and Drug Administration based on a phase II trial in 166 patients with relapsed follicular or low-grade NHL.[11,33] Analysis of the pharmacokinetics from this trial demonstrated that this dose achieved antibody excess in most patients.[30] Most patients experienced a steady increase in the serum levels of rituximab after each dose of the antibody, with a serum half-life of 76 hours after the first and 206 hours after the fourth infusion. Antibody was identified in the serum at 3 months (median level, 20 μg/mL) and at 6 months (median, 1.3 μg/mL) in patients tested and was higher in responders than in nonresponders. Some patients had pharmacokinetics characterized by rapid clearance or consumption of the serum antibody such that each pretreatment serum level was nearly undetectable. Patients with this pattern were more likely to be nonresponders to the antibody therapy and to have small lymphocytic lymphoma histology. Interestingly, tumors with this histology frequently have a lower density of CD20. It remains unclear whether the reason that these patients had poor pharmacokinetics was a greater tumor burden or other factors, such as an altered disposition of the antibody-antigen complex from the cell surface.

Additional data suggest that there may be more rapid consumption of the antibody in patients with CLL. This has prompted clinical trials of higher doses (375–2250 mg/m²) administered once each week for four infusions and trials of decreased dosing interval (375–500 mg/m² three times a week for 4 weeks).[34,35] At this time, no pharmacokinetic data have been presented that have evaluated these approaches. Early data from the clinical trials suggest a higher response rate at the higher doses, although it is unclear whether the duration and the magnitude of response will justify the expense. Additional clinical trials reporting the pharmacokinetics of mAb in these different histologies are needed. One approach would be to design a trial with the goal of achieving antibody excess in all patients and determining whether this will convert nonresponding patients with poor pharmacokinetics into responding patients.

Most experience has been with 375 to 500 mg/m² dosing each week for four weekly infusions. Extending the duration of antibody exposure by administering eight weekly treatments was associated with a slightly higher response rate (~60%) and a longer time to tumor progression in one small trial.[36] Unfortunately, there was still a low response rate (1/7) in the patients with small lymphocytic lymphoma in this trial. Repeat administration to responding patients after they have experienced relapse was associated with a 40% response rate, interestingly with a longer median time to progression than was associated with the first treatment.[26] An alternative approach that has been adopted by several of the large cooperative group trials is evaluating treatment with the standard dose of 375 mg/m² each week for four doses. Responding patients are then treated with scheduled repeat courses of treatment at 6-month intervals for up to 2 years in an effort to increase the depth and the duration of remission and to prevent relapse.

SINGLE-AGENT THERAPY WITH RITUXIMAB IN RELAPSED LOW-GRADE NHL

Selected clinical trials of single-agent rituximab are shown in Table 11.3. Doses from 10 to 500 mg/m^2 were tolerated with minimal infusion-related side effects without dose-limiting toxicity.[32] Depletion of peripheral blood B cells was observed and persisted for several months after treatment. Weekly infusion of 125 to 375 mg/m^2 was not associated with any increase in toxicity, and infusional reactions were uncommon with the second and subsequent doses.[37] The dose of 375 mg/m^2 was selected from the phase I/II experience as a dose that achieved antibody excess in most patients and was associated with an approximate 50% response rate in patients with relapsed follicular or low-grade NHL histology.[33] This trial was used as the basis for the pivotal single-agent trial of rituximab in 166 patients entered from 31 centers in the United States and Canada with relapsed low-grade or follicular NHL.[11] Data from these two trials were presented to the United States Food and Drug Administration, leading to the approval of rituximab as the first anticancer antibody in November 1997. The results from the pivotal trial were identical to those from the earlier phase II trials of the drug.[11,33] Overall, at the 375 mg/m^2 dose weekly given four times, 48% of the patients responded with a partial response (PR) or a CR. Toxicity was minimal, and the treatment was well tolerated in both young and elderly patients, as well as in patients who had failed to respond to prior high-dose therapy and autologous stem cell transplantation. A lower response rate (14%) was observed in patients with small lymphocytic histology.[11]

Patients with a detectable *Bcl-2* translocation by polymerase chain reaction (PCR) in pretreatment peripheral blood cleared detectable tumor cells in 62%, and 56% cleared detectable signal from the bone marrow.[11] Interestingly, most patients were judged to have only partial remissions based on residual adenopathy by use of stringent criteria for determination of a CR (all nodes less than 1.0 × 1.0 cm^2 on computed tomography of the neck, chest, abdomen, and pelvis, persisting more than 30 days). This again demonstrated the ability of rituximab to clear tumor from the blood and bone marrow to a greater extent than nodal-based tumor. Patients with a CR and those with molecular clearance of PCR-detectable disease generally have had longer remissions.

Supportive clinical trials using the identical dose in patients with bulky adenopathy or tumor masses (> 10 cm) showed a response of 43%.[38] A retreatment trial demonstrated response in 40% of patients who had previously responded to rituximab.[26] This indicates that mechanisms of resistance were acquired. In rare cases, this has been documented to be due to the loss of expression of

TABLE 11.3 Selected Single-Agent Rituximab NHL Trials

Histology	Number	Dose/Frequency	Response	Duration	Reference
Relapsed low-grade	37	375 mg/m^2 × 4	46%	TTP 10.2 mo	33
Relapsed low-grade	166	375 mg/m^2 × 4	48%	TTP 13 mo	11
Relapsed low-grade	37	375 mg/m^2 × 8	57%	≥ 19.4 mo	36
Relapsed NHL		375 mg/m^2 × 4			51
Mantle cell	74		38%		
Immunocytoma	28		28%	1.2 years	
Small lymphocytic	29		14%		
Relapsed NHL					46
Follicular	78	375 mg/m^2 × 4	52%		
Mantle cell	42		22%		
Relapsed follicular	38	375 mg/m^2 × 4	47%	TTP 201 days	82
Relapsed follicular	70	375 mg/m^2 × 4	46%	11 mo	83
Untreated low-grade		375 mg/m^2 × 4		77% PFS at 12 mo	42
Follicular	26		52%		
Small lymphocytic	15		57%		
Untreated follicular	50	375 mg/m^2 × 4	79%	Ongoing	43
Aggressive NHL	54	375–500 mg/m^2 × 8		≥ 246 days	44
Large cell			37%		
Mantle cell			33%		

Abbreviations: NHL, non-Hodgkins lymphoma; PFS, progression-free survival.

CD20.[39-41] In most cases, however, the mechanism of resistance to the subsequent treatment is not known. Possible explanations include augmentation of complement resistance proteins or resistance to immune-based killing or loss of direct antiproliferative effects of the antibody. A better understanding of these mechanisms of resistance may provide insights into the mechanism of action and may lead to trials augmenting efficacy through combinations with cytokines or chemotherapy.

SINGLE-AGENT THERAPY WITH RITUXIMAB IN PREVIOUSLY UNTREATED LOW-GRADE NHL

After demonstration of clinical activity in patients with relapsed follicular or low-grade NHL, two trials have evaluated antibody therapy as initial treatment for these patients and have observed higher response rates with more CR. A recent report by Hainsworth et al[42] evaluated 375 mg/m^2 weekly for four doses in patients with low-grade or follicular NHL who required therapy. At 6 weeks after therapy, 54% had a PR or a CR and 36% had stable disease. Stable or responding patients then were eligible to receive repeat courses of treatment every 6 months for three doses. With longer follow-up, the response rate was 64% at a time when only 13 patients had received the second course of rituximab therapy. The 12-month progression-free survival for the 39 patients was 77%. Interestingly, in contrast to the previously discussed trials, patients with small lymphocytic histology responded as well as the follicular NHL patients.

The French group has also evaluated primary therapy with rituximab in patients with low-tumor-burden follicular NHL and have reported a response rate of 73% at day 50 after therapy (36/49 with 10 CR and three CR unconfirmed, 23 PR).[43] Only one of 13 CR patients experienced disease progression within one year, whereas nine of 23 PR patients and five of 10 stable-disease patients progressed. Patients became PCR negative in peripheral blood (57%) and bone marrow (31%) at day 50, and 62% were PCR negative in the blood at one year. Including late responses, the overall response rate to this single course of rituximab was 79%. In both of these trials, longer follow-up is necessary to determine the duration of the complete and partial remissions.

RITUXIMAB THERAPY FOR CLL

In the initial phase I/II clinical trials of rituximab, classic CLL was excluded. Patients with small lymphocytic NHL with a white blood cell count of less than 5000 lymphocytes were included, and the response in this subset disappointing (approximately 14%).[11,36] Pharmacokinetics derived from this trial suggested that there was a more rapid consumption and a shorter half-life of the antibody in these patients.[30] Subsequent trials in both classic CLL and in lymphomas with high numbers of circulating tumor lymphocytes have evaluated more aggressive dosing schedules. O'Brien and colleagues[35] at the M.D. Anderson Cancer Center performed a dose escalation trial to 2250 mg/m^2. Although true dose-limiting toxicity was not observed even at the highest dose, increased infusion-related side effects were observed, and further dose escalation was not attempted. At the higher dose levels, responses were observed in approximately 50% of patients. Byrd et al[34] have used an increased frequency of treatment, with a three times weekly schedule, and also reported preliminary results suggesting a higher response rate. Details of these studies and pharmacokinetic analysis is required before increased dosing or schedule is adopted into clinical practice.

SINGLE-AGENT RITUXIMAB FOR AGGRESSIVE-HISTOLOGY NHL

In vitro analysis of the effects of CD20 ligation on cell lines created from patients with aggressive B cell NHL suggest that the antibody may also have direct antiproliferative effects, including the induction of apoptosis. The early trials included few patients with aggressive NHL or transformed histology but suggested single-agent activity in some patients. Selected trials are shown in Table 11.3. Coiffier et al[44] initiated the first study of single-agent rituximab for patients with aggressive histology NHL (12 mantle cell, 30 diffuse large B cell, and 10 other aggressive histologies). Treatment was with either 375 mg/m^2 or 500 mg/m^2 for eight doses. There was no difference in the response rate. Overall, 31% of patients responded, with 33% of patients with mantle cell and 37% of patients with diffuse large B-cell NHL attaining a PR or a CR. Although this trial did not suggest that rituximab should be used as a single agent in patients with aggressive NHL, it did establish that rituximab is active against these histologies and provides a rationale for studies in combination or in sequence with chemotherapy.

Foran et al[45] also treated a series of 87 patients with mantle cell lymphoma. Most patients received the 375 mg/m^2 × 4 dose schedule. This trial included patients without prior therapy and those who had experienced relapse. The overall response rate was 34% with a median duration of response of 1.2 years with a roughly equal response rate in relapsed patients and in patients without prior therapy. Ghielmini et al[46] also reported on 43 relapsed mantle cell lymphoma patients treated in a larger trial and observed a 22% response rate with the same dose and schedule. Subsequent trials have evaluated treatment with combinations of chemotherapy.

SINGLE-AGENT RITUXIMAB THERAPY FOR OTHER CD20+ MALIGNANCIES

Rituximab has been used for the treatment of patients with a variety of other hematopoietic malignancies believed to express the CD20 antigen. To date, however, these data are usually anecdotal rather than published series of patients.

CD20 is expressed from the late pre–B-cell stage throughout B-cell development and then lost on differentiation into the terminal plasma cell stage. Among B-cell malignancies, most lymphomas are CD20 positive, but only approximately 20% of myeloma cases continue to express the antigen. Most marrow-based lymphoplasmacytic tumors, such as Waldenström's, express significant levels of CD20. Rituximab therapy of these tumors induces objective response rates of approximately 35%; however, a higher percentage of patients have improvement in bone marrow function and lessening of transfusion requirements.[47-50] Foran et al[51] reported on treatment of immunocytoma with rituximab and observed a 28% response rate.

Several groups are exploring the use of rituximab in patients with myeloma. Despite the fact that in only approximately 20% of myeloma cases do the plasma cells express the CD20 antigen, a case has been made to use CD20-directed therapy to eliminate earlier-stage B cells that may contribute to the malignancy.[48,49,52] In early reports of these trials, rituximab treatment was active in cases only in which the plasma cell actually expressed the CD20 antigen, supporting the argument that the elimination of these B cells does not appear to have significant consequence for the malignancy. It remains to be determined whether rituximab will have a significant effect in the rare myeloma cases that express CD20. Alternatively, it may be possible to use cytokines to up-regulate the expression of CD20 on the myeloma cell. In vitro exposure of primary myeloma cells to IFN-γ increases expression of CD20 on the plasma cell and augments rituximab binding.[52] Combination of cytokines and rituximab may also increase immune-mediated killing through enhanced ADCC. Clinical trials evaluating these combinations are underway.

Minimal experience has been reported in B-cell ALL, acquired immunodeficiency deficiency syndrome–related lymphoma, primary central nervous system lymphoma, and lymphocyte-predominant Hodgkin's disease. Anecdotal and small series have demonstrated that two thirds of cases of relapsed childhood B acute lymphoblastic leukemia or Burkitt's lymphoma had a CR.[53] Some response has been observed in human immunodeficiency virus–related B-cell NHL, including a case associated with tumor lysis.[54] Interestingly, in a small series, two thirds of patients with refractory primary brain NHL had radiographic improvement after rituximab therapy.[55] Most lymphocyte-predominant Hodgkin's disease cases express the CD20 antigen, and preliminary reports suggest a very high response rate to rituximab therapy.[56] In rare cases of classical Hodgkin's disease, the Reed-Sternberg cell expresses CD20, and a few case reports have indicated some activity.

Posttransplantation lymphoproliferative disorders are serious complications of T-cell–depleted stem cell transplants and of organ transplantation requiring severe posttransplantation immunosuppression. Rituximab has shown activity in treating and preventing this complication and is now often given at the first sign of unchecked Epstein-Barr virus proliferation.[57-63] In the larger studies, long-term disease control has been documented with response rates of from 63% to 85%.[61] This treatment likely removes the B-cell population necessary to support Epstein-

Barr virus proliferation. Earlier use of therapy, rather than treatment of refractory clonal disease, appears to have greater efficacy.

IN VIVO B-CELL PURGING

The initial clinical trial of rituximab observed that B cells were rapidly and specifically depleted from the peripheral blood in nearly all patients after the first dose of antibody.[32] This B-cell depletion was observed for several months after administration of a single dose and for 6 to 9 months after multiple doses. A logical extension of this observation was to use antibody treatment before stem cell mobilization to eliminate B cells and tumor from peripheral blood stem cell collections. It appears that this can be accomplished safely and that the stem cells that are collected engraft with normal kinetics.[64–66] Multiple studies are now ongoing to determine whether the elimination of tumor cells from the stem cell graft will decrease the risk of relapse after autologous stem cell transplantation.

COMBINATION TREATMENT: RITUXIMAB WITH CYTOKINES

There are several reasons to pursue administration of rituximab with cytokines. It is likely that cytokines such as granulocyte macrophage colony stimulating factor, IFN, IL-2, and IL-12 may augment immune effector cells that are capable of eliminating antibody-coated tumor cells through ADCC. These and other cytokines may cause activation and increased number of these effector cells. In addition, preliminary data suggest that cytokines may up-regulate the expression of the CD20 antigen, and thus possibly augment clinical activity. Thus far, the most convincing data have been with the use of IFN-γ to induce and increase CD20 expression on myeloma cells.[48,52] Other cytokines (granulocyte macrophage colony stimulating factor, tumor necrosis factor-α, IL-4, and IFN-α) have been reported to slightly increase CD20 expression on CLL cells.[67,68] On the basis of these observations, multiple combination trials have been initiated and a few have now been reported.

Rituximab (four doses of 375 mg/m^2) in combination with a 3-month course of IFN-α (1 million U, three times a week) appeared to induce an identical response rate in patients with relapsed low-grade or follicular NHL, although the median duration of responding patients was nearly twice as long.[69] Preliminary reports from additional trials suggest that IFN-α may augment the response rate to rituximab alone or to retreatment with a second cycle.[70]

Combinations with G-CSF have also been reported. One trial used the standard dose of rituximab and included 3 days of treatment with G-CSF, starting 2 days before each antibody dose. The response rate from this trial did not appear to be different from that with rituximab treatment alone; however, there was an increased number of CRs with long duration.[71] A randomized study is required to determine whether this is different from rituximab alone. Although G-CSF has not been described to influence antigen expression, there have been some reports that neutrophils may mediate ADCC-like activity.[72]

Multiple other trials with cytokines are ongoing. A trial of rituximab and IL-12 observed increases in serum IFN-γ and a response rate of 70% in 32 patients.[73] A similar trial with rituximab and IL-2 documented an increase in natural killer cells and a response rate of 61% in 13 patients.[74] All of these studies are very preliminary but suggest that these approaches have merit. It is hoped that a better understanding of the mechanism of tumor cell kill by the antibody will allow rational combinations of the antibody with cytokines to augment antitumor activity without increasing toxicity.

COMBINATION TREATMENT: CHEMOTHERAPY WITH RITUXIMAB

The evidence of single-agent activity against a variety of relapsed B-cell lymphoma histologies, the different mechanism of action (including both immune and direct anti-tumor effects), and the modest nonoverlapping toxicity profile provide a strong rationale for combination treatments with standard chemotherapy. Multiple trials are ongoing, and a few selected trials are shown in Table 11.4. There is some evidence that rituximab may be at least additive and possibly synergistic, with many chemotherapeutic agents using in vitro tests on malignant B-cell lines.[28,29] However, it is difficult to clarify the interactions of chemotherapy and rituximab with the tumor cell and immune effector functions. Randomized clinical trials will likely be required to prove the superiority of any combination or schedule.

Combination studies may be performed by administering the antibody either simultaneously with the chemotherapy or in sequence after chemotherapy. The long serum half-life of rituximab generally ensures that antibody is present for a long duration after the initial infusion. Thus, treatments with the antibody given before the chemotherapy will result in antibody levels throughout the chemotherapy course. Minor variations in the timing are not likely to result in significant differences. However, the issue of synergy or additive effects with chemotherapy would suggest simultaneous rather than sequential therapy. In contrast, if the chemotherapy had an adverse effect on the immune system or on cells that were important in clearing antibody coated tumor cells, separating the two treatments may be more beneficial. In addition, administration after chemotherapy may allow the antibody to eliminate a minimal disease burden. Both approaches have been undertaken, and no current data prove that either course is superior.

Indolent Lymphoma

Czuczman et al[31] combined six doses of rituximab with six cycles of standard-dose CHOP chemotherapy for the treatment of patients with low-grade or follicular

TABLE 11.4 Selected Chemoimmunotherapy Combination NHL Trials with Rituximab

Histology	No.	Chemotherapy	Rituximab Dose/Frequency	Response	Duration	Reference
Low-grade	40	CHOP × 6	375 mg/m^2 × 6	95% OR	74% PFS at ≥ 29 mo	31
Low-grade	39	Fludabarine × 6 (25mg/m^2 × 5)	375 mg/m^2 × 6	92% OR	≥ 15 mo	77
Aggressive	33	CHOP × 6	375 mg/m^2 × 6	94% OR	29/33 PFS at ≥ 26 mo	79
Elderly aggressive NHL	169	CHOP × 6	375 mg/m^2 × 6	76% CR	69% 12 mo EFS	1

CHOP, cylcophosphamide, hydroxydaunomycin, Oncovin, prednisone; CR, complete response; EFS, event-free survival; NHL, non-Hodgkins lymphoma; OR, overall response; PFS, progression-free survival.

lymphoma. Two doses of rituximab (375 mg/m^2) were given before the first cycle and after the sixth cycle. One dose was also given before the third and fifth cycles. This dosing strategy was chosen to saturate tumor sites with the antibody before the administration of CHOP and to then sustain levels throughout the chemotherapy. The two doses at the end of treatment were to clear any potential residual disease. Thirty-eight patients were treated, and most were newly diagnosed, previously untreated patients with either follicular or small lymphocytic lymphoma. This trial demonstrated that the toxicity of combination therapy was that expected with CHOP alone and with relatively minor infusion-related side effects from the rituximab infusions. There was no increase in marrow toxicity or other adverse events. All patients responded with a high percentage of CR (55%). Most of a small subset of patients tested (6/7) who had detectable PCR product for a *Bcl-2* rearrangement cleared detectable tumor from the blood and from bone marrow. Overall, after more than 4 years of follow-up, approximately 70% of patients remain progression free. Encouragingly, patients with small lymphocytic lymphoma responded as well as the follicular histology patients did. Although the numbers of patients are small, this trial represents a lead that will be compared with standard CHOP for newly diagnosed, advanced-stage follicular NHL patients in the Southwest Oncology Group trial S0016.

The ability of rituximab to consolidate CHOP chemotherapy was evaluated in Southwest Oncology Group S9800. This trial evaluated six cycles of CHOP followed by four doses of rituximab for patients with advanced-stage, newly diagnosed follicular NHL. The results of this trial will be reported in the fall of 2001. In a similar trial in the Eastern Cooperative Oncology Group, rituximab is being evaluated after CVP (cyclophosphamide, vincristine, prednisone) chemotherapy.

The M.D. Anderson Cancer Center is exploring treatment with the FND regimen (fludarabine, mitoxantrone, dexamethasone) with rituximab and with maintenance IFN plus dexamethasone for stage IV indolent lymphoma. The treatment includes eight cycles of FND with 1 year of maintenance IFN plus dexamethasone. Rituximab is either given simultaneously with the first five cycles of FND or as an adjuvant starting at month 12. Thus, the trial will evaluate the risks and benefits of antibody sequence. Endpoints of the trial include standard clinical endpoints as well as clearance of molecular detectable disease as measured by PCR for *Bcl-2* gene rearrangements. One issue being carefully monitored in this trial is whether there may be increased immunodeficiency caused by the depletion of both B and T cells from the combination. Preliminary results from this trial suggest that the treatment is well tolerated, although there was slightly more neutropenia in patients receiving concurrent therapy.[75] There was a higher rate of molecular response in the peripheral blood at 6 months in the simultaneous-treatment group but no difference between the two groups at 1 year, indicating that the sequential treatment also induced a high rate of clearance of disease from the blood and bone marrow.[76] Czuczman et al[77] reported on the combination of rituximab with a standard 5-day course of fludarabine and also noted increased myelosuppression, especially in patients treated with trimethoprim/sulfamethoxazole (Bactrim) for pneumocystis prevention. Longer follow-up from both of these trials is required before these combinations are adopted.

Trials in CLL have also incorporated rituximab with fludarabine and cyclophosphamide. In preliminary reports, the regimen has been well tolerated and associated with rapid decreases in lymphocytosis. Based on the M.D. Anderson Cancer Center experience, a higher complete remission rate with some patients experiencing molecular resolution of their disease has been observed when compared with prior trials of fludarabine alone or fludarabine-cyclophosphamide combination.[78] Again, these results are preliminary but reflect the enthusiasm for these possible combinations. Longer follow-up of these trials are needed.

Aggressive NHL

As discussed earlier, Coiffier et al[44] demonstrated in a phase I clinical trial that approximately one third of patients with relapsed diffuse large cell aggressive NHL responded to single-agent rituximab, setting the stage for combination trials. Vose et al[79] recently reported a phase II trial of therapy with rituximab and CHOP in patients with aggressive NHL. Six cycles of CHOP were given with six doses of rituximab. Each antibody infusion was given 2 days before standard-dose CHOP. The response rate was 94% (61% CR, 33% PR) in this trial, with 29 of 31 patients who responded remaining in remission at a median observation time of 26 months. Toxicity was as expected from the antibody and from the chemotherapy. Howard et al[80] also combined rituximab with CHOP for the treatment of newly diagnosed mantle cell NHL. A high response rate was observed, and a large number of patients cleared detectable tumor from the blood and bone marrow. Unfortunately, the median duration of response was only 16 months. Although this may be better than results of CHOP alone, additional strategies are needed. One approach has been to use this as preparation to harvest autologous stem cells to support subsequent high-dose therapy. The M.D. Anderson group is evaluating more aggressive therapy with the combination of rituximab and fractionated cyclophosphamide, vincristine, doxorubicin, and dexamethasone (HCVAD) alternating with high-dose methotrexate and cytosine arabinoside for patients with mantle cell NHL and have reported a 97% response rate.[81] In all of these trials, longer follow-up and subsequent randomized phase III trials are necessary.

The first demonstration that antibody combined with CHOP may be better than CHOP alone for elderly patients with aggressive NHL was recently presented in the plenary session at the American Society of Hematology 2000 meeting.[1] This study by the French GELA group was a randomized trial comparing eight cycles of CHOP with eight cycles of rituximab-CHOP (R-CHOP) in 400 patients. A dose of rituximab was added to each cycle of CHOP in the R-CHOP group.

The groups were balanced in prognostic factors. The treatment was all given on the same day. Patients randomly assigned to R-CHOP received steroids, followed by rituximab, followed by the remaining chemotherapy—all on day 1. G-CSF was routinely given to all patients. Coiffier et al[1] reported on the first 328 patients enrolled in the trial with 1 year of follow-up. The CR rates from R-CHOP and CHOP were 76% and 60%, the 12-month event-free survival rates were 69% and 49%, and the 12-month overall survivals were 83% and 68%, respectively. All were statistically significant at $P < 0.01$. Infusion-related side effects were observed in the patients receiving R-CHOP, but otherwise, the adverse events reported were similar. There were more discontinuations of therapy in the CHOP group as a result of tumor progression on therapy (18 vs 5).

There is also a ongoing study by the Eastern Cooperative Oncology Group/ CALGB that is evaluating six to eight cycles of CHOP versus R-CHOP for elderly patients with aggressive NHL. Some differences from the GELA trial include the following: (1) rituximab is given before the chemotherapy, (2) responding patients are subsequently randomly assigned to maintenance courses of rituximab, and (3) G-CSF is not routinely given with each cycle. It is hoped that the encouraging data presented by the GELA group will be confirmed in the American trial and will establish a new standard for aggressive NHL in the elderly.

The preliminary report of the GELA trial has halted several ongoing trials in the United States that were evaluating the addition of rituximab to CHOP chemotherapy in younger patients. It is important that confirmatory trials are performed and that the results of this trial are not translated without data to the treatment of patients with other B-cell histologies.

CONCLUSION

Rituximab has revived interest in immunotherapy and has demonstrated that targeted treatments have anti-tumor activity with less toxicity to the host. The initial clinical trials demonstrated safety and anti-tumor activity in numerous B-cell histologies. Current trials are now combining this new therapy with standard chemotherapy. The early results from the randomized GELA trial demonstrate that this targeted approach, when added to CHOP chemotherapy, is better than CHOP alone for the treatment of elderly patients with aggressive NHL. Ongoing clinical trials are needed to confirm these results and thus establish a new standard for therapy in this clinical situation, and additional trials are needed to establish the role of targeted therapy for other tumor types. It is hoped that this will just be the beginning as targeted therapies provide increased tumor kill with limited toxicity to patients with lymphoma.

REFERENCES

1. Coiffier B, Lepage E, Herbrecht R et al. MABTHERA (rituximab) plus CHOP is superior to CHOP alone in elderly patients with diffuse large B-cell lymphoma (DLCL): interim results of a randomized GELA trial. Blood 2000;96:950.

2. Nadler LM, Ritz J, Hardy R et al. A unique cell surface antigen identifying lymphoid malignancies of B cell origin. J Clin Invest 1981;67:134–140.
3. Einfeld DA, Brown JP, Valentine MA et al. Molecular cloning of the human B cell CD20 receptor predicts a hydrophobic protein with multiple transmembrane domains. EMBO J 1988;7:711–717.
4. Bubien JK, Bell PD, Frizzell RA et al. B3.2 CD20 directly regulates transmembrane ion flux in B-lymphocytes. In: Knapp W, Dorken B, Gilks WR, eds. Leukocyte Typing IV. White Cell Differentiation Antigens. Oxford: Oxford University Press, 1989:51–54.
5. Tedder TF, Engel P. CD20: a regulator of cell-cycle progression of B lymphocytes. Immunol Today 1994;15:450–454.
6. Bubien JK, Zhou LJ, Bell PD et al. Transfection of the CD20 cell surface molecule into ectopic cell types generates a Ca2+ conductance found constitutively in B lymphocytes. J Cell Biol 1993; 121:1121–1132.
7. Press OW, Howell CJ, Anderson S et al. Retention of B-cell-specific monoclonal antibodies by human lymphoma cells. Blood 1994;83:1390–1397.
8. Reff ME, Carner K, Chambers KS et al. Depletion of B cells in vivo by a chimeric mouse human monoclonal antibody to CD20. Blood 1994;83:435–445.
9. Clynes RA, Towers TL, Presta LG et al. Inhibitory Fc receptors modulate in vivo cytoxicity against tumor targets. Nat Med 2000;6:443–446.
10. Janakiramen N, McLaughlin P, White CA et al. Rituximab: Correlation between effector cells and clinical activity in NHL. Blood 1998;92:337a (abstract).
11. McLaughlin P, Grillo-Lopez AJ, Link BK et al. Rituximab chimeric anti-CD20 monoclonal antibody therapy for relapsed indolent lymphoma: half of patients respond to a four-dose treatment program. J Clin Oncol 1998;16:2825–2833.
12. Harjunpaa A, Junnikkala S, Meri S. Rituximab (anti-CD20) therapy of B-cell lymphomas: direct complement killing is superior to cellular effector mechanisms. Scand J Immunol 2000;51: 634–641.
13. Golay J, Zaffaroni L, Vaccari T et al. Biologic response of B lymphoma cells to anti-CD20 monoclonal antibody rituximab in vitro: CD55 and CD59 regulate complement-mediated cell lysis. Blood 2000;95:3900–3908.
14. Bannerji R, Pearson M, Flinn IW et al. Cell surface complement inhibitors CD55 and CD59 may mediate chronic lymphocytic leukemia (CLL) resistance to Rituximab therapy. Blood 2000;96: 164a.
15. Schwaner I, von Engelhardt LV, Jordanova M et al. Rituximab induced complement cascade activation is related to adverse events and bone marrow involvement. Blood 2000;96:507a.
16. Dyer MJ, Hale G, Hayhoe FG et al. Effects of CAMPATH-1 antibodies in vivo in patients with lymphoid malignancies: influence of antibody isotype. Blood 1989;73:1431–1439.
17. Idusogie EE, Presta LG, Gazzano-Santoro H et al. Mapping of the C1q binding site on rituxan, a chimeric antibody with a human IgG1 Fc. J Immunol 2000;164:4178–4184.
18. Maloney D, Smith B, Appelbaum F. The anti-tumor effect of monoclonal anti-CD20 antibody (mAb) therapy includes direct antiproliferative activity and induction of apoptosis in CD20 positive non-Hodgkin's lymphoma (NHL) cell lines. Blood 1996;88:637a.
19. Taji H, Kagami Y, Okada Y et al. Growth inhibition of CD20-positive B lymphoma cell lines by IDEC-C2B8 anti-CD20 monoclonal antibody. Jpn J Cancer Res 1998;89:748–756.
20. Deans JP, Schieven GL, Shu GL et al. Association of tyrosine and serine kinases with the B cell surface antigen CD20: induction via CD20 of tyrosine phosphorylation and activation of phospholipase C-gamma 1 and PLC phospholipase C-gamma 2. J Immunol 1993;151:4494–4504.
21. Deans JP, Kalt L, Ledbetter JA et al. Association of 75/80-kDa phosphoproteins and the tyrosine kinases Lyn, Fyn, and Lck with the B cell molecule CD20: evidence against involvement of the cytoplasmic regions of CD20. J Biol Chem 1995;270:22632–22638.

22. Deans JP, Robbins SM, Polyak MJ et al. Rapid redistribution of CD20 to a low density detergent-insoluble membrane compartment. J Biol Chem 1998;273:344–348.
23. Shan D, Ledbetter JA, Press OW. Signaling events involved in anti-CD20-induced apoptosis of malignant human B cells. Cancer Immunol Immunother 2000;48:673–683.
24. Shan D, Ledbetter JA, Press OW. Apoptosis of malignant human B cells by ligation of CD20 with monoclonal antibodies. Blood 1998;91:1644–1652.
25. Hofmeister JK, Cooney D, Coggeshall KM. Clustered CD20 induced apoptosis: src-family kinase, the proximal regulator of tyrosine phosphorylation, calcium influx, and caspase 3-dependent apoptosis. Blood Cells Mol Dis 2000;26:133–143.
26. Davis TA, Grillo-Lopez AJ, White CA et al. Rituximab anti-CD20 monoclonal antibody therapy in non-Hodgkin's lymphoma: safety and efficacy of re-treatment. J Clin Oncol 2000;18:3135–3143.
27. Alas S, Bonavida B, Emmanouilides C. Potentiation of fludarabine cytotoxicity on non-Hodgkin's lymphoma by pentoxifylline and rituximab. Anticancer Res 2000;20:2961–2966.
28. Demidem A, Lam T, Alas S et al. Chimeric Anti-Cd20 (Idec-C2b8) monoclonal antibody sensitizes a B cell lymphoma cell line to cell killing by cytotoxic drugs. Cancer Biother Radiopharm 1997;12:177–186.
29. Golay J XY, DiGaetano N, Dastoli G et al. Fludarabine synergizes with anti-CD20 monoclonal antibody rituximab in complement mediated cell lysis. Blood 2000;96:339a.
30. Berinstein NL, Grillo-Lopez AJ, White CA et al. Association of serum rituximab (IDEC-C2B8) concentration and anti-tumor response in the treatment of recurrent low-grade or follicular non-Hodgkin's lymphoma. Ann Oncol 1998;9:995–1001.
31. Czuczman MS, Grillo-Lopez AJ, White CA et al. Treatment of patients with low-grade B-cell lymphoma with the combination of chimeric anti-CD20 monoclonal antibody and CHOP chemotherapy. J Clin Oncol 1999;17:268–276.
32. Maloney DG, Liles TM, Czerwinski DK et al. Phase I clinical trial using escalating single-dose infusion of chimeric anti-CD20 monoclonal antibody (IDEC-C2B8) in patients with recurrent B-cell lymphoma. Blood 1994;84:2457–2466.
33. Maloney DG, Grillo-Lopez AJ, White CA et al. IDEC-C2B8 (rituximab) anti-CD20 monoclonal antibody therapy in patients with relapsed low-grade non-Hodgkin's lymphoma. Blood 1997;90:2188–2195.
34. Byrd JC, Grever MR, Davis B et al. Phase I/II study of thrice weekly rituximab in chronic lymphocytic leukemia/ small lymphocytic lymphoma: a feasible and active regimen. Blood 1999;94[suppl 1]:704a.
35. O'Brien S, Thomas DA, Freireich EJ et al. Rituxan has significant activity in patients with CLL. Blood 1999;94[suppl 1]:603a.
36. Piro LD, White CA, Grillo-Lopez AJ et al. Extended rituximab (anti-CD20 monoclonal antibody) therapy for relapsed or refractory low-grade or follicular non-Hodgkin's lymphoma. Ann Oncol 1999;10:655–661.
37. Maloney DG, Grillo-Lopez AJ, Bodkin DJ et al. IDEC-C2B8: results of a phase I multiple-dose trial in patients with relapsed non-Hodgkin's lymphoma. J Clin Oncol 1997;15:3266–3274.
38. Davis TA, White CA, Grillo-Lopez AJ et al. Single-agent monoclonal antibody efficacy in bulky non-Hodgkin's lymphoma: results of a phase II trial of rituximab. J Clin Oncol 1999;17:1851–1857.
39. Davis TA, Czerwinski DK, Levy R. Therapy of B-cell lymphoma with anti-CD20 antibodies can result in the loss of CD20 antigen expression. Clin Cancer Res 1999;5:611–615.
40. Kinoshita T, Nagai H, Murate T et al. CD20-negative relapse in B-cell lymphoma after treatment with rituximab. J Clin Oncol 1998;16:3916.
41. Schmitz K, Brugger W, Weiss B et al. Clonal selection of CD20-negative non-Hodgkin's lymphoma cells after treatment with anti-CD20 antibody rituximab. Br J Haematol 1999;106:571–572.

42. Hainsworth JD, Burris HA, Morrissey LH et al. Rituximab monoclonal antibody as initial systemic therapy for patients with low-grade non-Hodgkin's lymphoma. Blood 2000;95:3052–3056.
43. Colombat P, Salles G, Brousse N et al. Rituximab (anti-CD20 monoclonal antibody) as single first-line therapy for patients with follicular lymphoma with a low tumor burden: clinical and molecular evaluation. Blood 2001;97:101–106.
44. Coiffier B, Haioun C, Ketterer N et al. Rituximab (anti-CD20 monoclonal antibody) for the treatment of patients with relapsing or refractory aggressive lymphoma: a multicenter phase II study. Blood 1998;92:1927–1932.
45. Foran JM, Cunningham D, Coiffier B et al. Treatment of mantle-cell lymphoma with rituximab (chimeric monoclonal anti-CD20 antibody): analysis of factors associated with response. Ann Oncol 2000;11:117–121.
46. Ghielmini M, Schmitz SF, Burki K et al. The effect of rituximab on patients with follicular and mantle-cell lymphoma. Swiss Group for Clinical Cancer Research (SAKK). Ann Oncol 2000;11: 123–126.
47. Weide R, Heymanns J, Koppler H. Induction of complete haematological remission after monotherapy with anti-CD20 monoclonal antibody (RITUXIMAB) in a patient with alkylating agent resistant Waldenstrom's macroglobulinaemia. Leuk Lymphoma 1999;36:203–206.
48. Treon SP, Raje N, Anderson KC. Immunotherapeutic strategies for the treatment of plasma cell malignancies. Semin Oncol 2000;27:598–613.
49. Treon SP, Shima Y, Preffer FI et al. Treatment of plasma cell dyscrasias by antibody-mediated immunotherapy. Semin Oncol 1999;26:97–106.
50. Byrd JC, White CA, Link B et al. Rituximab therapy in Waldenstrom's macroglobulinemia: preliminary evidence of clinical activity. Ann Oncol 1999;10:1525–1527.
51. Foran JM, Rohatiner AZ, Cunningham D et al. European phase II study of rituximab (chimeric anti-CD20 monoclonal antibody) for patients with newly diagnosed mantle-cell lymphoma and previously treated mantle-cell lymphoma, immunocytoma, and small B-cell lymphocytic lymphoma. J Clin Oncol 2000;18:317–324.
52. Treon SP, Shima Y, Grossbard ML et al. Treatment of multiple myeloma by antibody mediated immunotherapy and induction of myeloma selective antigens. Ann Oncol 2000;11:107–111.
53. Veerman AJP, Nuijens JH, Van der Schoot CE et al. Rituximab in the treatment of childhood B-ALL and Burkitt's lymphoma, report on three cases. Blood 1999;94[suppl 1]:296b.
54. Barrett JC, Linn CA, Arani RB et al. A pilot study of anti-CD20 MoAb rituximab in AIDS-associated non-Hodgkin's lymphoma. Blood 1999;94[suppl 1]:258b.
55. Raizer JJ, Lisa DM, Zelenetz AD et al. Activity of rituximab in primary central nervous system lymphoma. Proc ASCO 2000;19:166a.
56. Lucas JB, Hoppe R, Clark B et al. Rituximab therapy of lymphocyte predominance Hodgkin's disease. Proc AACR 2000;41:760.
57. Cook RC, Connors JM, Gascoyne RD et al. Treatment of post-transplant lymphoproliferative disease with rituximab monoclonal antibody after lung transplantation. Lancet 1999;354:1698–1699.
58. Faye A, Van Den Abeele T, Peuchmaur M et al. Anti-CD20 monoclonal antibody for post-transplant lymphoproliferative disorders. Lancet 1998;352:1285.
59. Ifthikharuddin JJ, Mieles LA, Rosenblatt JD et al. CD-20 expression in post-transplant lymphoproliferative disorders: treatment with rituximab. Am J Hematol 2000;65:171–173.
60. McGuirk JP, Seropian S, Howe G et al. Use of rituximab and irradiated donor-derived lymphocytes to control Epstein-Barr virus-associated lymphoproliferation in patients undergoing related haplo-identical stem cell transplantation. Bone Marrow Transplant 1999;24:1253–1258.

61. Milpied N, Vasseur B, Parquet N et al. Humanized anti-CD20 monoclonal antibody (rituximab) in post transplant B-lymphoproliferative disorder: a retrospective analysis on 32 patients. Ann Oncol 2000;11:113–116.
62. Oertel SH, Anagnostopoulos I, Bechstein WO et al. Treatment of posttransplant lymphoproliferative disorder with the anti-CD20 monoclonal antibody rituximab alone in an adult after liver transplantation: a new drug in therapy of patients with posttransplant lymphoproliferative disorder after solid organ transplantation? Transplantation 2000;69:430–432.
63. Zompi S, Tulliez M, Conti F et al. Rituximab (anti-CD20 monoclonal antibody) for the treatment of patients with clonal lymphoproliferative disorders after orthotopic liver transplantation: a report of three cases. J Hepatol 2000;32:521–527.
64. Buckstein R, Imrie K, Spaner D et al. Stem cell function and engraftment is not affected by "in vivo purging" with rituximab for autologous stem cell treatment for patients with low-grade non-Hodgkin's lymphoma. Semin Oncol 1999;26:115–122.
65. Magni M, Di Nicola M, Devizzi L et al. Successful in vivo purging of CD34-containing peripheral blood harvests in mantle cell and indolent lymphoma: evidence for a role of both chemotherapy and rituximab infusion. Blood 2000;96:864–869.
66. Voso MT, Pantel G, Weis M et al. In vivo depletion of B cells using a combination of high-dose cytosine arabinoside/mitoxantrone and rituximab for autografting in patients with non-Hodgkin's lymphoma. Br J Haematol 2000;109:729–735.
67. Venugopal P, Sivaraman S, Huang XK et al. Effects of cytokines on CD20 antigen expression on tumor cells from patients with chronic lymphocytic leukemia. Leuk Res 2000;24:411–415.
68. Sivaraman S, Venugopal P, Ranganathan R et al. Effect of interferon-alpha on CD20 antigen expression of B-cell chronic lymphocytic leukemia. Cytokines Cell Mol Ther 2000;6:81–87.
69. Davis TA, Maloney DG, Grillo-Lopez AJ et al. Combination immunotherapy of relapsed or refractory low-grade or follicular non-Hodgkin's lymphoma with rituximab and interferon-alpha-2a. Clin Cancer Res 2000;6:2644–2652.
70. Kimby E, Geisler C, Hagberg H et al. Rituximab as single agent and in combination with interferon-alpha 2a as treatment of untreated and first relapse follicular or other low-grade lymphomas: a randomized phase II study M 39035. Blood 2000;96:577a.
71. Van der Kolk LE, Grillo-Lopez AJ, Baars JW et al. Treatment of relapsed B-cell non-Hodgkin's lymphoma with a combination of chimeric anti-CD20 monoclonal antibodies (rituximab) and G-CSF: final report on safety and efficacy. Blood 2000;96:732a.
72. Ottonello L, Morone P, Dapino P et al. Monoclonal Lym-1 antibody-dependent lysis of B-lymphoblastoid tumor targets by human complement and cytokinine-exposed mononuclear and neutrophilic polymorphonuclear leukocytes. Blood 1996;87:5171–5178.
73. Ansell SM, Witzi TE, Kurtin PJ et al. Phase I study of IL-12 in combination with rituximab in patients with B cell non-Hodgkin's lymphoma (NHL). Blood 2000;96:577a.
74. Friedberg JW, Neuberg D, Gribben JG et al. Phase II study of combination immunotherapy with interleukin2 (IL-2) and rituximab in patients with relapsed or refractory follicular non-Hodgkin's lymphoma. Blood 2000;96:730a.
75. McLaughlin P, Hagemeister FG, Rodriguez MA et al. Safety of fludarabine, mitoxantrone, and dexamethasone combined with rituximab in the treatment of stage IV indolent lymphoma. Semin Oncol 2000;27(suppl 12):37–41.
76. Cabanillas F, McLaughlin P, Hagemeister F et al. Molecular responses with FND plus rituximab chemoimmunotherapy for stage IV indolent follicular non-Hodgkin's lymphoma. Blood 2000;96:331a.
77. Czuczman M, Fallon A, Scarpace A et al. Phase II study of rituximab in combination with fludarabine in patients with low-grade or follicular B-cell lymphoma. Blood 2000;96:729a.

78. Keating MJ, O'Brien S, Lerner S et al. Combination chemo-antibody therapy with fludarabine, cyclophosphamide, and rituximab achieves a high CR rate in previously untreated chronic lymphocytic leukemia. Blood 2000;96:514a.
79. Vose JM, Link BK, Grossbard ML et al. Phase II study of rituximab in combination with CHOP chemotherapy in patients with previously untreated, aggressive non-Hodgkin's lymphoma. J Clin Oncol 2001;19:389–397.
80. Howard O, Gribben J, Neuberg D, et al. Rituxan/CHOP induction therapy in newly diagnosed patients with mantle cell lymphoma. Blood 1999;94:631a.
81. Romaguera JE, Dang NH, Hagemeister F et al. Preliminary report of rituximab with intensive chemotherapy for untreated aggressive mantle cell lymphoma. Blood 2000;96:733a.
82. Feuring-Buske M, Kneba M, Unterhalt M et al. IDEC-C2B8 (rituximab) anti-CD20 antibody treatment in relapsed advanced-stage follicular lymphomas: results of a phase-II study of the German Low-Grade Lymphoma Study Group. Ann Hematol 2000;79:493–500.
83. Foran JM, Gupta RK, Cunningham D et al. A UK multicentre phase II study of rituximab (chimaeric anti-CD20 monoclonal antibody) in patients with follicular lymphoma, with PCR monitoring of molecular response. Br J Haematol 2000;109:81–88.

Graft versus Tumor Reactions: Mobilizing Allografting as a Treatment for Cancer

Bimalangshu R. Dey

Thomas R. Spitzer

Allogeneic hematopoietic stem cell transplantation (allo-HSCT) has been increasingly used for the treatment of various malignancies ranging from leukemias, lymphomas, and multiple myeloma to breast cancer. However, the full therapeutic (curative) potential of allo-HSCT is limited, mainly because of a high relapse rate and graft-versus-host disease (GVHD). Considerable clinical data clearly indicate that residual disease is often seen after the high-dose preparative regimen, the eradication of which is left to the immunocompetent cells contained in the graft. This immunologic component, which is an important part of the cure mediated by allo-HSCT, arises from a graft-versus-host reaction (GVHR) and is known as graft-versus-leukemia (GVL) or, more broadly, graft-versus-tumor (GVT) effect. Further intensification of the transplantation conditioning regimen in order to reduce the relapse rate results in increased morbidity and mortality. Consequently, the manipulation of GVT responses is being extensively explored as an alternative strategy both to prevent and to treat post-transplantation relapse.

In their original report of the treatment of murine leukemia by HSCT in 1956, Barnes et al[1] suggested that a reaction of the engrafted marrow against the leukemia might be required for elimination of the disease. Initially, indirect evidence for the existence of a GVT effect in humans was demonstrated from retrospective analyses of the risk of leukemia recurrence after human leukocyte antigen (HLA)–matched related donor allo-HSCT.[2] The role of donor-derived immune response on the GVT effect was subsequently better appreciated by the observation that patients with leukemia receiving T-cell–depleted (TCD) marrow transplantation designed to prevent GVHD had a significantly increased risk of posttransplantation relapse. GVL activity occurs in patients with myeloid[3] and lymphoid leukemias,[4] and analogous GVT responses have been observed in patients with other malignancies, such as multiple myeloma,[5,6] renal cell carcinoma,[7] and breast cancer.[8] The most striking and direct evidence supporting the concept of GVL/GVT came first from Kolb et al,[9] who showed that patients with chronic myelogenous leukemia (CML) in relapse after allo-HSCT could achieve a complete remission by simply infusing donor leukocytes. This has opened up an avenue for the clinical use of adoptive cellular immunotherapy with donor leukocyte infusion (DLI) for preventing or treating leukemic recurrence after allo-HSCT.

Although the association between GVHD and reduced incidence of leukemic relapse, that is, the GVL effect, is well established, the precise relationship between these two entities remains controversial. Studies in animal models and, subsequently, clinical experience have shown that the antileukemic response is achievable in the absence of GVHD, suggesting that the GVL effect and GVHD may be, at least partly, separable. This has now become a major challenge and the focus of intensive investigation, both in basic and clinical research arenas, to separate the beneficial GVL/GVT effect from the detrimental manifestations of GVHD.

In this chapter, we briefly summarize the GVT response in animal models; review the clinical trials for the existence of a GVL effect in clinical HSCT; analyze the therapeutic impact, that is, GVT response after DLI for various malignancies; describe the possible mechanisms of the GVT effect and elaborate on attempts to induce or enhance the GVL effect; and discuss nonmyeloablative approaches to allografting as a way to maximize the GVT effects while reducing transplantation-related toxicity. Although stimulation of effector cells after autologous HSCT (i.e., induction of "autologous" GVHD) is being explored by several investigators, the role of this strategy remains to be determined and is not discussed in this chapter.

PRECLINICAL MODELS OF GVT RESPONSES

About 46 years ago, Barnes and Loutit[10] proposed that allogeneic marrow infused into leukemic mice has antileukemic reactivity and contributes to cure of leukemia. In their studies,[1,10] lethally irradiated leukemic mice were transplanted with normal syngeneic or allogeneic marrow. Recipients of syngeneic marrow died of recurrent leukemia, whereas those receiving histoincompatible marrow survived for longer periods but ultimately died of GVHD and wasting without evidence of leukemia. Years later, Boranic et al[11,12] coined the term *graft-versus-leukemia* to describe the adoptive immunotherapeutic effect of transplanted immunocompetent cells against leukemia. This principle has been confirmed in multiple animal models with transplantable tumors.[11,13,14] It has also been shown subsequently that alloimmunization is capable of inducing a GVL effect without enhancing GVHD, suggesting that GVL effects and GVHD can be functionally separated.[15-20]

IMPORTANT LESSONS FROM CLINICAL OBSERVATION

Mathe et al[21] rationalized early efforts of marrow transplantation by invoking a GVL reaction and suggested that one might exploit the GVHR against the tumor but then control the GVHD and save the cured host. It was not possible, however, to separate the curative impact of total body irradiation from the reaction of the graft against leukemic cells. The real evidence for a GVT effect in human HSCT has been derived mostly from retrospective statistical analyses of the risk of leukemia relapse after HLA-matched HSCT. The important lessons obtained from these observational studies not only provide crucial clinical evidence for the GVL (GVT) effect but also suggest potential mechanisms of GVT reactivity.

Relapse in Syngeneic HSCT vs Allogeneic HSCT

In an updated analysis from the Seattle bone marrow transplantation (BMT) program, it was shown that the rate of leukemic relapse for 785 recipients of HLA-matched sibling HSCT was 62%, compared with 75% in 53 patients receiving syngeneic HSCT ($P < 0.001$).[22] In another multicenter study of HSCT recipients with AML in first remission,[3] the relapse rate in the twins was 59 ± 20%, compared with 18 ± 4% in non-twin siblings. These retrospective analyses from both a single institution[22,23] and the International Bone Marrow Transplant Registry (IBMTR)[2,24,25] strongly suggest that allo-HSCT mediates an important antileukemic effect (Fig. 12.1).

Relapse in Allogeneic Marrow Recipients without GVHD vs. with GVHD

There is now ample evidence that patients who have GVHD after allo-HSCT have a lower rate of relapse than similar patients who do not exhibit GVHD. Multivariate analyses from several reports demonstrate that GVHD is the most significant factor associated with decreased incidence of leukemia relapse and improved survival (Table 12.1).[22,23,26-29] Figure 12.1 presents the probability of relapse as a function of the development of acute or chronic GVHD in patients after allo-HSCT for acute lymphocytic leukemia (ALL) in first remission, acute myelocytic leukemia (AML) in first remission, and CML in a chronic phase.[2] GVHD is also protective against relapse for patients with advanced leukemia.[22,23,39] The apparent antileukemic effect associated with GVHD was suggested to be roughly proportional to the extent of clinically evident GVHD by the observation that patients with subclinical chronic GVHD (i.e., positive blind skin and oral biopsy) have

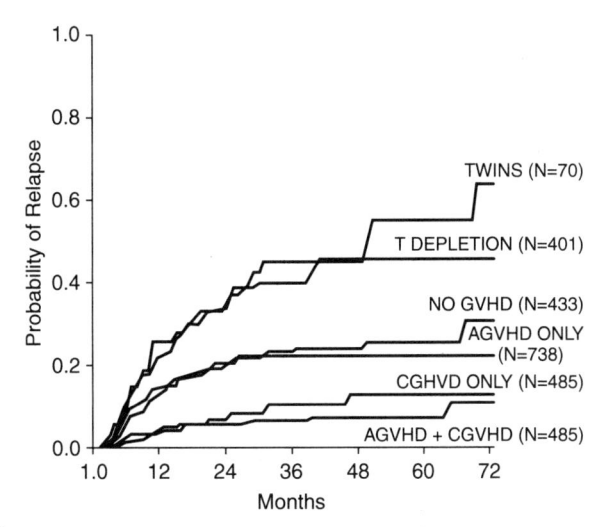

FIGURE 12.1 Actuarial probability of leukemic relapse after bone marrow transplantation for acute lymphocytic leukemia (ALL) in first remission, acute myelocytic leukemia (AML) in first remission, and chronic myelogenous leukemia (CML) in chronic phase as a function of type of graft and development of acute (AGVHD) or chronic (CGVHD) graft-versus-host disease. (Reproduced by permission from Horowitz MM, Gale RP, Sondel PM et al. Graft-versus-leukemia reactions after bone marrow transplantation. Blood 1990;75:555-562.)

a twofold higher relapse rate than patients with both clinical and histologic manifestations of GVHD.[30] However, attempts to harness the GVHR and enhance the beneficial GVT response by either reducing the intensity of GVHD prophylaxis or infusing buffy coat cells immediately after allo-HSCT were unable to manipulate GVL to a clinical advantage.[31] The relapse rate was unchanged, and there was substantial mortality resulting from transplantation-related toxicity and GVHD.

Association Between GVHD Flare or Cessation of Immunosuppression and Disease Remission

There have been case reports in which recurrent leukemia after allo-HSCT went into remission after a flare of clinically evident GVHD.[32] A similar observation was made when patients with AML,[33] ALL,[34] CML,[35] and chronic lymphocytic leukemia (CLL)[4,36] had a relapse after allografting and achieved a complete remission after discontinuation of immunosuppression. These reports provide the rationale for withdrawal of GVHD prophylaxis to induce a GVT response in patients who have recurrent disease after HSCT, although experience has shown that either the remission is very short-lived or most patients will not achieve remission.

TABLE 12.1 GVHD is Associated with a Reduced Relative Risk (RR) of Leukemic Relapse After Allogeneic SCT

Study Group	ALL in 1st CR RR	ALL in 1st CR P	AML in 1st CR RR	AML in 1st CR P	CML in CP RR	CML in CP P	All Patients RR	All Patients P
Allogeneic, non–T-cell depleted								
No GVHD	1.00	—	1.00	—	1.00	—	1.00	—
Acute GVHD only	0.36	0.004	0.78	0.26	1.15	0.75	0.68	0.03
Chronic GVHD only	0.44	0.16	0.48	0.12	0.28	0.16	0.43	0.01
Acute and chronic GVHD	0.38	0.02	0.34	0.0003	0.24	0.03	0.33	0.0001
Syngeneic SCT	0.99	0.99	2.58	0.008	2.95	0.08	2.09	0.005
Allogeneic, T-cell depleted								
No GVHD	1.48	0.33	1.57	0.12	6.91	0.0001	2.14	0.0001
Acute and/or Chronic GVHD	0.98	0.97	0.80	0.60	4.45	0.003	1.32	0.25

ALL, acute lymphocytic leukemia; AML, acute myelocytic leukemia; CML, chronic myelogenous leukemia; GVDH, graft-versus-host disease; SCT, stem cell transplantation.
Reproduced with permission from reference 2.

Relapse in Recipients of T-Cell-Depleted Allogeneic HSCT vs. Unmodified HSCT

Immune-competent cells (T and non-T cells) contained in the donor graft are instrumental in the pathogenesis of GVHD. Ex vivo T-cell depletion of the donor graft successfully reduces the incidence and severity of acute GVHD after HSCT,[37-41] but this approach is associated with an increased risk of leukemia relapse and engraftment failure.[39,42-45] This observation provides strong, albeit indirect, evidence that the reaction of donor T cells against normal host cells that results in GVHD might also induce a GVT effect. In patients with CML in chronic phase, Goldman et al[43] demonstrated that the posttransplantation leukemic relapse was 10% in recipients of unmodified (non–T-cell depleted) marrow who had moderate-to-severe GVHD, compared with 50% in recipients of TCD marrow who had no or mild GVHD. A similar loss of GVT effect was experienced when patients with accelerated-phase CML underwent transplantation with TCD marrow.[46]

GVT Effects Independent of Clinical GVHD

Earlier studies suggested that GVHD and GVL effects are tightly linked and that GVHD is likely a prerequisite for a GVL response.[22] However, IBMTR analysis of patients with AML and ALL in first remission and chronic-phase CML noted that recipients of allogeneic marrow in whom clinical GVHD did not develop had lower rates of leukemia relapse than recipients of syngeneic marrow,[25] suggesting that allogeneic marrow can induce a GVT response that is independent of clinical GVHD. An updated analysis of these data showed that recipients of TCD marrow had an increased rate of relapse even after adjustment for GVHD, suggesting an additional antileukemia effect independent of GVHD.[2] Patients with CML who developed GVHD after a TCD marrow transplantation had a substantially higher risk of relapse than patients who received non-TCD marrow and did not develop GVHD. These results indicate that a GVT effect can occur in the absence of GVHD, that is, GVHD and GVT response may be separable.

ADOPTIVE CELLULAR IMMUNOTHERAPY VIA DONOR LEUKOCYTE INFUSIONS

Relapse after allo-HSCT remains a major cause of treatment failure. The important clinical observations that suggested strong but indirect evidence for a GVT response in allo-HSCT also provided the basis for the development of rational approaches to manipulate and enhance the GVT response for therapeutic purposes, and hence the introduction of adoptive cellular immunotherapy, in other words, DLIs for the management of recurrent leukemia after allo-HSCT.

The most striking and direct evidence that allogeneic immune-competent cells can induce a GVT response in human malignancies came first from Kolb et al,[47] who demonstrated that three patients with relapsed CML achieved complete cytogenetic remission after treatment with interferon-α and buffy coat cells obtained by leukapheresis from the original donor. These preliminary results have been confirmed in several larger trials.[9,48-52] Updated results from the European Group for Blood and Marrow Transplantation (EBMT)[53,54] regarding their use of DLI in patients with relapsed leukemia after allo-HSCT are summarized in Table 12.2. Although the details of the treatment protocols vary slightly between institutions, the results have been highly consistent. Eighty percent of patients with relapsed CML achieved complete cytogenetic and molecular remissions when treated in early relapse (*Bcr/Abl* positive or Philadelphia chromosome positive) or in hematologic relapse (chronic phase). The response in patients with more advanced CML (accelerated or blastic phase) was less dramatic. Intermediate response rates were seen in patients with AML, myelodysplastic syndrome, and multiple myeloma, and poor results were noted in patients with ALL. It is possible that in more advanced, rapidly progressive leukemias, insufficient time was available for the antitumor effects of the DLI to be realized. Disease-free survival in those patients who achieve complete remission after DLI was favorable (Fig. 12.2). For example, disease-free survival of CML patients in cytogenetic relapse could be as high as 80% at 5 years.

Complications of DLI

Adoptive immunotherapy with DLI has been associated with significant GVHD and marrow aplasia. Almost 60% of evaluable patients have experienced acute GVHD and 61% have had chronic GVHD, with 22% of patients experiencing grade III to IV acute GVHD and 32% extensive chronic GVHD.[53] Although the toxicity from GVHD may be significant, it has generally been mild to moderate and perhaps less severe than one might anticipate considering that the dose of T cells administered has been up to 10 times higher than that typically contained in an unmodified allogeneic marrow graft and that it was administered without the use of GVHD prophylaxis. Moreover, the DLI-associated GVHD has typically responded to immunosuppressive therapy. The other major complication of DLI has been marrow aplasia, noted in 20% of patients, often requiring transfusions and associated with bleeding and infectious complications. Myelosuppression has been observed in patients with predominantly host-type hematopoiesis. In hematologic relapse of CML myeloid cells are either a mixture of host- and donor-derived cells or host-type exclusively.[47,55] It is possible that during the conversion to complete donor chimerism as a result of a host-reactive donor T-cell response, these donor immune cells also ablate the host hematopoiesis in a time period when donor stem cells are inadequate to allow recovery of normal hematopoiesis. This is probably best explained by a phenomenon observed in transfusion-associated GVHD.[56] This hypothesis is supported by the observation that patients in an early relapse of CML (cytogenetic or molecular relapse) rarely experience pancytopenia after DLI, because hematopoiesis is predominantly of donor-type

TABLE 12.2 Graft-Versus-Tumor Effect of Donor Leukocyte Infusion

Study	Diagnosis	No. of Patients Studied	Evaluable[a]	Complete Remission No. (%)
Kolb et al[9]	CML			
	Cytogenetic relapse	57	50	40 (80)
	Hematologic relapse	124	114	88 (77)
	Transformed phase relapse	42	36	13 (36)
	AML/MDS	97	59	15 (25)
	ALL	55	18	2 (11)
	Multiple myeloma	25	17	5 (29)
Collins et al[53]	CML			
	Cytogenetic relapse	3	3	3 (100)
	Hematologic relapse	35	34	25 (73.5)
	Transformed phase relapse	18	18	5 (27.7)
	AML/MDS	52	44	8 (18)
	ALL	15	11	2 (18)
	Multiple myeloma	5	4	2 (50)

ALL, acute lymphocytic leukemia; AML, acute myelocytic leukemia; CML, chronic myelogenous leukemia; DLI, donor leukocyte infusion; MDS, myelodysplastic syndrome.
[a] Patients surviving less than 30 days after DLI were excluded by Kolb et al. but included by Collins et al in the response calculation

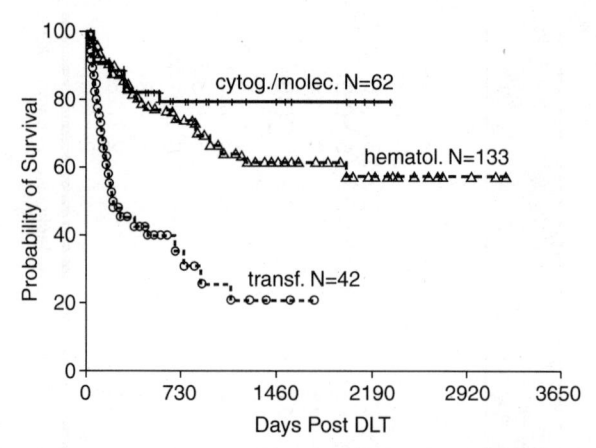

FIGURE 12.2 Survival of patients treated with donor leukocyte infusions for recurrent chronic myelogenous leukemia (CML) after allogeneic bone marrow transplantation. Cytog./molec., cytogenetic and molecular relapse; hematol., hematologic relapse; transf., relapse in transformed phase of CML. Data from the European Group for Blood and Marrow Transplantation as of February 1999. (Reproduced by permission from American Society of Hematology. Kolb H. Allogeneic Stem Cell Transplantation for CML: Update of Results and New Strategies. American Society of Hematology Education Program Book. Washington DC: American Society of Hematology, 1999:159–168.)

cells.[9] Marrow aplasia can occasionally be prolonged, but hematopoietic function can be successfully restored with the infusion of additional donor stem cells without further conditioning.[9,48,50] The complications of DLI have resulted in a treatment-related mortality rate of approximately 20%, which is quite high but compares favorably with the anticipated mortality rate of 40% or higher associated with a second HSCT.[57] The mortality rate from DLI-associated GVHD has been 5% to 8%,[53,58] and another 7% to 12% of patients have died from infectious complications, either related to marrow aplasia or to immunosuppressive therapy for GVHD.

Association of GVHD with Disease Response

Acute and chronic GVHD post-DLIs are highly correlated with disease remission[9,53] (Table 12.1). In the EBMT study, there was a close association of the GVT response with either GVHD or myelosuppression, or both. CML patients with any evidence of GVHD, marrow aplasia, or both had a high rate of complete remission (42 patients of 46, 91%). In the North American survey, in almost all complete responders, acute or chronic GVHD developed. However, 13 of 29 (45%) CML patients in the EBMT group and three of 23 patients in the North American group entered complete remission without experiencing clinical GVHD, suggesting that in some cases, a GVT response independent of GVHD can be attained with DLI.

T-Cell Dose

The appropriate cell dose for DLI for optimal immunotherapeutic effect remains an unresolved issue. The mean cell dose was noted to be approximately 4×10^8 mononuclear cells/kg, the range being 0.25 to 16.4×10^8 in most reports.[9,53] A recent clinical trial studying the effect of DLI in patients with relapsed multiple myeloma demonstrated that a T-cell dose of more than 1×10^8 cells/kg was correlated with the response.[6] It is possible that responses may occur at a lower cell dose. CML in cytogenetic relapse may respond to a T-cell dose as low as 1.0×10^7 cell/kg,[59] whereas other CML patients may require a T-cell dose as high as 5×10^8 cells/kg. The T-cell dose in DLI using mismatched family members or unrelated donors raises a special issue. Several studies have suggested that infusion from these donors of cell doses comparable to the doses used in HLA-matched sibling donors may cause fatal GVHD, mainly because of HLA disparity.[47,51,53] Thus, additional strategies are required to best determine the safe doses of DLI when the clinician is faced with an HLA disparity.

Timing of Chimerism Conversion and Anti-Tumor Response

The GVT effect may develop within 4 weeks after DLI, but the cytogenetic and molecular remission may not occur until several months after intervention.[9,51] In one report, the time to documentation of complete remission varied from 28 to 241 days, with a median time of 85 days.[53] In a recent study, it was demonstrated that the time for clonal expansion of infused donor immune cells may vary according to the host tumor burden and donor T-cell repertoire and that a critical effector/target ratio of T cells has to be reached before an overwhelming GVT response can take place.[55] This critical time period can be as short as 5 weeks in patients with CML in cytogenetic relapse or as long as 13 weeks in hematologic relapse.[55]

Factors that May Predict a Response

Several investigators have attempted to determine the characteristics that would predict a positive response to DLI, and they are (1) the pre-DLI status of the disease, for example, in patients with relapsed CML, early relapse as opposed to advanced disease[9,53]; (2) time interval between original HSCT to DLI of less than 2 years[53]; (3) TCD marrow grafting and lack of GVHD with the original transplant[9]; (4) presence of more than 40% donor-type T cells in the patients at the time of DLI [60]; and (5) T-cell dose in DLI of more than 1×10^8 cells/kg.[6]

SEPARATION OF GVT EFFECT FROM GVHD: STRATEGIES TO PREVENT GVHD WHILE PRESERVING THE GVT EFFECT

A fundamental question in HSCT is how to maximize the GVT effect in the post-HSCT period when tumor load has been minimized by the conditioning therapies and residual tumor eradication is left to the host-reactive donor immune response, while minimizing the deleterious effects of GVHD. In a series of studies in AKR mice bearing a syngeneic transplanted lymphocytic leukemia, Bortin et al[15] were among the first to demonstrate that GVH and GVT reactivity could be separated with the use of H-2 compatible and incompatible allogeneic donors of different strains. By selective alloimmunization to minor histocompatibility antigens (mHags), they were able to achieve GVT response in major histocompatibility complex (MHC)–matched allo-HSCT in mice without increasing the rate of GVHD-related mortality.[16] Although the precise mechanism of this selective GVT response was unclear, the primary GVT effector cells in this murine model were later characterized as CD8+ T cells reactive against host mHags.[61] In a fully MHC-mismatched murine BMT model, Sykes et al[18] showed that a course of interleukin-2 (IL-2) inhibited CD4-dependent GVHD, whereas CD8-mediated GVT effect against EL4 leukemia/lymphoma was well-preserved. In a similar model, they recently also demonstrated that mice treated with a single dose of IL-12 on the day of allo-HSCT from MHC-mismatched donors could be cured of leukemia, whereas GVHD was markedly abrogated.[20,62] These experimental results clearly indicate that GVHD and GVT effects are functionally separable.

In human allo-HSCT, the GVT response is often associated with the development of GVHD. It is possible that GVHD and GVT effects are governed by overlapping, but not identical, subsets of donor lymphocytes. The presence of GVHD does not always ensure a GVT response, and the lack of clinically evident GVHD does not indicate the absence of a GVT effect. Furthermore, the treatment of patients with DLI for relapsed hematologic malignancies (acute or chronic leukemia, multiple myeloma) after allo-HSCT has made it clear that there are patients who enter remission without clinical GVHD, suggesting that a separation of GVHD from GVT effects is also possible in humans. GVH-associated GVT response is found more commonly in patients with ALL than in patients with CML or AML, but GVT reactivity without evidence of GVHD appears to be greater in CML and AML than in ALL.[2,63]

Lower T-Cell Dose

Several strategies to prevent GVHD without losing the GVT effect have been developed in clinical HSCT. One approach is to administer lower doses of donor mononuclear cells (MNCs) in hopes of retaining the GVT effect while minimizing GVHD. Two groups of investigators suggest that in recipients of TCD transplants,[59] and also in recipients of unmodified marrow,[64] one can start with a small dose of CD3+ T cells, then increase the T-cell dose in stepwise fashion until the disease responds or GVHD develops. In many patients, there might be a "threshold" under which a GVT response occurs without clinical GVHD. For example, in a patient with CML in cytogenetic relapse after allo-HSCT, a particular cell dose may be high enough to induce a GVL effect yet low enough not to cause significant

GVHD. In patients in cytogenetic relapse of CML, remission can be induced with as low a mononuclear cell dose as 0.1 to 0.3 × 10^8 cells/kg.[9,59]

Selective Depletion of Donor T Cells

In another effort, donor mononuclear cells depleted of CD8+ T cells and administered to patients with relapsed CML were shown to mediate effective GVT effect with minimal GVHD.[65-67] In contrast, however, a recent study using CD4+ T-cell DLI revealed that all patients with response had GVHD.[68] Another novel method for the treatment of GVHD while exploiting the power of the GVT effect is the insertion of a "suicide" gene (thymidine kinase gene from herpes simplex virus: *HSV-TK* gene) into the genome of donor lymphocytes by retroviral transduction before allo-HSCT.[69-71] The activated lymphocytes transduced with *HSV-TK* gene can be killed by treatment with ganciclovir. Ideally, the transduced lymphocytes first eradicate the tumor, then are destroyed by treatment with ganciclovir if the patients show evidence of GVHD. Although pilot studies in patients with relapsed CML are promising, each of these elegant strategies is preliminary, and the effect of these manipulations on the overall GVT reactivity and the duration of clinical response must await further confirmatory trials.

Delayed DLI

GVHD can be considered an exaggerated manifestation of a normal inflammatory mechanism in which a host-reactive donor T-cell response occurs in a proinflammatory state marked by higher levels of cytokines, adhesion molecules, and MHC antigens, induced mainly by the toxic effects of conditioning regimen.[72,73] In murine BMT models, a mixed chimeric state, that is, the coexistence of both donor and host-derived lymphohematopoietic cells, can be achieved after TCD allo-HSCT. Sykes et al[74] and Pelot et al[75] demonstrated that when nontolerant DLIs are given to these mixed chimeras several months after BMT, they convert to full donor-type chimeras as a result of lymphohematopoietic GVHRs, but GVHD does not occur. Johnson et al[19] showed that delayed infusions of donor leukocytes can have a powerful antileukemic effect in mice without causing GVHD. In dogs, allogeneic lymphocytes can be safely administered to mixed chimeras 2 months after conditioning and BMT, with the resultant conversion to full donor chimerism in the absence of GVHD.[76,77] The strategy of "prophylactic" delayed DLI is being tried in several clinical trials, in which incremental lymphocyte infusions are given to patients after TCD allo-HSCT for hematologic malignancies.[78-80] Unlike in animal models, infusions of donor lymphocytes led to an increase in acute GVHD, and there was no statistically significant impact on leukemia-free survival (LFS).[78,79] Although it is difficult to draw conclusions on the basis of the mixed outcomes from these studies, their results have confirmed that the timing and the dose of DLI are instrumental in the induction of GVHD.[80] This also provides an opportunity to refine our thinking about the pathophysiology of GVHD in humans because by delaying DLI, the resultant GVHD can be studied in the absence of toxicity associated with the conditioning regimen.

STRATEGIES TO AUGMENT THE GVT EFFECT

Strategies have been designed to augment GVHD in an effort to enhance the GVT effect by reducing or withholding GVHD prophylaxis at the time of allogeneic stem cell transplantation or by administering DLI early after transplantation. Sixteen leukemic patients underwent HLA-matched sibling donor HSCT without posttransplantation immunosuppression.[81] The incidences of acute and hyperacute GVHD and GVHD-related mortality were extremely high in these patients, without a detectable impact on the LFS. In another approach, patients were given buffy coat cells from the marrow donors within 11 days after HSCT in an attempt to reduce the rate of posttransplantation leukemic relapse.[31] Severe GVHD increased from 25% in the control group who did not receive early DLI after transplantation to 82% in the treatment group. There was no significant reduction in leukemic relapse, mainly because of the very high rates of fatal GVHD. Because IL-2 stimulates both T and natural killer (NK) cells and it is also known to be one of many critical cytokines involved in the effector functions of a GVT response, investigators have attempted to use IL-2 in leukemic patients undergoing TCD marrow transplants in order to reduce the risk of relapse.[82] Patients treated with IL-2 were those who had no evidence of clinical GVHD after GVHD prophylaxis was stopped. Initial reports suggested that IL-2–treated patients had a lower incidence of leukemic relapse than similar patients who did not receive IL-2. The mean number of circulating NK cells in the IL-2–treated patients was increased 10-fold without any remarkable change in T-cell number, and the incidence of GVHD was essentially unaffected by IL-2 treatment.[82] Although the initial results appear promising, the optimal dose and timing of IL-2 administration need to be defined in further studies. Slavin et al[52] described five patients who failed to respond to DLI administered for relapsed leukemia after allogeneic HSCT, but who entered remission when treated with donor lymphocytes plus IL-2. The administration of DLI along with IL-2 at a later time point after allo-HSCT may have the potential to eliminate the residual tumor without inducing GVHD,[19,83] and this merits evaluation in prospective clinical trials.

GVT EFFECT IN DISEASES OTHER THAN CML

Acute Myeloid Leukemia

Both single and multi-institutional studies[2,84,85] have shown that LFS in patients with AML who are treated with allo-HSCT is superior to LFS in those treated with autologous or syngeneic HSCT, illustrating the role of a GVT effect in eliminating AML. Although the rate of remission after the treatment of recurrent

AML with DLI is less impressive when compared with CML in early relapse, occasionally patients achieve durable LFS[9,53] after DLI, indicating that DLI may be modestly effective in the treatment of relapsed AML after HSCT.

Acute Lymphoid Leukemia

The most compelling evidence for a GVL effect in ALL comes from both single-institution and IBMTR data.[2,86] However, the responses to DLI are very rare in patients with recurrent ALL after allo-HSCT.[2,86] In patients with ALL, a GVT response occurs in association with GVHD more commonly than with CML or AML, but a GVT reactivity without the evidence of GVHD appears to be greater in CML and AML than in ALL.[2,63] In one study, the actuarial risk of posttransplantation ALL relapse for patients without significant GVHD approached 80%, compared with 40% for those with grade II or greater GVHD.[87] The results of studies using DLI for patients with relapsed ALL are extremely poor, and durable responses to DLI in ALL patients are uncommon.[9,88] This poor outcome may reflect the inability of ALL cells to present antigens to donor immune cells, a decreased frequency of donor T-cell precursors reactive with minor antigens presented by ALL cells, or an inadequate expression by ALL cells of critical surface molecules, such as adhesion molecules, co-stimulatory molecules, and class I and II MHC molecules.[89-91] It is also likely that patients die from rapid disease progression before GVT effects have a chance to evolve. However, in a recent study, the administration of chemotherapy before DLI failed to improve outcomes in patients with relapsed ALL after transplantation.[88] Alternatively, it is possible that the failure of DLI to eradicate the rapidly expanding malignant clones is simply the result of administering too few T cells that are reactive with antigens expressed by tumor cells. In a murine leukemia model, the infusion of leukemia-reactive T-cell clones completely eliminated the leukemia, whereas the simple infusion of polyclonal lymphocytes not enriched in leukemia-reactive T cells was ineffective against the disease.[92]

Multiple Myeloma

Although a review of the outcomes of allo-HSCT in multiple myeloma from several centers, including the EBMT group, IBMTR,[93-95] the Seattle group,[96,97] the Dana-Farber Cancer Institute,[98,99] and the University of Arkansas,[100] demonstrated that small numbers of the patients are likely cured, a GVT (graft-versus-myeloma) effect in these studies was not clearly identified. Because of the extremely high transplantation-related mortality, it is often difficult to appreciate the curative potential of allo-HSCT for patients with multiple myeloma. However, multiple case reports in some small series have indicated that DLI from the original donors can induce remission in up to 50% of patients with relapsed multiple myeloma after transplantation, demonstrating that a GVT effect does exist in patients with multiple myeloma.[5,53,68,101,102] In a recent larger study,[6] 14 of 27 patients (52%)

receiving DLI for relapsed multiple myeloma after allo-HSCT showed response, including six patients (22%) who achieved a complete remission. Many patients in this study received chemotherapy before DLI. Although most of the responders had GVHD, in six of 14 patients with response to DLI, this occurred without clinical GVHD. The factors that were correlated with response were a T-cell dose of higher than 1×10^8 cells/kg, response to chemotherapy before DLI, and chemotherapy-sensitive disease before allo-HSCT.[6] These data clearly confirm the potential GVT effect of allogeneic immune cells in patients with multiple myeloma.

Chronic Lymphocytic Leukemia

Allogeneic HSCT can lead to durable disease-free survival in 20% to 55% of patients with CLL.[103-107] Although patients with lower tumor burden and chemotherapy-sensitive disease are likely to benefit the most, this approach may also be effective in patients who are heavily pretreated and are resistant to chemotherapy. At the M.D. Anderson Cancer Center, allo-HSCT performed for advanced CLL produced a superior 3-year disease-free survival to that of purged auto-HSCT (57% versus 24%). The difference in LFS likely reflects a GVT response, although tumor contamination may be responsible, at least partly, for the increased relapse risk in the autologous group. Recently, there has been demonstration of this graft-induced antileukemia effect in a patient who achieved complete remission after DLI for relapsed CLL after allo-HSCT.[4]

Lymphoma

The retrospective analyses of many single and multi-institutional studies show that allo-HSCT for patients with most types of NHL is associated with a lower rate of relapse than auto-HSCT.[98,104,105,108-112] These analyses included a few institutions that used ex vivo purged marrow. This trend of improved disease-free survival in patients undergoing allogeneic HSCT was recently confirmed by a prospective study comparing allogeneic with autologous HSCT for the treatment of lymphoma.[110] Allo-HSCT has generally been used for patients with advanced or chemotherapy-resistant lymphoma. The response rates have varied depending on the histologic subtype of lymphoma, with low-grade lymphoma faring the best. In one study, the rate of progression-free survival at 2 years in patients with advanced low-grade lymphoma was 68% in the allotransplantation group and 22% in the autologous transplantation group. However, there was no statistically significant difference in the overall survival because of the very high treatment-related mortality in the allograft group. Similarly, relapse rates for patients with intermediate- or high-grade lymphoma are lower after allotransplantation.[109] A graft-versus-lymphoma effect is likely playing a role in the reduced rate of relapse in patients who undergo transplantation with an allograft. The strong evidence for a GVT effect in patients with lymphoma came from a recent study in which six of nine patients achieved remission of their recurrent lymphoma after treatment with DLI or withdrawal of GVHD immunoprophylaxis.[113] One study demonstrated a strong correlation between the incidence of GVHD and the GVT response,[109] whereas other studies found no such association.[114] Although allografting and DLI have been confirmed to have a GVT effect, the general application of these approaches to the treatment of lymphoma has been questioned because of the poor results in some series, especially in patients with intermediate- and high-grade lymphoma; these results have mainly been due to a very high treatment-related mortality and relapse.

The outcomes of allo-HSCT in patients with Hodgkin's disease have thus far been very disappointing. Retrospective studies from both single and multi-institutional groups[115,116] have shown a less than 20% survival after allografting for advanced Hodgkin's disease and have failed to demonstrate any advantage over autologous HSCT. In contrast, two groups were able to show lower rates of relapse in patients receiving an allograft than in patients undergoing autologous or syngeneic HSCT.[98,117] However, most reports have not demonstrated the presence of a significant GVT response in patients with Hodgkin's lymphoma; these results could be due, at least in part, to the very high treatment-related mortality associated with myeloablative conditioning regimens. Alternative strategies, such as nonmyeloablative chemotherapy and allo-HSCT followed by DLI, need to be evaluated, with the aim of increasing the response rate while reducing transplantation-related toxicity.

Solid Malignancies

Recently, Childs et al[7] were able to show GVT effects in patients with metastatic renal cell cancer who underwent nonmyeloablative allogeneic peripheral blood stem cell transplantation. In 10 of 19 patients, metastatic disease regressed; seven had a partial response, and three had a complete response that was durable. The GVT response was mostly notable after the withdrawal of GVHD prophylaxis and the establishment of complete donor T-cell chimerism. In most cases, the response was associated with clinically evident GVHD. Although the response rate was not overly impressive, it clearly demonstrated a GVT effect in the treatment of solid malignancy and thus deserves serious consideration for further clinical application. Some case reports have suggested that a similar immune-mediated anti-tumor response can be achieved with allo-HSCT in patients with metastatic breast[8] and ovarian cancers.[118] However, clinical experience on a larger scale will be required to determine the overall clinical efficacy of GVT effects in patients with solid malignancies.

MECHANISM OF THE GRAFT-VERSUS-TUMOR RESPONSE

For a GVT response to occur, the presence of functional effector cells within the marrow/peripheral blood stem cell graft, as well as tumor cells susceptible to the effector cells, is required. "Allospecific" effector cells recognize antigens expressed by both normal host and neoplastic cells and "tumor-specific" effector cells recognize antigens that are exclusively or preferentially expressed by tumor cells.

Effector Cells and Their Cytokines

T cells are the major mediators of GVT responses, based on the evidence that (1) allo-HSCT with TCD marrow is associated with higher rates of leukemia relapse,[39,43,119] (2) DLI that contain large numbers of T cells can reverse relapse,[6,9,48,53] and (3) human T-cell clones can lyse leukemic cells in vitro.[120-122] CD4+ T cells recognize antigens presented in the context of class II MHC molecules and mediate their effector actions by direct cytolytic activity or through secretion of the Th1 type of cytokines, such as IL-2, which induces clonal expansion of CD8+ cytotoxic T lymphocytes (CTLs) and activates NK cells, and interferon-γ, which up-regulates expression of MHC class I molecules on neoplastic cells. CD8+ T cells recognize antigens in association with class I MHC molecules and mediate their effector activity by a direct cytolytic (CTL) response. Although both CD4+ and CD8+ T cells have been shown to induce GVT response in animal models,[123-126] CD8+ T cells appear to be the proximal T-cell mediators of the GVT reactivity. CD8+ T cells are able to mediate a GVT effect in the absence of CD4+ T cells. CD4+ T cells appear to promote the GVT response primarily by helping CD8+ cells undergo clonal expansion through secretion of IL-2. The relative importance of CD4+ and CD8+ T cells to GVT reactivity depends on the donor-host histoincompatibility and the nature of the target antigens expressed on the neoplastic cells. Thus, donor CD8+ T cells might be the primary mediators of GVT response against tumors expressing class I MHC molecules, and CD4+ T cells might be the mediators against tumors with presentation of MHC class II antigens. $\alpha\beta$TCR+ CD4+ T cell lines isolated from some patients have been generated that can specifically lyse cryopreserved leukemic cells.[120] Falkenburg et[127] showed recently that it is possible to establish both MHC class I– and class II–restricted CTL clones by stimulating the donor cells with irradiated leukemic cells from patients.

Although donor T cells probably dominate GVT responses, studies have also identified NK cells as being involved in antitumor activity[128,129] by MHC-nonrestricted direct cytolysis or through the production of cytokines such as IL-2, tumor necrosis factor-α, and interferon-γ. Studies in mice have confirmed that NK cells from allogeneic mismatched donors have anti-tumor effects without causing GVHD and are well tolerated.[130,131] NK cells are capable of lysing K562, a cell line derived from CML patients that is usually resistant to apoptosis because of *Bcr/Abl* expression,[132] and they are among the earliest cells to reappear after allo-HSCT.[133] Patients with CML who relapsed after allo-HSCT have lower numbers of blood NK cells than patients who remain in remission,[128] and the risk of relapse after allo-HSCT is reduced if NK/lymphokine-activated killer cell cells can induce lysis of autologous CML cells in vitro.[134] IL-2 has been well-known to increase NK cell or lymphokine-activated killer cell activity after marrow grafting, and it can be administered after TCD marrow transplantation without exacerbation of GVHD.[135,136] Various cytokines secreted by T and non-T cells can kill or induce apoptosis of tumor cells, up-regulate antigen expression on tumor cells, or retard their growth through cytostatic mechanisms.

Target Antigens for GVT Response

Three classes of peptides are thought to be present on host neoplastic cells that are required for the donor-derived anti-tumor effect. These include (1) MHC and mHag molecules, present on both normal host and neoplastic cells; (2) cellular proteins present in both normal host and neoplastic cells but overexpressed in the latter; and (3) proteins encoded by mutated genes and expressed exclusively by tumor cells. The first two groups of proteins can be grouped as allospecific and the third one as tumor-specific antigens. Peptides such as mHag molecules have been identified and cloned.[137,138] These minor antigens can be presented either to CD4+ T cells in association with MHC class II molecules or to CD8+ cells in the context of MHC class I molecules. Recently, it has been confirmed that in the setting of HLA-matched donor allo-HSCT, the host-reactive donor immune response that results in GVHD is mainly directed at the donor-host mHag disparity.[139] Some mHags can elicit a strong GVHR by activating CD4+ cells, whereas others induce the immune response by stimulating CD8+ T cells, and there are minor antigens that activate both subsets of T cells. The preferential activation of CD4+ and CD8+ T cells might account for the "immunodominance" of certain minor antigens.[140] In the absence of any tumor-specific antigens, GVT reactivity mediated by donor immune cells is limited to recognition of host alloantigens, either MHC or minor antigens, or both, and as a result, a GVT response would likely be related to GVHD. Because of the existence of distinct but separate mHags in various host tissues and because mHags may be expressed at varying levels in different host tissues, a preferential activation of T-cell subsets may occur that destroys tumor cells, but not those that cause GVHD, thus explaining the observation that a GVT response is possible in the absence of clinically evident GVHD. The reverse could also happen, which would explain why the presence of GVHD, even its most severe form, does not always ensure a GVT response. Some of the mHags are restricted to lymphohematopoietic cells but are absent in nonhematopoietic epithelial cells, such as HA-1 and HA-2, whereas others, like H-Y and HA-3, show a broad tissue distribution.[141,142] Thus, some mHags, such as the HA-2 determinant, can, because their expression is limited to hematopoietic cells, potentially serve as tumor cell targets for donor T cells with minimal risk of GVHD.[143] In patients with relapsed CML after allo-HSCT, although the lymphoid cells are predominantly of donor type, a minority of nonmalignant host T cells persist in a state of mixed T-cell chimerism that disappears in complete remission after DLI,[9,55] suggesting a broader allospecific target than a leukemia-specific target for the GVL effect. There are normal proteins that are overexpressed in tumor cells. HER-2/NEU protein is overexpressed in a proportion of breast and ovarian cancers and has been identified by tumor-specific cytotoxic T lymphocyte lines.[144-146] In melanoma, multiple T-cell lines reactive against tumor-specific antigens have been established, including both HLA class I–restricted CD8+ CTLs and class II–restricted CD4+ CTL clones against various tumor-specific targets. These targets include tyrosinase, gp100, gp75, and MART1, which are associated with melanocyte differentiation,[147-149] and MAGA 1 and 3, which have limited expression in normal tissues.[150-151] For an exclusive GVT response, the tumor cells must express a unique antigen or antigens that are absent in normal tissues and are immunogenic enough to induce an immune response against it. The demonstration that some patients with leukemia enter remission after allo-HSCT or DLI without evidence of GVHD supports the existence of true leukemia-specific antigens,[2,9,53] although alternatively, this may reflect nonspecific effects of subclinical GVHD directed at mHags. For example, fusion proteins resulting from chromosomal translocations, including p210 in *Bcr/Abl+* CML [t(9;22)] and RAR-α in AML-M3 [t(15;17)], could potentially be processed and presented to T cells for a specific immune response. These fusion peptides can bind to both MHC class I and class II molecules and induce specific CTLs.[152-154] Although indirect clinical evidence for leukemia-antigen–specific anti-leukemia reactivity does exist, it has not yet been proved whether such tumor-specific CTL clones are the essential effector cells for the GVT response after allo-HSCT or DLI.

EFFECT OF DONOR-RECIPIENT HISTOCOMPATIBILITY ON GVT RESPONSE

Given the shortage of suitably HLA-matched allogeneic-related bone marrow donors and the increased risk of transplantation-related mortality associated with alternative donor transplants, new strategies are needed to improve the outcomes of transplantations from HLA-mismatched related or HLA-matched unrelated donors. Besides significantly expanding the available donor pool, a potential advantage of successful allogeneic transplantation across HLA barriers is an improved anti-tumor effect, owing to enhanced graft-versus-host alloresponses that also eliminate malignant cells.[50,110,111,155] In general, it appears that with respect to histocompatibility differences between donors other than HLA-matched siblings, there is an increased incidence of acute GVHD, with the risk correlating with the degree of histoincompatibility. However, the overall disease-free survival is not always adversely affected; a GVT effect may counterbalance the increased death rate from GVHD.[156,157] Experience from Seattle and the IBMTR has shown that HSCT performed with the use of either HLA-matched or single-antigen–mismatched related donors is associated with statistically similar survival probabilities,[158,159] probably because the increased risks of graft rejection and GVHD associated with non–HLA-matched donor transplantations are offset by a reduced probability of relapse, likely caused by an increased GVT effect. With the use of HLA two or three antigen from disparate family donors, however, survival probabilities are significantly decreased due to increased transplantation-related mortality.[158] Hessner et al[160] have shown that patients with CML in chronic phase who receive HLA-matched TCD unrelated marrow had significantly lower rates of relapse than those who underwent HLA-matched TCD sibling marrow transplantation, suggesting that an augmented GVT effect attributable to increased histoincompatibility in unrelated HSCT compensates for reduced GVT reactivity associated with TCD marrow transplantation.

INDUCTION OF A GRAFT-VS-TUMOR RESPONSE USING A NONMYELOABLATIVE PREPARATIVE REGIMEN AND DONOR LEUKOCYTE INFUSIONS

Because of the substantial toxicity associated with the high-dose chemoradiotherapy preparative regimens, the use of conventional allo-HSCT is usually restricted to young patients without comorbid medical illnesses. This myeloablative treatment modality is also associated with a high incidence of severe acute and chronic GVHD.[73,161] Large numbers of malignant diseases typically affect older, often debilitated, patients, and only a minority of these patients are eligible for standard allo-HSCT. Recently, attempts have been made to diminish transplantation-related mortality by administering relatively nontoxic, nonmyeloablative doses of chemotherapy or radiation therapy before allo-HSCT.[155,162-165] Donor engraftment is feasible, even after nonmyeloablative conditioning therapy.[166-169] Importantly, a mixed donor-host chimeric state can be achieved after nonmyeloablative conditioning treatment, which has the potential for inhibiting GVHD, presumably because of the persistence of host immunoregulatory cells, and thus provides a platform for the later delivery of DLI in order to convert the mixed chimeric state to full donor hematopoiesis and to capture the maximal anti-tumor effect. In animal models, these goals have been reached with the achievement of maximum GVT effect in the absence of evident GVHD.[75] We have performed approximately 60 HLA-matched or HLA-mismatched donor HSCTs in patients with chemotherapy-refractory hematologic malignancies. We used a nonmyeloablative preparative regimen consisting of cyclophosphamide, peritransplantation antithymocyte globulin, thymic irradiation, cyclosporine, and "prophylactic" DLI beginning 5 to 6 weeks after HSCT. Patients exhibiting evidence of GVHD did not receive DLI. Although grade II or greater GVHD is seen in almost 30% of the HLA-matched recipients after the transplantation, in most cases, the GVHD is manageable with low-dose immunosuppressive therapy; and the overall treatment-related mortality is less than 10%.[165] The following cases highlight some of the important observations from this pilot transplantation strategy. One patient underwent HLA-matched donor stem cell transplantation for recurrent multiple myeloma after two previous autologous SCTs; his serum immunoglobulin G level was 8000 mg/dL with 20% plasma cells in the bone marrow at the time of allo-HSCT; although he experienced mucocutaneous GVHD after a prophylactic DLI given 5 weeks after transplantation, he remains in complete remission 7 months after the allo-HSCT. Another patient received an HLA-2 Ag-mismatched HSCT for chemotherapy-refractory NHL/CLL; he remains in complete remission 8 months after allo-HSCT and is receiving low-dose immunosuppressive therapy for grade II (mainly mucocutaneous) GVHD. A third patient received an HLA-matched donor HSCT for chemotherapy-refractory NHL; he is in complete remission 3 years after the transplantation and has never had GVHD, despite a potent lymphohematopoietic anti-host response after his prophylactic DLI, which converted his mixed chimerism to a state of full donor hematopoiesis. These three cases demonstrate the striking anti-tumor effects that have been observed in many of our patients with chemotherapy-refractory disease; the second case also illustrates the feasibility of this approach even across HLA barriers; the third case demonstrates the fact that lymphohematopoietic GVHR can induce a powerful anti-tumor effect without inducing GVHD, indicating that GVT response can be separable from GVHD. Nonmyeloablative approaches are generally better tolerated, thus allowing for treatment of older patients and patients with comorbid diseases. However, the effectiveness of these approaches, in terms of durable disease control, and the optimal timing and dosing of delayed DLI in order to maximize a GVT effect while minimizing GVHD remain to be determined.

CONCLUSION

Donor-mediated immunologic anti-tumor effects can be exceptionally potent, as evidenced by the apparent cure of certain hematologic malignancies in relapse after allo-HSCT by DLI. The separation of this desired outcome from the deleterious effects of epithelial GVHD remains a major challenge. As our understanding of the mechanism of the GVT and GVHD responses grows, the potential for manipulation of the host:donor cellular environment by, for example, infusing donor cells directed against tumor-specific antigens into GVHD-free mixed chimeras, seems limitless. Given what is known about the broad range of anti-tumor activity of allogeneic stem cell therapy, it is hoped that these strategies will have wide-reaching applications for neoplastic disease.

REFERENCES

1. Barnes D, Corp M, Loutit J et al. Treatment of murine leukemia with x-rays and homologous bone marrow. BMJ 1956;2:626–627.
2. Horowitz M, Gale RP, Sondel PM et al. Graft-versus-leukemia reactions after bone marrow transplantation. Blood 1990;75:555–562.

3. Gale R, Champlin RE. How does bone-marrow transplantation cure leukaemia? Lancet 1984;2: 28–30.
4. Rondon G, Giralt S, Huh Y et al. Graft-versus-leukemia effect after allogeneic bone marrow transplantation for chronic lymphocytic leukemia. Bone Marrow Transplant 1996;18:669–672.
5. Tricot G, Vesole D, Jagannath S et al. Graft-versus-myeloma effect: proof of principle. Blood 1996;87:1196–1198.
6. Lokhorst H, Schattenberg A, Cornelissen JJ et al. Donor lymphocyte infusions for relapsed multiple myeloma after allogeneic stem-cell transplantation: predictive factors for response and long-term outcome. J Clin Oncol 2000;18:3031–3037.
7. Childs R, Chernoff A, Contentin N et al. Regression of metastatic renal-cell carcinoma after nonmyeloablative allogeneic peripheral-blood stem-cell transplantation. N Engl J Med 2000; 343:750–758.
8. Eibl B, Schwaighofer H, Nachbaur D et al. Evidence of a graft-versus-tumor effect in a patient treated with marrow ablative chemotherapy and allogeneic bone marrow transplantation for breast cancer. Blood 1996;88:1501–1508.
9. Kolb H, Schattenberg A, Goldman JM et al. Graft-versus-leukemia effect of donor lymphocyte transfusions in marrow grafted patients. European Group for Blood and Marrow Transplantation Working Party Chronic Leukemia. Blood. 1995;86:2041–2050.
10. Barnes D, Loutit J. Treatment of murine leukemia with x-rays and homologous bone marrow: II. Brit J Haematol 1957;3:241–252.
11. Boranic M. Delayed mortality in sublethally irradiated mice treated with allogeneic lymphoid and myeloid cells. J Natl Cancer Inst 1968;41:439–450.
12. Bortin MM, Rimm AA, Saltzstein EC. Graft versus leukemia: quantification of adoptive immunotherapy in murine leukemia. Science 1973;179:811–813.
13. Cheever M, Greenberg PD, Fefer A. Specificity of adoptive chemoimmunotherapy of established syngeneic tumors. J Immunol 1980;125:711–714.
14. Truitt R, Shih CC, LeFever AV. Manipulation of graft-versus-host disease for a graft-versus-leukemia effect after allogeneic bone marrow transplantation in AKR mice with spontaneous leukemia/lymphoma. Transplantation 1986;41:301–310.
15. Bortin M, Rimm AA, Saltzstein EC et al. Graft versus leukemia. 3. Apparent independent antihost and antileukemia activity of transplanted immunocompetent cells. Transplantation 1973;16: 182–188.
16. Bortin M, Truitt RL, Rimm AA, Bach FH. Graft-versus-leukaemia reactivity induced by alloimmunisation without augmentation of graft-versus-host reactivity. Nature 1979;281:490–491.
17. Moscovitch M, Kaufmann Y, Berke G. Memory CTL-hybridoma: a model system to analyze the anamnestic response of cytolytic T lymphocytes. J Immunol 1984;133:2369–2374.
18. Sykes M, Romick ML, Sachs DH. Interleukin 2 prevents graft-versus-host disease while preserving the graft-versus-leukemia effect of allogeneic T cells. Proc Natl Acad Sci USA 1990;87:5633–5637.
19. Johnson B, Drobyski WR, Truitt RL. Delayed infusion of normal donor cells after MHC-matched bone marrow transplantation provides an antileukemia reaction without graft-versus-host disease. Bone Marrow Transplant 1993;11:329–336.
20. Yang Y, Sergio JJ, Pearson DA et al. Interleukin-12 preserves the graft-versus-leukemia effect of allogeneic CD8 T cells while inhibiting CD4-dependent graft-versus-host disease in mice. Blood 1997;90:4651–4660.
21. Mathe G, Amiel J, Schwarzenberg J et al. Successful allogeneic bone marrow transplantation in man: chimerism, induced specific tolerance and possible anti-leukemic effects. Blood 1965;25: 179–189.

22. Weiden P, Flournoy N, Thomas ED et al. Antileukemic effect of graft-versus-host disease in human recipients of allogeneic-marrow grafts. N Engl J Med 1979;300:1068–1073.
23. Weiden P, Flournoy N, Sanders J et al. Antileukemic effect of graft-versus-host disease contributes to improved survival after allogeneic marrow transplantation. Transplant Proc 1981;13:248–251.
24. Butturini A, Bortin MM, Gale RP. Graft-versus-leukemia following bone marrow transplantation. Bone Marrow Transplant 1987;2:233–242.
25. Ringden O, Horowitz MM. Graft-versus-leukemia reactions in humans. The Advisory Committee of the International Bone Marrow Transplant Registry. Transplant Proc 1989;21:2989–2992.
26. Sanders J, Flournoy N, Thomas ED et al. Marrow transplant experience in children with acute lymphoblastic leukemia: an analysis of factors associated with survival, relapse, and graft-versus-host disease. Med Pediatr Oncol 1985;13:165–172.
27. Kersey J, Weisdorf D, Nesbit ME et al. Comparison of autologous and allogeneic bone marrow transplantation for treatment of high-risk refractory acute lymphoblastic leukemia. N Engl J Med 1987;317:461–467.
28. Weisdorf D, Nesbit ME, Ramsay NK et al. Allogeneic bone marrow transplantation for acute lymphoblastic leukemia in remission: prolonged survival associated with acute graft-versus-host disease. J Clin Oncol 1987;5:1348–1355.
29. Sullivan K, Weiden PL, Storb R et al. Influence of acute and chronic graft-versus-host disease on relapse and survival after bone marrow transplantation from HLA-identical siblings as treatment of acute and chronic leukemia. Blood 1989;73:1720–1728.
30. Sullivan K, Witherspoon R, Storb R. Alternating-day cyclosporine and prednisone for treatment of high-risk chronic graft-versus-host disease. Blood 1988;72:555–561.
31. Sullivan K, Storb R, Buckner CD et al. Graft-versus-host disease as adoptive immunotherapy in patients with advanced hematologic neoplasms. N Engl J Med 1989;320:828–834.
32. Odom L, August CS, Githens JH et al. Remission of relapsed leukaemia during a graft-versus-host reaction: a "graft-versus-leukaemia reaction" in man? Lancet 1978;2:537–540.
33. Higano C, Brixey M, Bryant EM et al. Durable complete remission of acute nonlymphocytic leukemia associated with discontinuation of immunosuppression following relapse after allogeneic bone marrow transplantation: a case report of a probable graft-versus-leukemia effect. Transplantation 1990;50:175-177.
34. Sullivan KM, Witherspoon RP, Storb R et al. Long term results of allogeneic bone marrow transplantation. Transplant Proc 1989;21:2926–2928.
35. Collins RJ, Rogers ZR, Bennett M et al. Hematologic relapse of chronic myelogenous leukemia following allogeneic bone marrow transplantation: apparent graft-versus-leukemia effect following abrupt discontinuation of immunosuppression. Bone Marrow Transplant 1992;10:391–395.
36. deMagalhaes-Silverman M, Donnenberg A, Hammert L et al. Induction of graft-versus-leukemia effect in a patient with chronic lymphocytic leukemia. Bone Marrow Transplant 1997;20:175–177.
37. Waldmann H, Polliak A, Hale G et al. Elimination of graft-versus-host disease by in-vitro depletion of alloreactive lymphocytes with a monoclonal rat anti-human lymphocyte antibody (CAMPATH-1). Lancet 1984;2:483–486.
38. Martin P, Hansen JA, Vitetta ES. A ricin A chain-containing immunotoxin that kills human T lymphocytes in vitro. Blood 1985;66:908–912.
39. Mitsuyasu R, Champlin RE, Gale RP et al. Treatment of donor bone marrow with monoclonal anti-T-cell antibody and complement for the prevention of graft-versus-host disease: a prospective, randomized, double-blind trial. Ann Intern Med 1986;105:20–26.
40. Antin J, Bierer BE, Smith BR et al. Selective depletion of bone marrow T lymphocytes with anti-CD5 monoclonal antibodies: effective prophylaxis for graft-versus-host disease in patients with hematologic malignancies. Blood 1991;78:2139–2149.

41. Young J, Papadopoulo EB, Cunningham I et al. T-cell-depleted allogeneic bone marrow transplantation in adults with acute nonlymphocytic leukemia in first remission. Blood 1992;79: 3380–3387.
42. Goldman J, Apperley JF, Jones L et al. Bone marrow transplantation for patients with chronic myeloid leukemia. N Engl J Med 1986;314:202–207.
43. Goldman J, Gale RP, Horowitz MM et al. Bone marrow transplantation for chronic myelogenous leukemia in chronic phase: increased risk for relapse associated with T-cell depletion. Ann Intern Med 1988;108:806–814.
44. Apperley J, Mauro FR, Goldman JM et al. Bone marrow transplantation for chronic myeloid leukaemia in first chronic phase: importance of a graft-versus-leukaemia effect. Br J Haematol 1988;69:239–245.
45. Marmont A, Horowitz MM, Gale RP et al. T-cell depletion of HLA-identical transplants in leukemia. Blood 1991;78:2120–2130.
46. Martin P, Hansen J, Torok-Storb B et al. Graft failure in patients receiving T-cell-depleted HLA-identical allogeneic bone marrow transplants. Bone Marrow Transplant 1988;3:445-456.
47. Kolb H, Mittermuller J, Clemm C et al. Donor leukocyte transfusions for treatment of recurrent chronic myelogenous leukemia in marrow transplant patients. Blood 1990;76:2462–2465.
48. Drobyski W, Keever CA, Roth MS et al. Salvage immunotherapy using donor leukocyte infusions as treatment for relapsed chronic myelogenous leukemia after allogeneic bone marrow transplantation: efficacy and toxicity of a defined T-cell dose. Blood 1993;82:2310–2318.
49. Hertenstein B, Wiesneth M, Novotny J et al. Interferon-alpha and donor buffy coat transfusions for treatment of relapsed chronic myeloid leukemia after allogeneic bone marrow transplantation. Transplantation 1993;56:1114–1118.
50. Porter D, Roth MS, McGarigle C et al. Induction of graft-versus-host disease as immunotherapy for relapsed chronic myeloid leukemia. N Engl J Med 1994;330:100–106.
51. Van Rhee F, Feng L, Cullis J et al. Relapse of chronic myeloid leukemia after allogeneic bone marrow transplantation: the case for giving donor leukocyte infusions before the onset of hematologic relapse. Blood 1994;83:3377–3383.
52. Slavin S, Naparstek E, Nagler A et al. Allogeneic cell therapy with donor peripheral blood cells and recombinant human interleukin-2 to treat leukemia relapse after allogeneic bone marrow transplantation. Blood 1996;87:2195–2204.
53. Collins RJ, Shpilberg O, Drobyski WR et al. Donor leukocyte infusions in 140 patients with relapsed malignancy after allogeneic bone marrow transplantation. J Clin Oncol 1997;15: 433–444.
54. Kolb H. Allogeneic Stem Cell Transplantation for CML: Update of Results and New Strategies. American Society of Hematology Education Program Book. Washington DC: American Society of Hematology 1999:159–168.
55. Baurmann H, Nagel S, Binder T et al. Kinetics of the graft-versus-leukemia response after donor leukocyte infusions for relapsed chronic myeloid leukemia after allogeneic bone marrow transplantation. Blood 1998;92:3582–3590.
56. Anderson K, Weinstein HJ. Transfusion-associated graft-versus-host disease [review]. N Engl J Med 1990;323:315–321.
57. Mrsic M, Horowitz MM, Atkinson K et al. Second HLA-identical sibling transplants for leukemia recurrence. Bone Marrow Transplant 1992;9:269–275.
58. Porter D, Antin JH. Adoptive immunotherapy for relapsed leukemia following allogeneic bone marrow transplantation. Leuk Lymphoma 1995;17:191–197.
59. Mackinnnon S, Papadopoulos EB, Carabasi MH et al. Adoptive immunotherapy evaluating escalating doses of donor leukocytes for relapse of chronic myeloid leukemia following bone

marrow transplantation: separation of graft-versus-leukemia responses from graft-versus-host disease. Blood 1995;86:1261–1268.
60. Schattenberg A, Schaap N, Van De Wiel-Van Kemenade E et al. In relapsed patients after lymphocyte depleted bone marrow transplantation the percentage of donor T lymphocytes correlates well with the outcome of donor leukocyte infusion. Leuk Lymphoma 1999;32:317–325.
61. Truitt R, Shih CY, Lefever AV et al. Characterization of alloimmunization-induced T lymphocytes reactive against AKR leukemia in vitro and correlation with graft-vs-leukemia activity in vivo. J Immunol 1983;131:2050–2058.
62. Dey B, Yang YG, Szot GL et al. Interleukin-12 inhibits graft-versus-host disease through an Fas-mediated mechanism associated with alterations in donor T-cell activation and expansion. Blood 1998;91:3315–3322.
63. Marmont AM. The graft versus leukemia (GVL) effect after allogeneic bone marrow transplantation for chronic myelogenous leukemia (CML). Leuk Lymphoma 1993;11[suppl 1]:221–226.
64. Olavarria E, Dazzi F, Craddock C et al. Donor lymphocyte infusions (DLI) for treatment of CML in relapse after allogeneic BMT: low incidence of GVHD using an escalation dose protocol. Blood 1990;90:589a.
65. Champlin R. Immunobiology of bone marrow transplantation as treatment for hematologic malignancies. Transplant Proc 1991;23:2123–2127.
66. Giralt S, Hester J, Huh Y et al. CD8-depleted donor lymphocyte infusion as treatment for relapsed chronic myelogenous leukemia after allogeneic bone marrow transplantation. Blood 1995;86:4337.
67. Nimer S, Ireland P, Meshkinpour A et al. An increased HLA DR2 frequency is seen in aplastic anemia patients. Blood 1994;84:923–927.
68. Alyea E, Soiffer RJ, Canning C et al. Toxicity and efficacy of defined doses of CD4(+) donor lymphocytes for treatment of relapse after allogeneic bone marrow transplant. Blood 1998;91:3671–3680.
69. Mavilio F, Ferrari G, Rossini S et al. Peripheral blood lymphocytes as target cells of retroviral vector-mediated gene transfer. Blood 1994;83:1988–1997.
70. Bonini C, Ferrari G, Verzeletti S et al. HSV-TK gene transfer into donor lymphocytes for control of allogeneic graft-versus-leukemia. Science 1997;276:1719–1724.
71. Cohen J, Boyer O, Salomon B et al. Prevention of graft-versus-host disease in mice using a suicide gene expressed in T lymphocytes. Blood 1997;89:4636–4645.
72. Antin JH, Ferrara JL. Cytokine dysregulation and acute graft-versus-host disease. Blood 1992;80:2964-2968.
73. Ferrara JLM, Deeg HJ. Graft-versus-host disease. N Engl J Med 1991;324:667–674.
74. Sykes M, Bukhari Z, Sachs DH. Graft-versus-leukemia effect using mixed allogeneic bone marrow transplantation. Bone Marrow Transplant 1989;4:465–474.
75. Pelot M, Pearson DA, Swenson K et al. Lymphohematopoietic graft-vs.-host reactions can be induced without graft-vs.-host disease in murine mixed chimeras established with a cyclophosphamide-based nonmyeloablative conditioning regimen. Biol Blood Marrow Transplant 1999;5:133–143.
76. Weiden P, Storb R, Tsoi MS et al. Infusion of donor lymphocytes into stable canine radiation chimeras: implications for mechanism of transplantation tolerance. J Immunol 1976;116:1212–1219.
77. Kolb H, Holler E. Adoptive immunotherapy with donor lymphocyte transfusions. Curr Opin Oncol 1997;9:139–145.

78. Slavin S, Naparstek E, Nagler A et al. Graft vs leukemia (GVL) effects with controlled GVHD by cell mediated immunotherapy (CMI) following allogeneic bone marrow transplant (BMT). Blood 1993;82:423a.
79. Naparstek E, Or R, Nagler A et al. T-cell-depleted allogeneic bone marrow transplantation for acute leukaemia using Campath-1 antibodies and post-transplant administration of donor's peripheral blood lymphocytes for prevention of relapse. Br J Haematol 1995;89:506–515.
80. Barrett A, Mavroudis D, Molldrem J et al. Optimizing the dose and timing of lymphocyte add-back in T-cell depleted BMT between HLA-identical siblings. Blood 1996;88:460a.
81. Sullivan K, Deeg H, Sanders J et al. Hyperacute graft-versus-host disease in patients not given immunosuppression after allogeneic marrow transplant. Blood 1986;67:1172–1175.
82. Soiffer R, Murray C, Gonin R et al. Effect of low-dose interleukin-2 on disease relapse after T-cell-depleted allogeneic bone marrow transplantation. Blood 1994;84:964–971.
83. Johnson B, Truitt RL. Delayed infusion of immunocompetent donor cells after bone marrow transplantation breaks graft-host tolerance allows for persistent antileukemic reactivity without severe graft-versus-host disease. Blood 1995;85:3302–3312.
84. Shaw P, Bergin ME, Burgess MA et al. Childhood acute myeloid leukemia: outcome in a single center using chemotherapy and consolidation with busulfan/cyclophosphamide for bone marrow transplantation. J Clin Oncol 1994;12:2138–2145.
85. Ravindranath Y, Yeager AM, Chang MN et al. Autologous bone marrow transplantation versus intensive consolidation chemotherapy for acute myeloid leukemia in childhood. Pediatric Oncology Group. N Engl J Med 1996;334:1428–1434.
86. Appelbaum FR. Graft versus leukemia (GVL) in the therapy of acute lymphoblastic leukemia (ALL). Leukemia 1997;11[suppl 4]:S15–S17.
87. Doney K, Fisher LD, Appelbaum FR et al. Treatment of adult acute lymphoblastic leukemia with allogeneic bone marrow transplantation: multivariate analysis of factors affecting acute graft-versus-host disease, relapse, and relapse-free survival. Bone Marrow Transplant 1991;7:453–459.
88. Collins R, Goldstein S, Giralt S et al. Donor leukocyte infusions in acute lymphocytic leukemia. Bone Marrow Transplant 2000;26:511–516.
89. Garrido F, Cabrera T, Concha A et al. Natural history of HLA expression during tumour development. Immunol Today 1993;14:491–499.
90. Guinan E, Gribben JG, Boussiotis VA et al. Pivotal role of the B7:CD28 pathway in transplantation tolerance and tumor immunity. Blood 1994;84:3261–3265.
91. Hirano N, Takahashi T, Takahashi T et al. Expression of costimulatory molecules in human leukemias. Leukemia 1996;10:1168–1176.
92. Greenberg P, Cheever MA, Fefer A. Detection of early and delayed antitumor effects following curative adoptive chemoimmunotherapy of established leukemia. Cancer Res 1980;40:4428–4432.
93. Gahrton G, Tura S, Ljungman P et al. Allogeneic bone marrow transplantation in multiple myeloma. European Group for Bone Marrow Transplantation N Engl J Med 1991;325:1267–1273.
94. Gahrton G, Tura S, Ljungman P et al. Prognostic factors in allogeneic bone marrow transplantation for multiple myeloma. J Clin Oncol 1995;13:1312–1322.
95. Gahrton G. Bone Marrow Transplantation In: Forman S, ed. Bone Marrow Transplantation. Boston: Blackwell Scientific Publication, 1999:887–891.
96. Bensinger W, Buckner CD, Clift RA et al. Phase I study of busulfan and cyclophosphamide in preparation for allogeneic marrow transplant for patients with multiple myeloma. J Clin Oncol 1992;10:1492–1497.
97. Bensinger WI, Buckner CD, Anasetti C et al. Allogeneic marrow transplantation for multiple myeloma: an analysis of risk factors on outcome. Blood 1996;88:2787–2793.

98. Anderson K, Andersen J, Soiffer R et al. Monoclonal antibody-purged bone marrow transplantation therapy for multiple myeloma. Blood 1993;82:2568–2576.
99. Seiden M, Schlossman R, Andersen J et al. Monoclonal antibody-purged bone marrow transplantation therapy for multiple myeloma. Leuk Lymphoma 1995;17:87–93.
100. Mehta J, Ayers D, Mattox S et al. Allogeneic bone marrow transplantation in multiple myeloma: single-center experience of 97 patients. Blood 1990;90:225a.
101. Verdonck L, Lokhorst HM, Dekker AW et al. Graft-versus-myeloma effect in two cases. Lancet 1996;347:800–801.
102. Aschan J, Lonnqvist B, Ringden O et al. Graft-versus-myeloma effect. Lancet 1996;348:346.
103. Montserrat E, Gale RP, Rozman C. Bone marrow transplants for chronic lymphocytic leukaemia [review]. Leukemia 1992;6:619–622.
104. Rabinowe S, Soiffer RJ, Gribben JG et al. Autologous and allogeneic bone marrow transplantation for poor prognosis patients with B-cell chronic lymphocytic leukemia. Blood 1993;82:1366–1376.
105. Khouri I, Keating MJ, Vriesendorp HM et al. Autologous and allogeneic bone marrow transplantation for chronic lymphocytic leukemia: preliminary results. J Clin Oncol 1994;12:748–758.
106. Michallet M, Archimbaud E, Bandini G et al. HLA-identical sibling bone marrow transplantation in younger patients with chronic lymphocytic leukemia. European Group for Blood and Marrow Transplantation and the International Bone Marrow Transplant Registry. Ann Intern Med. 1996;124:311–315.
107. Khouri I, Przepiorka D, van Besien KO et al. Allogeneic blood or marrow transplantation for chronic lymphocytic leukaemia: timing of transplantation and potential effect of fludarabine on acute graft-versus-host disease. Br J Haematol 1997;97:466–473.
108. Appelbaum F, Sullivan KM, Buckner CD et al. Treatment of malignant lymphoma in 100 patients with chemotherapy, total body irradiation, and marrow transplantation. J Clin Oncol 1987;5:1340–1347.
109. Chopra R, Goldstone AH, Pearce R et al. Autologous versus allogeneic bone marrow transplantation for non-Hodgkin's lymphoma: a case-controlled analysis of the European Bone Marrow Transplant Group Registry data. J Clin Oncol 1992;10:1690–1695.
110. Ratanatharathorn V, Uberti J, Karanes C et al. Prospective comparative trial of autologous versus allogeneic bone marrow transplantation in patients with non-Hodgkin's lymphoma. Blood 1994;84:1050.
111. Verdonck LF, Decker AW, Lokhorst HM et al. Allogeneic versus autologous bone marrow transplantation for refractory and recurrent low-grade non-Hodgkin's lymphoma. Blood 1997;90:4201.
112. van Besien K, Thall P, Korbling M et al. Allogeneic transplantation for recurrent or refractory non-Hodgkin's lymphoma with poor prognostic features after conditioning with thiotepa, busulfan, and cyclophosphamide: experience in 44 consecutive patients. Biol Blood Marrow Transplant 1997;3:150–156.
113. van Besien K, de Lima M, Giralt SA et al. Management of lymphoma recurrence after allogeneic transplantation: the relevance of graft-versus-lymphoma effect. Bone Marrow Transplant 1997;19:977–982.
114. van Besien K, Sobocinski KA, Rowlings PA et al. Allogeneic bone marrow transplantation for low-grade lymphoma. Blood 1998;92:1832–1836.
115. Gajewski J, Phillips GL, Sobocinsk KA et al. Bone marrow transplants from HLA-identical siblings in advanced Hodgkin's disease. J Clin Oncol 1996;14:572–578.
116. Milpied N, Fielding AK, Pearce RM et al. Allogeneic bone marrow transplant is not better than autologous transplant for patients with relapsed Hodgkin's disease. European Group for Blood and Bone Marrow Transplantation. J Clin Oncol 1996;14:1291–1296.

117. Jones R, Ambinder RF, Piantadosi S et al. Evidence of a graft-versus-lymphoma effect associated with allogeneic bone marrow transplantation. Blood 1991;77:649–653.
118. Bay J, Choufi B, Pomel C et al. Potential allogeneic graft-versus-tumor effect in a patient with ovarian cancer. Bone Marrow Transplant 2000;25:681–682.
119. Apperley J, Jones L, Hale G et al. Bone marrow transplantation for patients with chronic myeloid leukaemia: T-cell depletion with Campath-1 reduces the incidence of graft-versus-host disease but may increase the risk of leukaemic relapse. Bone Marrow Transplant 1986;1:53–66.
120. Sosman J, Oettel KR, Smith SD et al. Specific recognition of human leukemic cells by allogeneic T cells: II. Evidence for HLA-D restricted determinants on leukemic cells that are crossreactive with determinants present on unrelated nonleukemic cells. Blood 1990;75:2005–2016.
121. Faber L, van Luxemburg-Heijs SA, Willemze R et al. Generation of leukemia-reactive cytotoxic T lymphocyte clones from the HLA-identical bone marrow donor of a patient with leukemia. J Exp Med. 1992;176:1283–1289.
122. van Lochem E, de Gast B, Goulmy E. In vitro separation of host specific graft-versus-host and graft-versus-leukemia cytotoxic T cell activities. Bone Marrow Transplant 1992;10:181–183.
123. Weiss L, Weigensberg M, Morecki S et al. Characterization of effector cells of graft vs leukemia following allogeneic bone marrow transplantation in mice inoculated with murine B-cell leukemia. Cancer Immunol Immunother 1990;31:236–242.
124. Truitt R, Atasoylu AA. Contribution of CD4+ and CD8+ T cells to graft-versus-host disease and graft-versus-leukemia reactivity after transplantation of MHC-compatible bone marrow. Bone Marrow Transplant 1991;8:51–58.
125. Okunewick J, Kociban DL, Machen LL et al. The role of CD4 and CD8 T cells in the graft-versus-leukemia response in Rauscher murine leukemia. Bone Marrow Transplant 1991;8:445–452.
126. Korngold R, Leighton C, Manser T. Graft-versus-myeloid leukemia responses following syngeneic and allogeneic bone marrow transplantation. Transplantation 1994;58:278–287.
127. Falkenburg J, Faber LM, van den Elshout M et al. Generation of donor-derived antileukemic cytotoxic T-lymphocyte responses for treatment of relapsed leukemia after allogeneic HLA-identical bone marrow transplantation. J Immunother 1993;14:305–309.
128. Jiang Y, Barrett AJ, Goldman JM et al. Association of natural killer cell immune recovery with a graft-versus-leukemia effect independent of graft-versus-host disease following allogeneic bone marrow transplantation. Ann Hematol 1997;74:1–6.
129. Glass B, Uharek L, Zeis M et al. Graft-versus-leukaemia activity can be predicted by natural cytotoxicity against leukaemia cells. Br J Haematol 1996;93:412–420.
130. Zeis M, Uharek L, Glass B et al. Allogeneic MHC-mismatched activated natural killer cells administered after bone marrow transplantation provide a strong graft-versus-leukaemia effect in mice. Br J Haematol 1997;96:757–761.
131. Asai O, Longo DL, Tian ZG et al. Suppression of graft-versus-host disease and amplification of graft-versus-tumor effects by activated natural killer cells after allogeneic bone marrow transplantation. J Clin Invest 1998;101:1835–1842.
132. Roger R, Issaad C, Pallardy M et al. BCR-ABL does not prevent apoptotic death induced by human natural killer or lymphokine-activated killer cells. Blood 1996;87:1113–1122.
133. Rooney C, Wimperis JZ, Brenner MK et al. Natural killer cell activity following T-cell depleted allogeneic bone marrow transplantation. Br J Haematol 1986;62:413–420.
134. Hauch M, Gazzola MV, Small T et al. Anti-leukemia potential of interleukin-2 activated natural killer cells after bone marrow transplantation for chronic myelogenous leukemia. Blood 1990;75:2250–2262.
135. Verdonck L, van Heugten HG, Giltay J et al. Amplification of the graft-versus-leukemia effect in man by interleukin-2. Transplantation 1991;51:1120–1124.

136. Soiffer R, Murray C, Mauch P et al. Prevention of graft-versus-host disease by selective depletion of CD6-positive T lymphocytes from donor bone marrow. J Clin Oncol 1992;10:1191–1200.
137. den Haan J, Sherman NE, Blokland E et al. Identification of a graft versus host disease-associated human minor histocompatibility antigen. Science. 1995;268:1476–1480.
138. Wang W, Meadows LR, den Haan JM et al. Human H-Y: a male-specific histocompatibility antigen derived from the SMCY protein. Science 1995;269:1588–1590.
139. Goulmy E, Schipper R, Pool J et al. Mismatches of minor histocompatibility antigens between HLA-identical donors and recipients and the development of graft-versus-host disease after bone marrow transplantation. N Engl J Med 1996;334:281–285.
140. Korngold R WPJ. Immunodominance in the graft-vs-host disease T cell response to minor histocompatibility antigens. J Immunol 1990;145:4079–4088.
141. Goulmy E. Human minor histocompatibility antigens: new concepts for marrow transplantation and adoptive immunotherapy. Immunol Rev 1997;157:125–140.
142. de Bueger M, Bakker A, Van Rood JJ et al. Tissue distribution of human minor histocompatibility antigens: ubiquitous versus restricted tissue distribution indicates heterogeneity among human cytotoxic T lymphocyte-defined non-MHC antigens. J Immunol 1992;149:1788–1794.
143. Mutis T, Verdijk R, Schrama E et al. Feasibility of immunotherapy of relapsed leukemia with ex vivo-generated cytotoxic T lymphocytes specific for hematopoietic system-restricted minor histocompatibility antigens. Blood 1999;93:2336–2341.
144. Cheever M, Disis ML, Bernhard H et al. Immunity to oncogenic proteins [review]. Immunol Rev 1995;145:33–59.
145. Peoples G, Blotnick S, Takahashi K et al. T lymphocytes that infiltrate tumors and atherosclerotic plaques produce heparin-binding epidermal growth factor-like growth factor and basic fibroblast growth factor: a potential pathologic role. Proc Natl Acad Sci USA 1995;92:6547–6551.
146. Fisk B, Blevins TL, Wharton JT et al. Identification of an immunodominant peptide of HER-2/neu protooncogene recognized by ovarian tumor-specific cytotoxic T lymphocyte lines. J Exp Med 1995;181:2109–2117.
147. Yee C, Gilbert MJ, Riddell SR et al. Isolation of tyrosinase-specific CD8+ and CD4+ T cell clones from the peripheral blood of melanoma patients following in vitro stimulation with recombinant vaccinia virus. J Immunol 1996;157:4079–4086.
148. Kawakami Y, Eliyahu S, Delgado CH et al. Identification of a human melanoma antigen recognized by tumor-infiltrating lymphocytes associated with in vivo tumor rejection. Proc Natl Acad Sci U S A 1994;91:6458–6462.
149. Kawakami Y, Eliyahu S, Sakaguchi K et al. Identification of the immunodominant peptides of the MART-1 human melanoma antigen recognized by the majority of HLA-A2-restricted tumor infiltrating lymphocytes. J Exp Med 1994;180:347–352.
150. van der Bruggen P, Traversari C, Chomez P et al. A gene encoding an antigen recognized by cytolytic T lymphocytes on a human melanoma. Science 1991;254:1643–1647.
151. Gaugler B, Van den Eynde B, van der Bruggen P et al. Human gene MAGE-3 codes for an antigen recognized on a melanoma by autologous cytolytic T lymphocytes. J Exp Med 1994;179:921–930.
152. Chen W, Peace DJ, Rovira DK et al. T-cell immunity to the joining region of p210BCR-ABL protein. Proc Natl Acad Sci USA 1992;89:1468–1472.
153. Bocchia M, Korontsvit T, Xu Q et al. Specific human cellular immunity to bcr-abl oncogene-derived peptides. Blood 1996;87:3587–3592.
154. Bosch G, Joosten AM, Kessler JH et al. Recognition of BCR-ABL positive leukemic blasts by human CD4+ T cells elicited by primary in vitro immunization with a BCR-ABL breakpoint peptide. Blood 1996;88:3522–3527.

155. Sykes M, Preffer F, Saidman SL et al. Mixed lymphohematopoietic chimerism is achievable following non-myeloablative therapy and HLA-mismatched donor marrow transplantation. Lancet 1998;353:1755–1759.
156. Beatty PG. Results of allogeneic bone marrow transplantation with unrelated or mismatched donors. Semin Oncol 1992;19:13–19.
157. Davies S, Wagner JE, Weisdorf DJ et al. Unrelated donor bone marrow transplantation for hematological malignancies-current status. Leuk Lymphoma 1996;23:221–226.
158. Beatty PG, Clift FM, Mickelson BB et al. Marrow transplantation from related donors other than HLA-identical siblings. N Engl J Med 1985;313:765–771.
159. Bortin M. Bone marrow transplantation for leukemia using family donors other than HLA-identical siblings: a preliminary report from the International Bone Marrow Transplant Registry. Transplant Proc 1987;19:2629–2631.
160. Hessner M, Endean DJ, Casper JT et al. Use of unrelated marrow grafts compensates for reduced graft-versus-leukemia reactivity after T-cell-depleted allogeneic marrow transplantation for chronic myelogenous leukemia. Blood 1995;86:3987–3996.
161. Hagglund L, Bostom L, Remberger M et al. Risk factors for acute graft-versus-host disease in 291 consecutive HLA-identical bone marrow transplant recipients. Bone Marrow Transplant 1995;16:747–755.
162. Giralt S, Estey E, Albitar M et al. Engraftment of allogeneic hematopoietic progenitor cells with purine analog-containing chemotherapy: harnessing graft-versus-leukemia without myeloablative therapy. Blood 1997;89:4531–4536.
163. Khouri IF, Keating M, Korbling M et al. Transplant-lite: Induction of graft-versus-malignancy using fludarabine-based nonablative chemotherapy and allogeneic blood progenitor-cell transplantation as treatment for lymphoid malignancies. J Clin Oncol 1998;16:2817–2824.
164. Slavin S, Nagler A, Naparstek E et al. Nonmyeloablative stem cell transplantation and cell therapy as an alternative to conventional bone marrow transplantation with lethal cytoreduction for the treatment of malignant and nonmalignant hematologic diseases. Blood 1998;91:756–763.
165. Spitzer T, McAfee S, Sackstein R et al. Intentional induction of mixed chimerism and achievement of antitumor responses after nonmyeloablative conditioning therapy and HLA-matched donor bone marrow transplantation for refractory hematologic malignancies. Biol Blood Marrow Transplant 2000;6:309–320.
166. Sharabi Y, Abraham VS, Sykes M et al. Mixed allogeneic chimeras prepared by a non-myeloablative regimen: requirement for chimerism to maintain tolerance. Bone Marrow Transplant 1992;9:191–197.
167. Kawai T, Cosimi AB, Colvin RB et al. Mixed allogeneic chimerism and renal allograft tolerance in cynomolgus monkeys. Transplantation 1995;59:256.
168. Storb R, Yi C, Wagner JL et al. Stable mixed hematopoietic chimerism in DLA-identical littermate dogs given sublethal total body irradiation before and pharmacologic immunosuppression after bone marrow transplantation. Blood 1997;89:3048.
169. Sykes M, Szot GL, Swenson KA et al. Induction of high levels of allogeneic hematopoietic reconstitution and donor-specific tolerance without myelosuppressive conditioning. Nat Med 1997;3:783–787.

Radiofrequency Ablation for the Treatment of Liver Metastases

T. S. Ravikumar

Ronald Kaleya

Hepatic resection is the treatment of choice for patients with limited and discrete metastatic liver tumors, especially from colorectal primaries.[1-3] Curative resection of liver metastases yields reproducible, durable, long-term (5-year) survival in approximately 25%-35% of patients, accompanied by an excellent quality of life. However, only 5%–17% of patients presenting with liver tumors are amenable to curative resection due to extent of disease and/or comorbid conditions. Among the patients who are not candidates for liver resection, 90% die of liver failure caused by the local effects of the hepatic tumor rather than as a consequence of other sites of metastases.[4,5]

Standard treatment for unresectable metastatic liver tumors is well documented (Table 13.1). Untreated, the median survival for colorectal metastases is 3–21, months depending upon the extent of liver involvement at presentation.[4,6-8] Medical treatment of unresectable metastatic liver tumors marginally improves survival and is accompanied by significant toxicity. In contrast, regional chemotherapy has substantially higher response rates and lower toxicity as compared to systemic chemotherapy.[9,10] Survival, however, has been only modestly improved.

Because the immediate cause of death of most patients with liver tumors is directly attributable to the extent of liver involvement, and chemotherapy has

TABLE 13.1 Liver Metastases from Colorectal Cancer: Patient Survival[a]					
	Time, years				Median
Rx Modality	1	3	4	5	(months)
No treatment	32%	10%	3%	<2%	9
Systemic Chemotherapy	45%	21%	3%	occasional	12
HAI Chemotherapy	64%	25%	5%	1%	16
Ablation (cryo and RFA)	90%	—	22%	10%	27
Resection	90%	—	48%	35%	33

[a]The patient cohorts are NOT comparable, but significant overlap exists between the groups.

limited effect on hepatic disease progression, efforts to improve survival and quality of life must be directed towards local ablation of the liver tumors. Ablation of such tumors can achieve a complete response by reliably destroying all apparent viable tumors during a single procedure, thus possibly altering the natural history for patients with unresectable liver tumors.

PATIENT POPULATION

Gastrointestinal malignancies frequently produce metastatic spread to the liver, but rarely without additional metastases at extrahepatic sites. In this setting, regional therapies—be they infusional, resectional, or ablative—are, for obvious reasons, unsuitable management stategies. In contrast, the pattern of recurrence for colorectal cancer differs from most other gastrointestinal tumors. Of the approximately 140,000 new cases expected in 2001,[11] half will develop liver metastases within five years of diagnosis, and approximately 20% (14,000) of these patients will develop metastatic disease confined to the liver. Because only a quarter (3000–4000) of these patients are amenable to hepatic metastasectomy with curative intent, there are about 10,000 patients with liver-only colorectal metastases each year that might be candidates for regional therapies. As illustrated in an audit of all patients treated for colorectal cancer who were followed at a regional cancer center and developed hepatic metastases, 25.3% were resectable.[2] Therefore, most of the patients with metastatic disease localized to the liver were not eligible for curative resection but would be candidates for operative tumor ablation.

Similarly, patients with metastatic gastrointestinal neuroendocrine tumors die, not as a result of diffuse systemic metastases, but rather because of liver failure due to extensive liver involvement or from the sequella of associated paraneoplastic syndromes. Cytoreductive procedures (debulking resection or ablation) may provide local hepatic tumor control and reduce the incidence and/or severity of the paraneoplastic symptoms. In addition, select subsets of patients with primary tumors from disparate sites (i.e. breast, sarcoma, lung, and gynecologic malignancies) develop liver metastases as the only site of recurrence. These highly selected patients may also benefit from ablation of the liver metastases.

RADIOFREQUENCY ABLATION

For centuries, hyperthermia has been a well-known anti-tumor modality. The classical definition of hyperthermia in mammalian systems is temperature between 42°C and 46°C. Most mammalian cells do not survive prolonged exposure to temperatures exceeding 42°C.[12] Irreversible cellular damage occurs within 45 minutes when tissues are heated to 46°C–48°C. Tissues exposed to 50°C–52°C develop coagulative necrosis in 4–6 minutes.[6] When the tissue is subjected to heating between 46°C–50°C, enzyme systems fail, and some proteins become denatured. Cell death ensues. Cells exposed to this level of hyperthermia for an adequate period of time experience both heat induced apoptosis and coagulative necrosis. Between 42°C and 50°C, the time required for certain cell death is inversely proportional to the temperature. The apoptotic cells may appear histologically and morphologically viable by routine hematoxylin and eosin stains however more sophisticated immunocytologic studies show non-viability. In contrast, instantaneous coagulative necrosis occurs at temperatures exceeding 60°C. At temperatures higher than 100°C, cellular membranes melt, intra- and extracellular water vaporizes, proteins denature, and tissue dessicates. Based on these principles, the hyperthermic technique, in this instance radiofrequency interstitial ablation, must achieve temperatures exceeding 50°C throughout the tumor for at least 6 minutes to assure certain cell death.

Mechanism of Radiofrequency Ablation

Radiofrequency ablation (RFA) is a relatively new method to induce precisely focused tissue hyperthermia. Based on investigative work credited to D'Arsonval in 1891,[13] electrocautery and medical diathermy were the first clinical applications of radiofrequency waves in surgery. Modern applications of radiofrequency energy to create focal thermal injuries in the liver were pioneered by McGahan[14] and Rossi.[15]

Radiofrequency generators produce low voltage current, which alternates rapidly at a frequency of approximately 400 KHz (within the frequency range used for radio transmission) at the treatment electrode. An electrical circuit is completed through the target tissue and a large dispersion grounding pad placed remotely on the patient. When current is applied, ions in proximity to the electrode move toward or away from the electrode, depending upon their charge. As the current alternates, the ions rapidly change direction (ionic agitation), which causes frictional heating (resistive heating) of the tissue.[14] Therefore, the targeted tissue, not the electrode itself, produces the heat. Tissue heating is proportional to the square of the current multiplied by the resistance of the tissue (heating I^2R). Since the current decreases to the inverse square of the distance from the electrode (current = $I \propto 1/D^2$), the heat generated in the target tissue falls off in proportion to the inverse fourth power of the distance from the electrode (heating $\propto I^2R \propto (I/D^2)^2 \propto R/D^4$).

These principles of heat induction by radiofrequency waves are based on static systems and have been modified for biologic systems. Thus, the hyperthermic effect in living tissues, or "bioheat", is the net result of energy deposition multiplied by tissue interactions minus the heat loss. Energy deposition—and therefore the diameter of coagulative necrosis—correlates with the electrode tip length, gauge of the electrode, duration of heating, and mechanisms minimizing tissue vaporization and dessication. Both vaporization and dessication near the electrode tip cause increased tissue resistance, decreasing current flow, and, ultimately, break the circuit through the target tissue. In addition, fluid filled structures such as blood vessels and bile ducts behave as low resistance pathways and, in effect, short-circuit the RF electrode resulting in less frictional heating. Several strategies have been used to enhance the energy deposition, such as multi-tyne electrical arrays, internally cooled electrodes, and pulsed energy delivery protocols. Additionally, injection of hypertonic saline into the target tissue minimizes dessication and increases tissue ionicity, which may improve thermocoagulation by this modality.[16] Similarly, tissue interactions affect the size and shape of the coagulative necrosis lesion. Tissue temperatures directly adjacent to the electrode are approximately 100°C. The contribution of resistive heating falls precipitously with increasing distance from the electrode (heating $\propto 1/D^4$). Therefore, tissue surrounding the electrode is warmed by conduction of the heat produced in the tissue directly adjacent to the electrode. The extent of conductive heating is influenced by the distance from the electrode and the thermal conductivity of the tissue. Furthermore, blood flow through the target tissue acts as a heat-sink, diminishing local heat conduction. Therefore, within the liver, the RFA lesion becomes deformed by areas of high and low resistance, blood flow through the tumor, and presence or absence of dessication. Transient inflow occlusion, within a narrow range of temperatures, can enhance the coagulation diameter by minimizimg thermal loss.[17]

In addition to coagulative necrosis, vessels smaller than 3 mm in diameter are obliterated following RFA, leading to local tissue hypoxia and more certain cell death in the target tissue. In vivo studies have shown that internally cooled RFA probes induce larger volumes of coagulative necrosis than the multi-tyne arrays; however, the lesions produced by the multi-tyne arrays are more uniform, spheric, and reproducible.[16]

RFA Methods

The current approaches to radiofrequency ablation of liver tumors include: (1) percutaneous RFA under ultrasound guidance; (2) percutaneous RFA with CT monitoring; (3) laparoscopic RFA using laparoscopic ultrasound guidance and monitoring; and (4) laparotomy with intraoperative ultrasound guidance. More recently, with the development of MRI-compatible electrodes, RFA has been performed using an open MRI to monitor and direct the ablation.

RFA Devices

Currently, three devices are approved for radiofrequency themoablation of liver tumors (Radionics, Burlington, MA; Radiotherapeutics, Mountain View, CA; and RITA Medical Systems, Mountain View, CA). All produce coagulative necrosis in the target tissue; however, they vary with respect to electrode type, geometry of the thermoablative lesion, wattage generated, and method of controlling energy delivery. The Radionics system uses an internally (saline) cooled, straight needle electrode, whereas the other two utilize deployable multi-tyne (7–10 tynes), umbrella shaped arrays to create the thermal lesion (Fig. 13.1). The newer iterations of these systems can create up to 4.5–5 cm ellipsoid to spherical shaped lesions using 14–15 gauge needle electrodes. The generators produce 50–200 watt alternating current which is modulated by the impedance of the heated tissue (Fig. 13.2). The parameters used for thermal ablation in general are target tissue temperatures of 105°C–110°C as monitored by thermocouples at the tip of the tynes. The intended target temperature is > 50°C for 5 minutes or more at the peripheral rim of the tumor plus a 1 cm rim of normal liver. Therefore, a typical ablation cycle is approximately 8 minutes for tumors 2 cm or less in diameter. For larger tumors, each ablation cycle can take up to 20 minutes. A single deployment and ablation cycle suffices for tumors less than 3 cm in diameter (Fig. 13.3) whereas multiple overlapping electrode placements and ablation cycles are required for larger lesions. The grounding pads, one or two, are placed on the patient's back or thigh. To eliminate "pad burns", one pad is placed on each thigh with the broad edge facing the abdomen to achieve maximal electrical dispersion.

CLINICAL PARAMETERS

Preoperative Evaluation

Potential candidates for RFA include patients with limited volume liver tumor burden, each tumor less than 5 cm in diameter, with no extra-hepatic spread, and who are deemed unresectable by conventional criteria. By far, the most common type of liver metastasis treated with RFA has been colorectal cancer; however, a variety of other histologic types, including neuroendocrine tumors, sarcomas, lung, breast, and pancreas, have been treated in this fashion. Preoperative studies should include cross-sectional imaging to evaluate the extent and number of liver lesions as well as to exclude extra-hepatic disease; tissue diagnosis

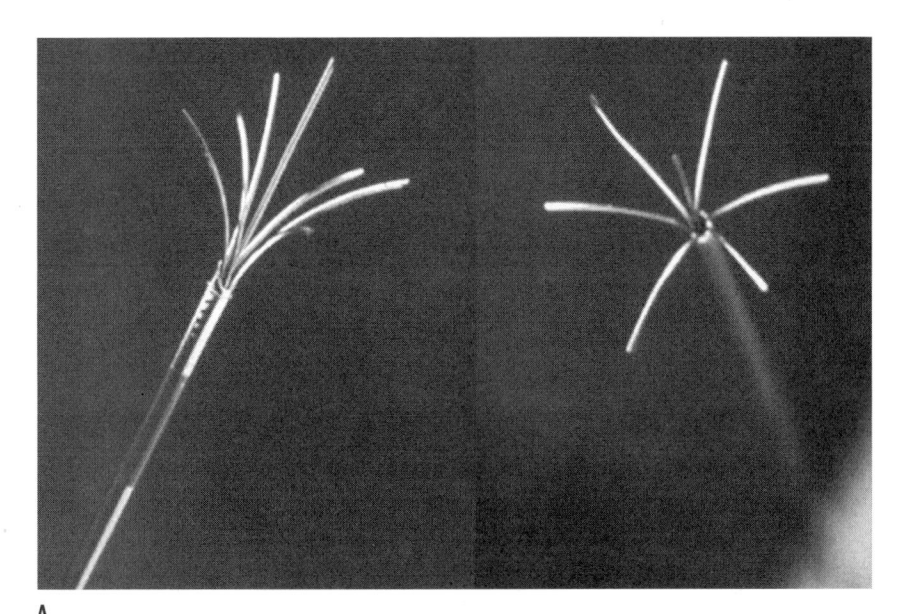

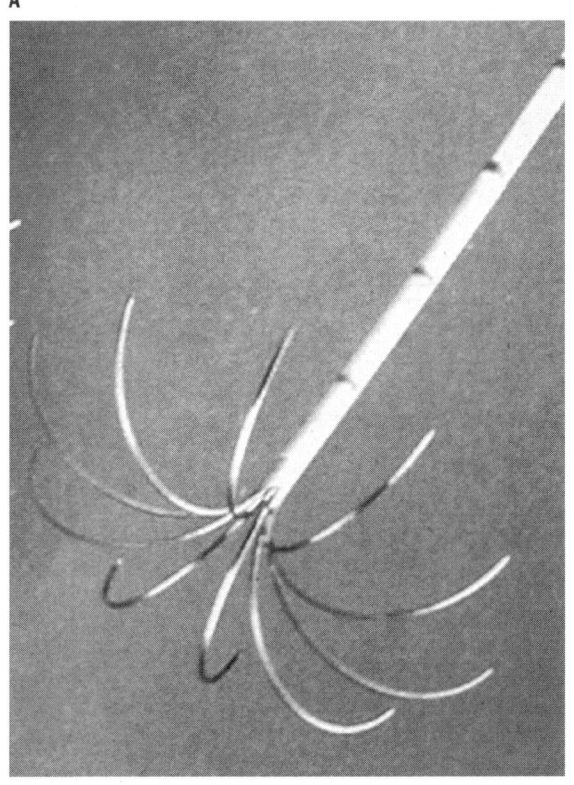

FIGURE 13.1 Examples of two radiofrequency electrodes currently available for use in RFA treatment. (A) RITA Medical Systems; (B) Radiotherapeutics.

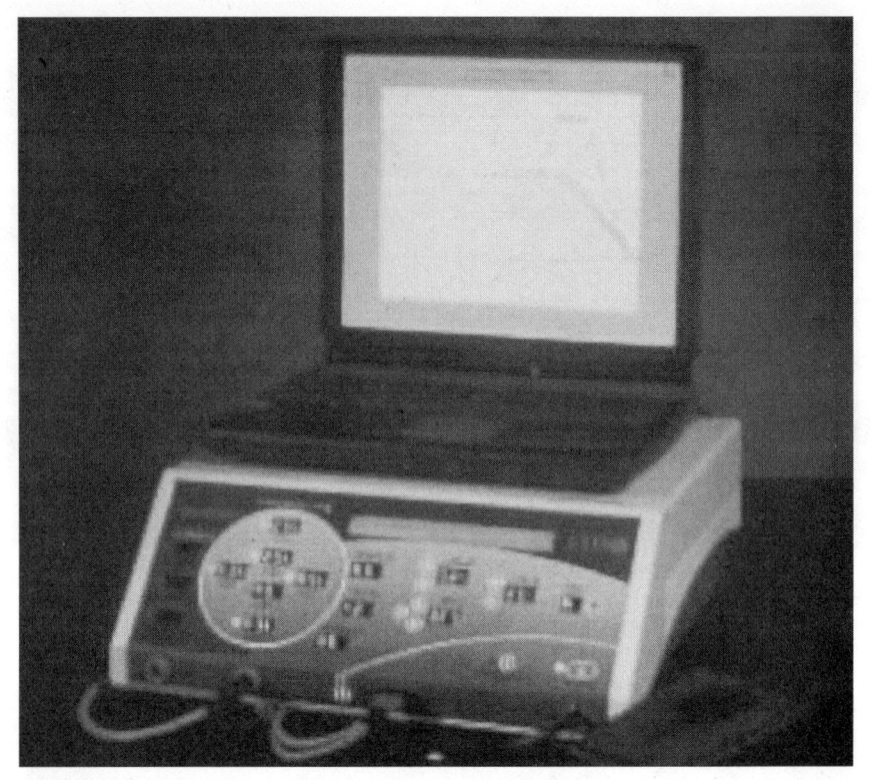

FIGURE 13.2 RITA Medical Systems radiofrequency generator.

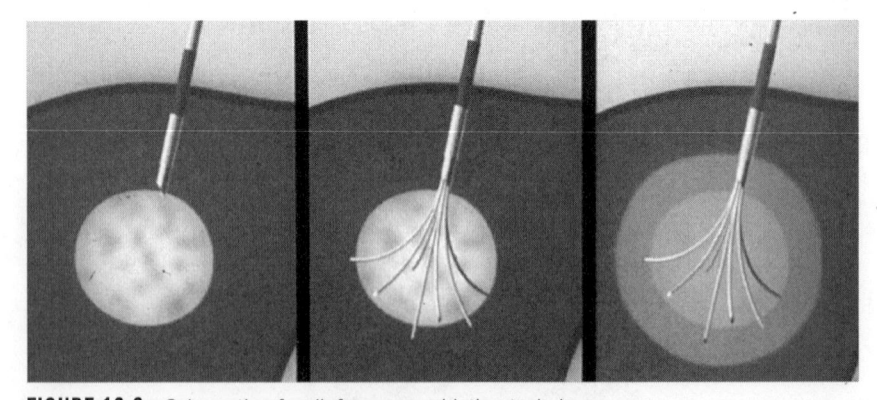

FIGURE 13.3 Schematic of radiofrequency ablation technique.

as clinically indicated; blood tests (hematology, coagulation studies, liver profile, and tumor markers); chest x-ray; and electrocardiogram.

Treatment Plan

The choice of the operative approach is, to a large degree, dependent upon the institution and local expertise. The percutaneous route is least invasive, can be performed on an outpatient or short-stay basis, allows multiple repeat treatments as needed, and is preferred for patients with significant medical co-morbidities. The laparoscopic approach is minimally invasive and requires only an overnight hospitalization. Laparoscopy has significant advantages over the percutaneous approach by allowing visualization of occult peritoneal disease, as well as detection of additional hepatic metastases using laparoscopic ultrasound. Furthermore, the lesions can be treated more effectively and precisely than with the percutaneous approach. The open laparotomy approach is the most flexible and most accurate in staging, and enables proper electrode placement and assessment of complete ablation. Its disadvantages are those of increased morbidity associated with open surgery, a 3–5 day hospitalization, and added expense. While these methods are interchangeable to an extent, caution must be exercised in the percutaneous treatment of multiple lesions and those adjacent to other organs and vital structures. Tumors close to the diaphragm or the hilum of the liver may require a laparoscopic or open approach to achieve safe ablations. Thermal injury to the diaphragm, bile ducts, major hepatic vascular structures, and abdominal viscera are best avoided by the laparoscopic and open methods.

Irrespective of the approach chosen, a treatment strategy must be established prior to needle placement, since RFA produces microbubbles from water vaporization in the ablated tissue that obscure anatomic landmarks during the procedure (Fig. 13.4). As indicated earlier, a single electrode placement may be sufficient to treat a 2–3 cm metastasis and achieve a zone coagulative necrosis measuring 4–5 cm in diameter. For larger lesions, overlapping ablations (overlapping thermal ellipsoid) are needed. During treatment of multiple liver lesions, the deepest and most posterior lesions should be treated initially in order to minimize artefacts induced by intraparenchymal microbubbles that interfere with the accuracy of subsequent ablations. In addition to gray-scale ultrasound, demonstration of loss of blood flow within the target tissue using power/color Doppler ultrasonography reliably confirms complete tumor ablation.[18]

Follow Up

The patients are examined by CT or MRI scan within one month of ablation to assess the completeness of the ablation (fig. 13.5). If no residual tumor is demonstrable, patients undergo repeat imaging studies at 3–6 months along with blood tests and tumor marker evaluations. Isolated liver recurrences can be treated with repeat RFA, commonly using a percutaneous approach. Positron emission

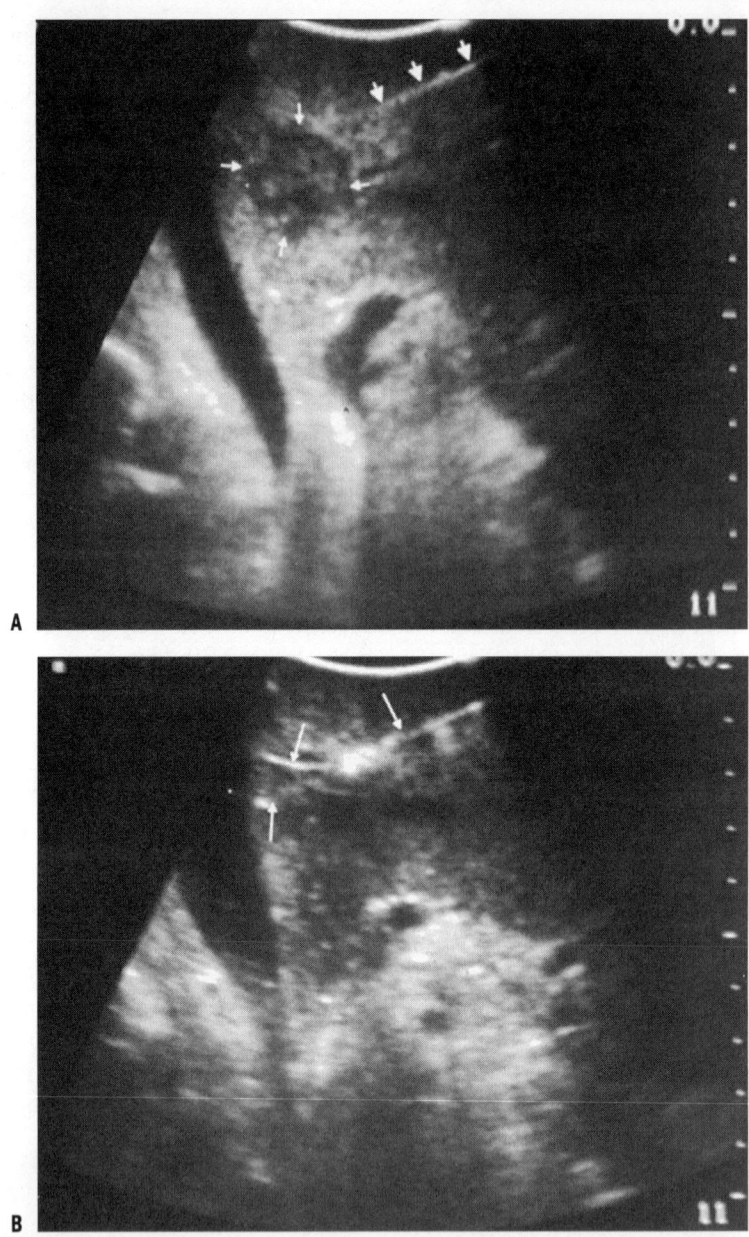

FIGURE 13.4 Intraoperative ultrasound of radiofrequency ablation. (A) tumor (small arrows) with undeployed RF electrode (large arrows). (B) Deployed RF electrode array in tumor. (C) Microbubble interference during ablation cycle. (D) Completed ablation with characteristic "lacrosse racket" appearance.

RF Ablation for Liver Metastases **267**

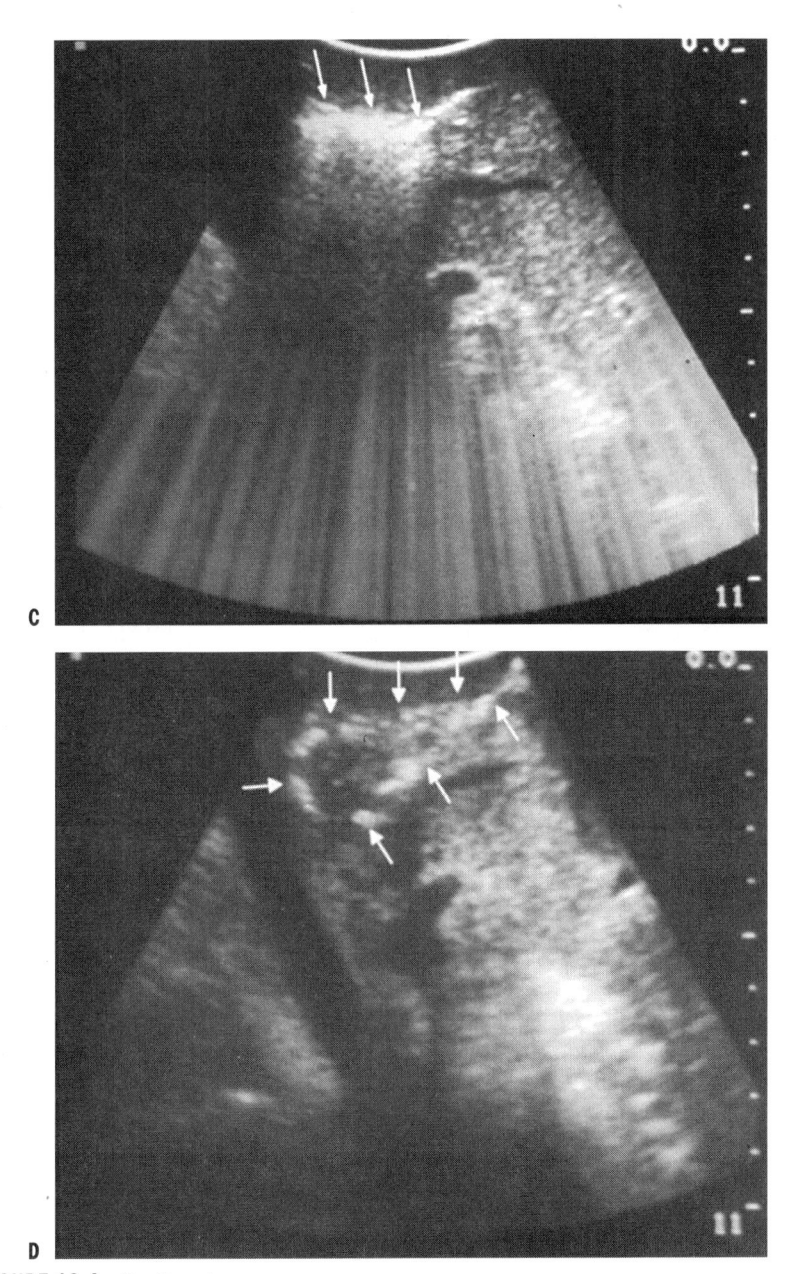

FIGURE 13.4 Continued

tomography (PET) may be a more accurate method to screen patients before treatment and to detect recurrences.[19] PET scans may be more sensitive in detection of residual or recurrent disease in previously ablated liver tissue. A persistent defect can be seen on both CT and MRI at the ablated site, confounding the detection of recurrent disease.

Complications

RFA is a relatively safe procedure with an extremely low rate of complications, as demonstrated by multiple published series. Minor complications include nausea, pain (incisional and peritoneal), and "post-ablation syndrome,"[20] which occurs after large volume ablations and consists of low grade fever (up to 101°F), lethargy, sweats, and "flu-like" symptoms. These are usually self-limited and resolve without treatment within 5 days. The rare serious complications that have been reported in the literature are compiled in Table 13.2. It should be noted that these complications are anecdotal and generally occur with a frequency of less than 5%. The complications can be classified as thermal injuries, liver trauma related complications, infectious problems, and general complications. While early studies reported dispersion pad skin burns, this complication has been all but eliminated by using multiple large surface area foil pads placed remotely from the treated liver and oriented with the longest surface edge facing the RF electrode.[21] Thermal injuries to bowel, bile ducts, and diaphragm are avoidable by adequate mobilization of the liver, insulation of perihepatic structures, and diligent monitoring during the ablation process.

RESULTS OF A COLLECTIVE REVIEW OF RFA FOR LIVER METASTASES

Because the clinical application of RFA to treat liver tumors is relatively recent, publications of results regarding tumor control started appearing in the literature

TABLE 13.2 Complications of Radiofrequency Ablation

Burn injuries
   Ground pad burn
   Diaphragm/bowel necrosis
Bleeding
   Subcapsular hematoma
   Intraperitoneal bleeding
Hepatic abscess
Liver failure
Pleural effusion
Hemothorax
Myocardial infarction
Mortality < 1%

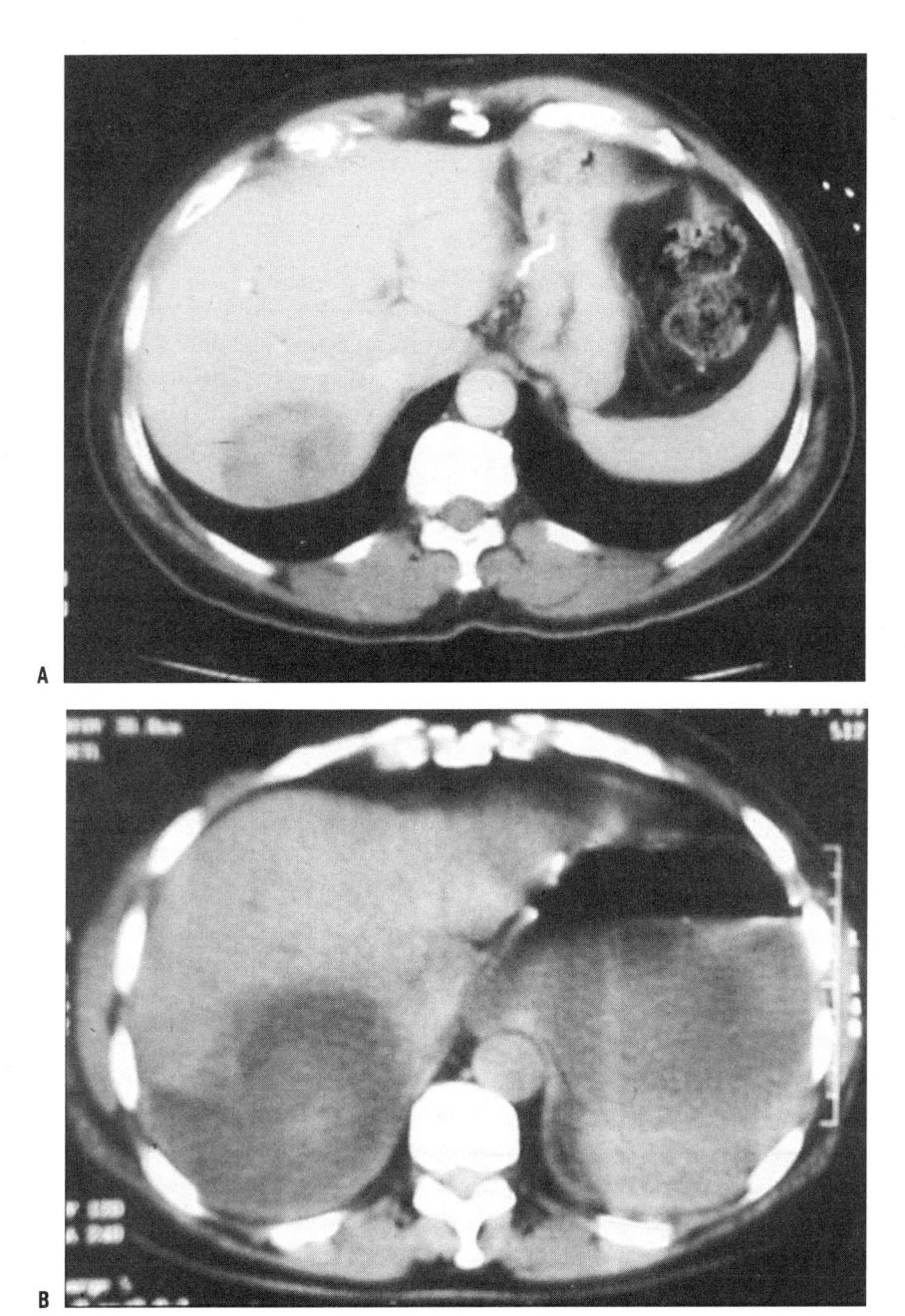

FIGURE 13.5 Computed tomography of liver metastasis pretreatment (A) and 1 week following RF ablation (B).

only 5 years ago. The earliest reports were from Italy, reported by Rossi[22] and Solbiati[23] in 1996 and 1997. While long-term results have yet to emerge, short-term results of local tumor control and intermediate-term results of survival have been forthcoming. We have made an attempt to compile the existing information extracted from English language publications to date (Table 13.3).[24-36] Although most of the studies are retrospective, a few are prospective. Reports concerning hepatocellular carcinoma were excluded because this update focuses on liver metastases. Publications that combine both primary and metastatic liver tumors are included in this collective review but only the metastatic lesions were included in the analysis. Data from some groups with multiple publications containing overlapping patient information have been parsed to include the most updated or largest series published by that group in this review. Lastly, this is not a "meta-analysis" since the studies are diverse, and most are retrospective and uncontrolled.

The most salient information is the collective data provided at the bottom of the Table 13.3. Based on the 621 patients included in this review from 1997–2000, tumors treated with RFA ranged from 0.5 cm to 12 cm, with a mean diameter of 2.8 cm. The duration of follow up ranges from 3 months to 28 months, with a mean of 12 months. There is enormous variability in the reported rates of recurrence, which probably reflects the evolution of the technique and the technology, the method of treatment (open vs percutaneous), and the intensity of evaluation for recurrent disease. Local recurrences range from 2%–55%, with a mean of 19%. Recurrence at non-treated sites (new liver lesions or extra-hepatic sites) account for 43% of recurrences at the average follow-up of one year. At this same duration of follow up, 86% of patient were alive and 53% were free of disease. It is very difficult to define the benefit of RFA alone from this collective review, since some of the studies report other concurrent treatments including chemotherapy, resection, cryotherapy, and repeat RFA. An in-depth analysis of factors affecting local recurrence is provided below because the impact of RFA in the treatment of liver metastases will be largely predicated on its ability to achieve local control within the liver.

Local Recurrence Following RF Ablation

Table 13.3 shows the spectrum of local recurrence rates reported in the published series from 1997–2000. The wide range of 2%–55% (mean: 19%) raises concern and several questions. Recurrence at the site of the ablated lesion in the liver is related to several factors: (1) tumor characteristics, (2) technique of ablation, (3) length of follow up, and (4) diligence/technique used for detection.

Tumor Characteristics The local recurrence rate post RF ablation seems to be directly proportional to the size of the treated lesion (Table 13.4). Solbiati et al[37] reported an overall recurrence rate of 25%, but the rates were 0%, 30%, and 42% for lesions < 2 cm, 2–3 cm, and > 3 cm respectively. Bilchik et al[38] noted that the local recurrence for tumors > 3 cm was 38% following RFA. In the same

TABLE 13.3 RFA for Liver Metastases: Collected Review[a]

Study	N	Cohort w/Mets	No. of Tumors Rx'd	Tumor size: mean, cm (range)	Mean F/U (mo)	Other Rx[b]	Survival DF	Survival Overall	Recurrence Local	Recurrence Other
Dodd et al, 1997	19	10	—	2.6 (0.5–8.0)	3	A	86%	—	—	—
Livraghi et al 1997	14	14	24	—	6	A	52%	—	—	—
Solbiati et al 1998	16	16	—	—	18	A	33%	89%	25%	65%
Lencioni et al 1998	29	29	—	3.0	7	A	52%	93%	12%	52%
Rossi et al 1998	37	14	—	2.5 (1.1–3.5)	10	A	46%	—	6%	54%
Kainuna et al 1999	9	9	—	—	15	A,C	—	66%	55%	44%
Curley et al 1999	123	75	—	3.4 (0.5–12.0)	15	A,C	70%	—	—	28%
Jiao et al 1999	35	27	—	—	10	A,B	—	80%	—	14%
Scudamore et al 1999	12	12	—	3.0 (2.0–4.0)	10	A	—	90%	—	—
Siperstein et al 2000	66	55	170	2.5 (1.0–10)	12	—	72%	—	—	—
Goldberg et al 2000	22	18	19	3.3 (0.8–8)	N/A	N/A	N/A	N/A	N/A	—
Wood et al 2000	84	73	213	2.0 (0.3–9)	9	A,B,C,D	43%	—	—	—
Gillams et al 2000	69	69	—	3.9 (1–8)	28	C	(median: 27 mos)	—	—	—
Goharin et al 2000	21	—	—	1.4 (0.5–5.2)	17	—	22%	95%	—	—
Collective Data	—	621	—	2.8 (0.5–12)	12	—	53%	86%	19%	43%

[a] Published reports of patient data following RFA for metastasis to the liver (predominantly colorecal). Reports of primary liver cancer only are not included. Those reports with both primary and metastatic are included and the cohort with metastatic disease to liver is analyzed.
[b] Other Rx: A, report RFA; B, Resection; C, chemotherapy; D, cryotherapy.
N/A: Not applicable; this study was for pathologic correlation.

TABLE 13.4 RF Ablation of Liver Metastases: Predictors of Local Failure

Tumor Size[a]			
Size	N	Local Recurrence	Compound Poor Prognostic Criteria[b]
NA	—	—	Lack of increased lesion size at 1 week
< 2 cm	12	0	Adenocarcinoma, sarcoma
2–3 cm	20	6 (30%)	Larger tumor volume (failures 18 cm^3; successes 7 cm^3)
> 3 cm	12	5 (42%)	Vascular invasion on real time ultrasound

[a]Adapted from Solbiati et al.[37]
[b]Adapted from Siperstein et al.[18]

report, the recurrence rate following cryosurgery was noted to be 17% for lesions > 3 cm in size. From the data in this study, RFA seems inferior to cryosurgery for larger lesions in terms of local control. A more objective quantification of lesion size should be obtained by volume determination. In Siperstein's study,[18] the volume was calculated using the equation for an ellipsoid (4/3 π (X/2) (Y/2) (Z/2); there were no local recurrences for tumors < 7.5 cm^3, while a significant number of tumors recurred if the volume was > 18 cm^3. Another tumor characteristic that may affect local recurrence pattern is the histologic type of tumor. Hepatocellular carcinoma, when encapsulated, tends to have the best control rate following RFA, while metastatic cancers to the liver seem to fare less well. Among the metastatic tumors, adenocarcinoma and sarcoma demonstrate higher than expected local recurrence rates compared with other histologic types. It is not known if colorectal metastases as a subset do better compared with other adenocarcinomas, since biologically they behave differently than pancreatic, gastric, breast, and lung cancers.

In addition to the size and histology, the location of tumors and the number of lesions treated per patient may have an impact on local recurrence. None of the studies published to date provides a definitive answer to this question. It seems intuitive to suggest that lesions close to the major vessels may not be treatable with an adequate tumor-free margin and thus will suffer from thermal sink effect at the center tumor rim, such that a higher local recurrence rate is to be expected. Further, the more numerous the lesions are in a given liver being subjected to RFA, the greater are the chances of microscopic and satellite lesions around the index tumor; therefore, the local recurrence rate will be high.

Technique of Ablation Two variables in the technique of ablation are the approach used (laparoscopic vs open vs percutaneous) and the expertise of the caregiver. There is insufficient information to make any definitive statements regarding these factors, but the early reports suggest that, at least, laparoscopic and open surgical approaches may be equivalent in terms of local tumor control.[38]

There have not been any comparisons between percutaneous and open/laparoscopic approaches. However, since 5%–10% more lesions are detected by laparoscopic/open intraoperative ultrasonography as compared with state-of-the-art preoperative imaging, it should follow that such occult lesions will increase "apparent" liver recurrence rates following percutaneous RFA when compared with the other two approaches where "occult" lesions would have been detected and treated. The expertise of the surgeon/radiologist performing image guided RFA is to be considered an important variable, especially as a quality assurance issue in future trials, be they single-institutional or multi-institutional.

Length of Follow Up   Demonstration of local recurrence will depend on the duration of follow up, at least in the intermediate term. Since the published reports have a range of mean follow up from 3 months to 28 months after RFA, the local recurrence rates mirror this disparity. While 3 months is too short a time to declare local control, long-term follow up of 2–5 years is not required either, to answer this question. Perhaps a minimum of 6–12 months is required for the demonstration of either local control or recurrence.

Diligence/Technique Used to Detect Recurrence   There is a high variability of the methods used to detect local recurrences post-RFA. Triphasic CT, gadolinium enhanced MRI, image guided biopsy, and positron emission tomography (PET) are the methods used for recurrence detection. In most studies, complete response was defined as a nonenhancing, treated area on follow up CT. Based on this criteria alone, a complete response was achieved in 76% of patients (range 52%-100%) in the collected review. However, a few studies have used histologic criteria to report efficacy. Scudamore et al[32] reported complete ablation by histologic criteria in 8 of 9 patients when tumors were resected following RFA; Rossi et al[28] reported complete necrosis in 4/5 tumors resected after RFA. These studies stand in contrast with the report of Solbiati et al,[23] wherein residual microscopic viable tumor was detected in all 4 patients who underwent resection following RFA. Although this discrepancy may reflect the technique and expertise of the caregiver, it is quite likely that the timing of resection, extent of scrutiny of excised tumor, and staining techniques (H&E stain, NADH, LDH) may play a role.

An experimental study in pigs has correlated the real time sonographic appearance of RFA and biphasic contrast enhanced helical CT 12–48 hours post RFA with histopathology.[39] This study suggested that real time ultrasound underestimated the true size of ablated lesions, while CT closely correlated with the size of ablated tissue. Quantitative CT criteria using HU density (lack of increase with contrast in necrotic tissue) add more validity. While CT is the current standard in assessing response during follow up, recent data suggest gadolinium enhanced MRI, or MRI using T2-weighted turbo spin-echo sequences (TSET2) and short T1 inversion recovery techniques (STIR) may be better techniques for assessment of thermal lesions.[40]

In addition to an analysis of all the factors listed above, local recurrences should be viewed in the context of both number of lesions as well as number of patients. For example, multiple recurrences in one patient should be viewed differently from recurrences at single sites in multiple patients. The former may be related to the biology of tumor and patient selection, while the latter may be relevant in addressing the technique or technology. In a report by Siperstein et al,[18] the recurrence rate was analyzed both as a function of lesion number as well as the number of patients as a denominator. In their study, recurrence was noted in 19% of lesions treated, while the rate increased to 39% when analyzed by the total number of patients in whom local recurrence was noted.

NEED FOR PROSPECTIVE CLINICAL TRIALS

With the burgeoning technology and the consumer-driven demand for RFA, it has become imperative to answer some questions germane to the utility of RFA in formal clinical trials. Some examples of the work already accomplished are those of Goldberg et al[33] in their phase I trial to obtain radiologic and pathologic correlation and that of Siperstein et al[18] in their phase II study defining the laparoscopic approach to RFA. Several new trials are emerging in phase II and phase III formats; these trials use comparison of RFA with regional, systemic, or combined regional and systemic chemotherapy. As in the upcoming strategies, our group has been interested in the design of a clinical trial to define how best to achieve an R0 ablation, what constitutes the best and most cost effective follow up regimen, and whether RF ablation makes a difference in quality and length of survival in the setting of metastatic colorectal cancer. We activated a phase II trial over a year ago with an expected accrual of 75 patients from multiple centers comparing RFA plus hepatic artery infusion and systemic chemotherapy versus RFA plus systemic chemotherapy. The primary outcome endpoints are local control, disease-free and overall survival, and patterns of failure. Secondary outcome measurements include length of hospitalization, cost of therapy, quality of life, and correlative molecular parameters.

SUMMARY AND FUTURE PROSPECTS

RFA of metastatic liver tumors is a promising and rapidly improving technology with which to produce focused thermal necrosis. It can be performed safely by a variety of approaches with minimal morbidity as an outpatient or short-stay procedure. Early reports of tumor control and intermediate-term survival rates are very encouraging, but have a wide range of successes and failures. Continued progress will be ensured by advances that (1) achieve greater volumes of ablated tissue; (2) shorten ablation cycle time for multiple lesions; (3) develop technology permitting more precise and sophisticated percutaneous and minimally invasive approaches (i.e. steerable electrodes); (4) refine real-time monitoring modalities (contrast-enhanced ultrasonography, open MRI); and (5) standardize post-ablation "damage assessment" protocols such that the data will become meaningful and comparable. With more standardized reporting, patterns of failure can be analyzed to optimized regional and systemic therapies. The use of PET scans may provide useful metabolic imaging data, which allows earlier retreatment or other multimodality approaches.[19] Furthermore, prospective evaluations of complementary modalities such as anti-angiogenic or embolic therapies, regional hepatic artery infusion chemotherapy, and other novel treatments based on apoptosis and heat shock are needed to maximize the benefit of this localized therapy. Lastly, cost effectiveness and quality-of-life outcome analyses should be included in all studies, enabling objective quantification of benefits of RFA. The need for prospective clinical trials must again be emphasized in order to make strides that are patient-centered rather than technology-driven.

REFERENCES

1. Steele G Jr, Ravikumar TS. Resection of hepatic metastases from colorectal cancer. Biologic perspective. Ann Surg 1989;210:127–138.
2. Scheele J, Stang R, Altendorf-Hofmann A, Paul M. Resection of colorectal liver metastases. World J Surg 1995;19:59–71.
3. Fong Y, Blumgart LH. Hepatic colorectal metastasis: current status of surgical therapy. Oncology (Huntingt) 1998;12:1489–1498; discussion 1498–1500, 1503.
4. Wagner JS, Adson MA, Van Heerden JA et al. The natural history of hepatic metastases from colorectal cancer. A comparison with resective treatment. Ann Surg 1984;199:502–508.
5. Nagorney DM, Gigot JF. Primary epithelial hepatic malignancies: etiology, epidemiology, and outcome after subtotal and total hepatic resection. Surg Oncol Clin N Am 1996;5:283–300.
6. LeVeen R. Laser hyperthermia and radiofrequency ablation of hepatic lesions. Semin Interven Radiol 1997;14:313–324.
7. Stangl R, Altendorf-Hofmann A, Charnley RM, Scheele J. Factors influencing the natural history of colorectal liver metastases. Lancet 1994;343:1405–1410.
8. Wood CB, Gillis CR, Blumgart LH. A retrospective study of the natural history of patients with colorectal metastases. Clin Oncol 1976;2:285–288.
9. Gallagher JT, Vauthey JN. Selective continuous intra-arterial chemotherapy for liver tumors. In: Clavien PA, ed. Malignant liver tumors: Current and Emerging therapies. Malden, MA: Blackwell Science, Inc, 1999:116–124.
10. Sanz-Altamira P, Spence L, Huberman M. Selective chemoembolization in the management of hepatic metastases in refractory colorectal carcinoma. Dis Colon Rect 1997;40:770–775.
11. Greenlee RT, Hill-Harmon MB, Murray T, Thun M. Cancer Statistics, 2001. CA Cancer J Clin 2001;51:15–36.
12. Dickson JA, Calderwood SK. Temperature range and selective sensitivity of tumors to hyperthermia: a critical review. Ann NY Acad Sci 1980;335:180–205.
13. D'Arsonval DM. Action physiologique des courants alternatifs. C R Soc Biol 1891;43:283–286.
14. McGahan JP, Browning PD, Brock JM, Tesluk H. Hepatic ablation using radiofrequency electrocautery. Invest Radiol 1990;25:267–270.

15. Rossi S, Fornari F, Pathies C, Buscarini L. Thermal lesions induced by 480 KHz localized current field in guinea pig and pig liver. Tumori 1990;76:54–57.
16. de Baere T, Denys A, Wood BJ et al. Radiofrequency liver ablation: experimental comparative study of water-cooled versus expandable systems. AJR Am J Roentgenol 2001;176:187–192.
17. Patterson EJ, Scudamore CH, Owen DA et al. Radiofrequency ablation of porcine liver in vivo: effects of blood flow and treatment time on lesion size. Ann Surg 1998;227:559–565.
18. Siperstein A, Garland A, Engle K et al. Local recurrence after laparoscopic radiofrequency thermal ablation of hepatic tumors. Ann Surg Oncol 2000;7:106–113.
19. Ravikumar TS, Jones M, Serrano M et al. The role of PET scanning in radiofrequency ablation of liver metastases from colorectal cancer. Cancer J 2000;6[suppl 4]:S330–S343.
20. McGhana JP, Dodd GD. Radiofrequency ablation of the liver: current status. AJR Am J Roentgenol 2001;176:3–16.
21. Goldberg SN, Solbiati L, Halpern EF, Gazelle GS. Variables affecting proper system grounding for radiofrequency ablation in an animal model. J Vasc Interv Radiol 2000;11:1069–1075.
22. Rossi S, Di Stasi M, Buscarini E et al. Percutaneous RF interstitial thermal ablation in the treatment of hepatic cancer. AJR Am J Roentgenol 1996;167:759–768.
23. Solbiati L, Goldberg SN, Ierace T et al. Hepatic metastases: percutaneous radio-frequency ablation with cooled-tip electrodes. Radiology 1997;205:367–373.
24. Dodd GD, Halff G, Rhim HC et al. Ultrasound guided radiofrequency thermal ablation of liver tumors, San Antonio Cancer Symposia, San Antonio, Texas, 1997.
25. Livraghi T, Goldberg SN, Monti F et al. Saline-enhanced radio-frequency tissue ablation in the treatment of liver metastases. Radiology 1997;202:205–210.
26. Solbiati L, Arsizio B, Goldberg SN et al. Long-term followup of liver metastases treated with percutaneous US-guided radiofrequency ablation using internally cooled electrodes, Radiologic Society of North America 84th Scientific Assembly, Chicago IL, December 3, 1998.
27. Lencioni R, Goletti O, Armillotta N et al. Radio-frequency thermal ablation of liver metastases with a cooled-tip electrode needle: results of a pilot clinical trial. Eur Radiol 1998;8:1205–1211.
28. Rossi S, Buscarini E, Garbagnati F et al. Percutaneous treatment of small hepatic tumors by an expandable RF needle electrode. AJR Am J Roentgenol 1998;170:1015–1022.
29. Kainuma O, Asano T, Aoyama H et al. Combined therapy with radiofrequency thermal ablation and intra-arterial infusion chemotherapy for hepatic metastases from colorectal cancer. Hepatogastroenterology 1999;46:1071–1077.
30. Curley SA, Izzo F, Delrio P et al. Radiofrequency ablation of unresectable primary and metastatic hepatic malignancies: results in 123 patients. Ann Surg 1999;230:1–8.
31. Jiao LR, Hansen PD, Havlik R et al. Clinical short-term results of radiofrequency ablation in primary and secondary liver tumors. Am J Surg 1999;177:303–306.
32. Scudamore CH, Lee SI, Patterson EJ et al. Radiofrequency ablation followed by resection of malignant liver tumors. Am J Surg 1999;177:411–417.
33. Goldberg SN, Gazelle GS, Compton CC et al. Treatment of intrahepatic malignancy with radiofrequency ablation: radiologic-pathologic correlation. Cancer 2000;88:2452–63.
34. Wood TF, Rose DM, Chung M et al. Radiofrequency ablation of 231 unresectable hepatic tumors: indications, limitations, and complications. Ann Surg Oncol 2000;7:593–600.
35. Gillams AR, Lees WR. Survival after percutaneous image-guided thermal ablation of hepatic metastases from colorectal cancer. Dis Colon Rect 2000;43:656–661.
36. Goharin ED, El-Otmany A, Taieb J et al. Usefulness of intraoperative radiofrequency thermoablation of liver tumors associated or not with hepatectomy. Eur J Surg Oncol 2000;26:763–769.

37. Solbiati L, Ierace T, Goldberg SN et al. Percutaneous US-guided radio-frequency tissue ablation of liver metastases: treatment and follow-up in 16 patients. Radiology 1997;202:195–203.
38. Bilchik AJ, Wood TF, Allegra D et al. Cryosurgical ablation and radiofrequency ablation for unresectable hepatic malignant neoplasms: a proposed algorithm. Arch Surg 2000;135:657–662; discussion 662–664.
39. Raman SS, Lu DS, Vodopich DJ et al. Creation of radiofrequency lesions in a porcine model: correlation with sonography, CT, and histopathology. AJR Am J Roentgenol 2000;175:1253–1258.
40. Aschoff AJ, Rafie N, Jesberger JA et al. Thermal lesion conspicuity following interstitial radiofrequency thermal tumor ablation in humans: A comparison of STIR, turbo spin-echo T2-weighted, and contrast-enhanced T1-weighted MR images at 0.2 T. J Magn Reson Imaging 2000;12:584–589.

Treatment of Prostate Cancer: Surgery

James A. Eastham, M.D.

Peter T. Scardino, M.D.

Prostate cancer remains the most common form of noncutaneous malignancy and the second leading cause of cancer death in American men.[1] Because prostate cancer incidence increases rapidly with age, the absolute number of diagnosed cases is destined to rise worldwide as life expectancy increases. Indeed, the number of men older than 65 years is likely to double from 1990 to 2020. Prostate cancer will cause the death of 3% of all men alive today who are over 50 years old. It will also cause many men to suffer serious complications from local tumor growth or distant metastases as well as from complications of treatment.

Despite its nearly epidemic proportions, prostate cancer evokes considerable controversy because of its unusual biologic features and because of the lack of firm data regarding the natural history of the disease. Patients diagnosed with a clinically localized prostate cancer face a daunting variety of treatment choices, including observation ("watchful waiting") and brachytherapy and/or external beam irradiation therapy with or without androgen deprivation therapy, as well as surgery. Because the disease often strikes older men with other co-morbid conditions, the risk to life and health posed by the cancer itself has been difficult to quantify.[2-4] Prospective, randomized trials, such as the National Cancer Institute's Prostate, Lung, Colorectal and Ovarian Cancer Screening Trial (PLCO) and the Prostate Cancer Intervention Versus Observation Trial (PIVOT), have not yet been completed; these trials have been undertaken to establish whether early detection (PLCO) or treatment (PIVOT) of localized prostate cancer will decrease the mortality rate from the disease.[5,6] Until such studies are concluded, patients and their physicians must make the decision whether to treat aggressively or manage conservatively with the best evidence available today.

RATIONALE FOR TREATMENT

Serum prostate-specific antigen (PSA), discovered in the late 1970s, has been shown to be effective in the early detection of prostate cancer through the work of Catalona and others.[7] Consequently, a dramatic shift in the stage of disease at diagnosis has occurred. Prior to the development of serum PSA testing, only 30% of patients were diagnosed with a cancer that was clinically confined to the prostate (stage A or B).[8] Today, 90% of cancers detected in screening trials are clinically confined (stage T1–T2 N0 M0).[9] The incidence of nodal metastases at pelvic lymphadenectomy has declined to 1%–3%.[10] In 60% of patients with clinically confined prostate cancer, the cancer is completely confined to the prostate pathologically. Some investigators, however, have questioned the routine use of serum PSA as a screening tool. Examination of the prostate gland at autopsy in men 50 years of age or older who had no clinical evidence of cancer identified adenocarcinoma in approximately 30% of cases,[11–13] but the lifetime risk of developing a clinically detected prostate cancer is about 16%.[1] This discrepancy between the high prevalence of prostate cancer found at autopsy and the lower incidence of clinically detected cancer raises the question concerning which prostate cancers might be best managed without immediate treatment. In other words, are cancers detected solely on the basis of an elevated serum PSA level clinically indolent, or are these cancers clinically active, but simply identified at an earlier stage?

To examine this question, we compared the pathologic features of three types of prostate cancer: (1) prostate cancers found incidentally at cystoprostatectomy for bladder cancer; (2) prostate cancers that were palpable on digital rectal examination; and (3) impalpable prostate cancers detected by an elevated serum PSA (stage T1c) (Table 14.1.1).[14] Prostate cancer was diagnosed in 209 men based solely on an elevated serum PSA level. While these tumors were often high grade (55% had a primary or secondary Gleason grade of 4 or 5) and frequently demonstrated extracapsular extension (40%), these tumors had a more favorable profile than tumors in a group of 468 men with palpable cancer. Only 25% of clinical stage T1c tumors had advanced pathologic features compared to 40% of palpable cancers, while the proportion of indolent tumors was similar (9%) in each group (Table 14.1.1).[14] This contrasts sharply with results from the cystoprostatectomy series in which none had advanced pathologic features and 78% were considered indolent. These results suggest that most prostate cancers detected solely on the basis of an elevated serum PSA level are clinically important and are more likely to be cured by radical prostatectomy than palpable tumors.

TABLE 14.1.1 Clinical and Incidental Detection of Cancers[a]

Cancer	N	Prognostic Category (%)		
		Indolent	Curable	Advanced
Cystoprostatectomy series	90	78	22	0
Radical prostatectomy series	759	10	56	34
Clinical stage T1a, b	73	19	59	22
Palpable tumor	468	9	52	40
Impalpable, elevated PSA level	209	9	66	25
Elevated PSA only, impalpable, not visible	110	12	69	19

Abbreviation: PSA, prostate-specific antigen.
Percentage of cancers detected clinically (radical prostatectomy series) and incidentally (cystoprostatectomy series) that were indolent, clinically important but curable, and advanced.
[a]Categories are defined by pathologic criteria. Indolent cancers are < 0.5g, confined to the prostate with no poorly-differentiated elements. Advanced cancers are those that are high grade (Gleason score > 6) and extend through the capsule (established extracapsular extension) to the margins of resection or those that invade the seminal vesicles or metastasize to the pelvic lymph node. Curable cancers are all others in the two series.
(Modified from Ohori et al,[14] and reprinted with permission)

The natural history of localized prostate cancer has only recently been documented.[15–18] Two large series have been published which document the risk of developing metastases and of death from prostate cancer in men with clinically localized disease managed conservatively. Chodak and associates analyzed the risk of metastases and of death from prostate cancer in a pooled analysis of 828 patients with clinical stage T1–T2 cancers managed conservatively from six medical centers around the world.[15] The risk of metastases at 10 years was 19% for well differentiated, 42% for moderately differentiated, and 74% for poorly differentiated cancers. While the confidence intervals were broad beyond 10 years, it is evident that when the primary tumor is not controlled, metastases continue to develop over long periods of time. The cancer-specific mortality rate (13%) at 10 years was identical for well and moderately differentiated tumors, which reflects the inadequacy of a 10-year time interval to assess the full impact of a localized prostate cancer on mortality. Of those patients with poorly differentiated tumors, 66% died of prostate cancer at 10 years.

Albertsen and colleagues[17] reported 15-year cancer mortality rates by age and by Gleason grade at diagnosis in a large, population-based study in Connecticut (Fig. 14.1.1). This study documented the profound impact on survival of high-grade cancers (Gleason score 7–10) when these cancers were not controlled. Few men (4%–7%; 18% of the study population) with tumors having a Gleason score of 2–4 that were identified from prostate biopsy specimens had progression leading to death from prostate cancer within 15 years. A majority of the younger patients are still alive but face the possibility of death from prostate cancer in

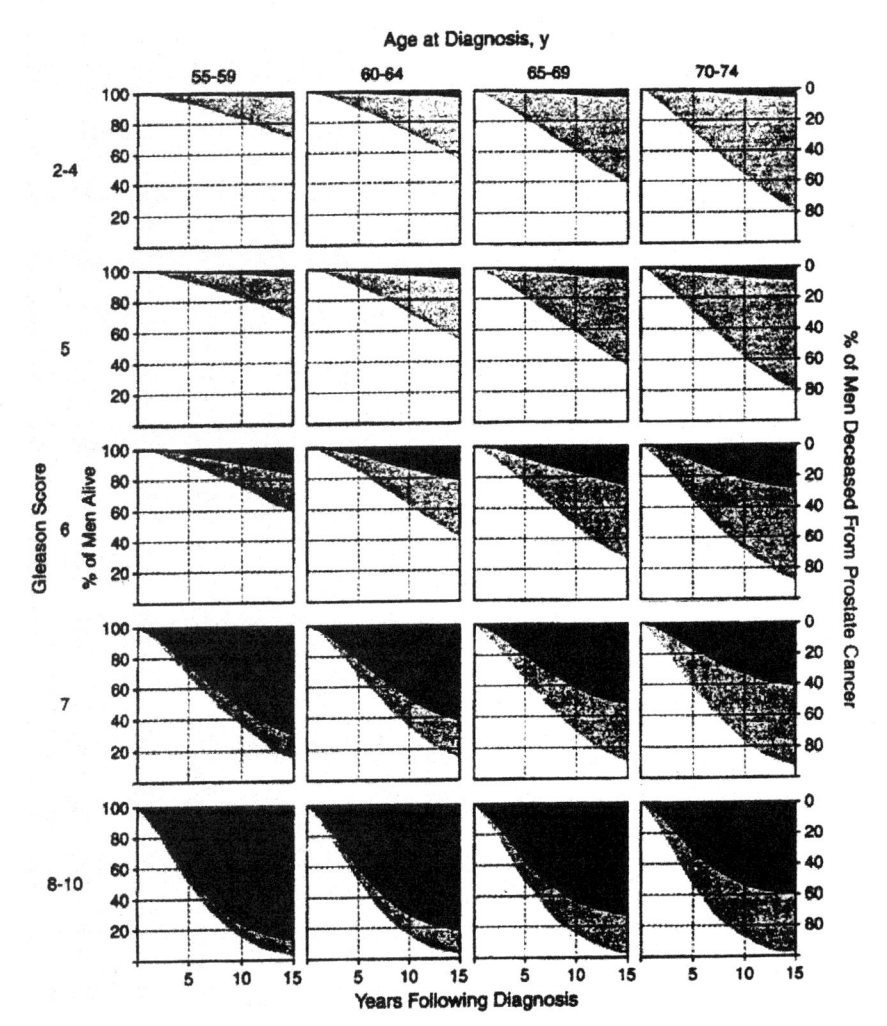

FIGURE 14.1.1 Competing risk survival rate compared with cause-specific survival rate for 767 men diagnosed with localized prostate cancer and managed conservatively, stratified by Gleason score. Cumulative mortality from prostate cancer is shown by the dark upper band; cumulative mortality from other causes is shown by the lighter middle band. The percentage of men surviving is shown by the lowest white band. (Reprinted with permission from Ref. 17)

the future. In contrast, most older men have died from competing medical risks rather than prostate cancer.

Compared with men with well-differentiated tumors, men with Gleason score 5 and 6 cancers identified on prostate biopsy have a higher risk of death from prostate cancer when managed conservatively (6%–11% and 18%–30%, respectively). Men with tumors of Gleason score 7 and 8–10 face a significant chance of dying from prostate cancer when treated conservatively even if the cancer is diagnosed as late as 74 years of age (42%–70% and 60%–87%, respectively). Certainly, these data convince us that cure is necessary in patients with clinical stage T1–T2 NX M0 prostate cancer that is high-grade when detected in the biopsy specimen. What, then, is the evidence that radical prostatectomy can cure such patients? In our series of 1368 patients with clinical stage T1–2 NX M0 cancers treated between 1983 and 1997, the 5-year progression-free probability (PFP) for all patients was 78%, and the 10-year PFP was 73% (Hull GW et al, unpublished data used with permission). Few patients with an undetectable serum PSA level at 6 years had recurrence of their disease.[19] The probability of disease progression was related to the Gleason score of the cancer in the initial biopsy specimen. For 235 patients whose cancer had a Gleason score of 7, 56% were free of progression at 5 years and 46% at 10 years. Even patients with a Gleason score 8–10 cancer fared well, with a 5-year PFP of 45%. These results at 5 and 10 years resemble data reported from other institutions[20,21] and are substantially lower than the 15-year cancer mortality rates reported by Albertsen and colleagues for patients with Gleason score 8–10 cancer.[17]

Because PSA progression precedes clinical progression by 3 to 6 years, it predates mortality from cancer by an even longer period. If patients with high-grade cancer do not experience PSA progression by 5 to 10 years, they are unlikely to die from prostate cancer within 15 years. It is reasonable to conclude, therefore, that radical prostatectomy in patients with these potentially lethal, clinical stage T1–2 NX M0, high-grade cancers can interrupt the natural history of the disease and reduce the chances that they will die of their cancer.[22] Actual 15-year, cancer-specific survival data adjusted for Gleason grade are available in few modern surgical series. Zincke et al[21] reported 10- and 15-year, cause-specific survival rates of 95% and 93%, respectively, for a Gleason score of 3 or less; 90% and 82%, respectively, for Gleason score 4 to 6; and 82% and 71%, respectively, for a Gleason score of 7 or more. These investigators stated that clinical stage did not significantly impact survival, but tumor grade was associated.[21]

Further evidence that surgery can alter the natural history of poorly differentiated cancers comes from a comparison of the pooled analyses of patients managed conservatively, reported by Chodak et al,[15] and those treated surgically, reported by Gerber et al (Table 14.1.2).[15,23–25] Both series report actuarial 10-year metastasis-free and cancer-specific survival rates. No significant differences were noted within this time period in survival rates for patients with well or moderately differentiated cancers (Gleason grading was not done). In those with poorly differentiated cancer, however, the 10-year probability of remaining metastasis free was only 26% for conservatively managed patients, compared to 43% for patients treated surgically. The corresponding 10-year, cancer-specific survival rates were 35% in

TABLE 14.1.2 Survival Rates for Conservatively Managed and Surgically Managed Cancers[a]

	Metastasis-free (%)				Cancer-specific (%)			
	5-Year		10-Year		5-Year		10-Year	
Grade	WW	RP	WW	RP	WW	RP	WW	RP
I	93	95	81	86	98	98	87	93
II	84	92	58	79	97	95	87	79
III	51	78	26	43	67	87	35	60

[a]Comparison of metastatis-free and cancer-specific survival rates in pooled analyses after "watchful waiting" conservative management (WW)[15] and radical prostatectomy (RP).[93] (Reprinted from Ref. 25 with permission).

conservatively managed patients and 60% for surgically treated patients, a highly significant difference (Table 14.1.2).[15,24,25]

These studies provide strong evidence that clinically localized prostate cancer, while slow growing, can affect patient morbidity and mortality (Table 14.1.3).[15–18] Some prostate cancers progress slowly and present little risk to the overall health of the patient. These cancers almost always fall into the T1a classification or the occasional T1b-T2 cancer that is focal, small, and well differentiated. Expectant management may be a reasonable option for these patients, especially if their life expectancy is less than 10 years. However, most clinically detected prostate cancers are not indolent and pose a significant threat to the health and life expectancy and should be treated with the intent to eradicate the primary tumor.

TABLE 14.1.3 Probability of Dying from Prostate Cancer Managed Conservatively According to Biopsy Tumor Grade

		Grade		
Investigators	N	Well (2–4)	Mod (5–7)	Poor (8–10)
Chodak et al, 1994[15] (10 years)	828	13	13	34
Albertsen et al, 1995[16] (15 years)	411	9	28	51
Johansson et al, 1997[18] (15 years)	642	6	17	56
Albertsen et al, 1998[17] (15 years)	767	4–7	6–70[a]	60–87

[a] Gleason 5 = 6–11%; Gleason 6 = 18–30%; Gleason 7 = 42–70%

PATIENT SELECTION: RADICAL PROSTATECTOMY

Radical prostatectomy remains a mainstay of treatment because it offers patients a high level of confidence that they can live out their lives free of cancer recurrence. Since the late 1970s, clear definition of periprostatic anatomy has allowed the development of an operative procedure more respectful of the intricate anatomy of the prostate. It is clear that outcomes following radical prostatectomy are exquisitely sensitive to fine details of the surgical technique. Technical refinements have resulted in less blood loss and fewer transfusions,[26] shorter hospital stays,[27,28] a lower rate of positive surgical margins,[29–32] lower rates of urinary incontinence,[33–36] and higher rates of recovery of erectile function.[34,37,38] A thorough understanding of periprostatic anatomy that emphasizes vascular control permits the safe performance of radical prostatectomy with reduced morbidity.

Age, Health, and Co-morbidity

Radical prostatectomy should be reserved for men who are likely to be cured and will live long enough to benefit from the cure. Mortality from an untreated, localized prostate cancer is not likely to occur for 8–10 years, yet the risk of death from cancer will continue to increase for at least 15–20 years or more. As well, the associated morbidity from local progression or metastases can be substantial.[17,39–42] In 1998, the average life expectancy of a 70-year-old man was 12.8 years, and for a 75-year-old man life expectancy was 10.0 years.[43] Thus, the potential benefits of treatment decrease as a man ages.

Chronological age, however, is only one factor that influences life expectancy. Prostate cancer is frequently diagnosed in older men with associated co-morbid conditions. Conversely, some older patients are in excellent health and have a life expectancy greater than the average for their age group. Therefore, an arbitrary age should not be set at which a patient would no longer be considered a surgical candidate. Clinical judgments based upon a thorough assessment of the life expectancy of the individual patient with prostate cancer will allow the physician to inform the patient fully about the risks and benefits of expectant management as well as active intervention, so that the patient can make a well-informed decision about managing his disease.

Clinical Prognostic Factors

Freedom from progression after radical prostatectomy is associated with several well-established clinical prognostic factors including clinical stage, Gleason score in the prostate biopsy specimen, and serum PSA levels (Table 14.1.4).[21,44,45] Figure 14.1.2 shows the actual non-progression rates in our series of 1,000 men with clinical stage T1–T2 prostate cancer followed for a mean of 53 months (range, 1 to 170 months) after radical prostatectomy. No patient received adjuvant therapy before relapse. Recurrence was defined as a rising PSA level ≥ 0.4 ng/mL.

TABLE 14.1.4 Actuarial (PSA-based) 5-Year Nonprogression Rates (%) After Radical Prostatectomy for Clinical Stage T1-2NXN0 Prostate Cancer

	Pound et al[33]	Catalona and Smith[34]	Zincke et al[35]	Hull et al*
No. Patients	1623	925	3170	1000
Clinical Stage				
T1a	100	89[a]		89[a]
T1b	89		85[e]	
T1c	86	99		85
T2a	85	85[b]	81	82
T2b	69		74[f]	67
T2c	63			70
Gleason Score				
2–4	100	91	93[g]	89
5	97		80[h]	84[j]
6	92	89[c]		
7	66		60[i]	60
8–10	41	74		49
Preoperative PSA Level				
0–4	94	95		94
4.1–10.0	82	93		86
10.1–20.0	72	71[d]		65
>20.0	54			41
Pathologic Stage				
Organ confined	—	91	—	95
Extracapsular extension	—	—	—	76
Seminal vesicle invasion	—	—	—	37
Positive lymph node(s)	—	—	—	18
Surgical Margin				
Negative				81
Positive				36

PSA, prostate-specific antigen.
[a] Includes T1a and T1b
[b] Includes T2a and T2b
[c] Includes Gleason scores 5–7
[d] Includes PSA >10
[e] Includes T1a, T1b, and T1c
[f] Includes T2b and T2c
[g] Includes Gleason scores ≤3
[h] Includes Gleason scores 4–6
[i] Includes Gleason score 7
[j] Includes Gleason scores 5–6
*Hull GW et al, unpublished data used with permission

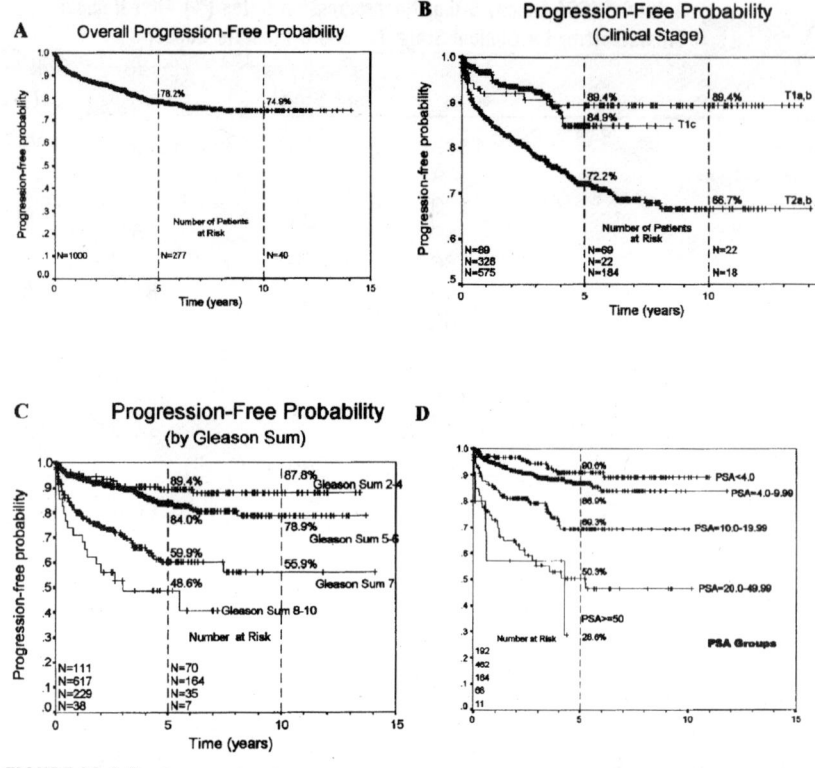

FIGURE 14.1.2 Progression-free probability for the overall population (A) and based on clinical stage (B), biopsy Gleason score (BxGS) (C), and preoperative serum prostate specific antigen (PSA) level (D). The number of patients is shown on the horizontal axis. (Modified from Hull GW et al, unpublished data, and reprinted with permission)

Clinical Stages In general, as clinical stage increases, so does the risk of disease recurrence (Table 14.1.4; Fig. 14.1.2).[21,44,45] Notice, however, that patients with cancers found solely on the basis of an elevated serum PSA level (clinical stage T1c, 328 patients) had an 85% PSA non-progression rate at 5 years in our series (Fig. 14.1.2B). Outcome after radical prostatectomy is influenced by clinical stage, but with the substages considered localized (cT1–T2), it has not proven to be a powerful independent prognostic factor. Between June 1993 and April 1998, we analyzed the progression-free probability after radical prostatectomy for clinically localized prostate cancer in 1,000 consecutive patients (Hull GW et al, unpublished data used with permission). Clinical stage was assigned preoperatively using the 1992 tumor nodal metastasis (TNM) system.[29] Among the clinical T stages, progression rates for T1c and T2a cancers were more favorable than T2b or T2c cancers, while T2b and T2c were similar. In a multivariate analysis of clinical parameters, clinical T stage was an independent predictor of progression, with T1c cancers having a better progression-free survival than T2 cancers. There was no significant difference among the T2 substages in this analysis (Hull GW et al, unpublished data used with permission).

The success of radical prostatectomy when treating clinical stage T3 disease relies on the presence of an intact barrier overlying the cancer as well as removal of all cancer-bearing tissue. No role exists for neurovascular bundle preservation when radical prostatectomy is performed for clinical stage T3 disease. The risk of a positive surgical margin may also be reduced if the plane posterior to Denonvilliers' fascia is entered, anterior to the smooth muscle layer of the rectal wall and inferior to the rectal fascia. In this way, both layers of Denonvilliers' fascia are completely removed with the prostate gland. Lerner et al recently reported the results of the Mayo Clinic experience with radical prostatectomy in men with clinical stage T3 prostate cancer.[46] Their series included 1,090 men with clinical stage T3a or T3b prostate cancer. Pathologically, organ-confined disease was identified in 26% of patients, whereas 30% had positive pelvic lymph nodes. Adjuvant hormonal therapy was used in 28% of cases. Overall non-progression rates (systemic and local) were 67% at 10 years and 61% at 15 years. These investigators concluded that clinical stage T3 disease could be treated successfully with surgery and result in little operative morbidity.

Gleason Score Identified in Biopsy Specimens While the Gleason score is an important prognostic factor, it cannot be used categorically to justify management. PSA nonprogressive rates at 5 years following radical prostatectomy according to the Gleason score identified in specimens from needle biopsy of the prostate are summarized in Table 14.1.4.[21,44,45] As the tumor becomes more poorly differentiated, the likelihood of disease recurrence increases. In our own series, a marked decrease was shown in the probability of non-progression with more poorly-differentiated cancers (Fig. 14.1.2C).

Of all localized prostate cancers, those that are poorly differentiated pose the greatest threat to the life of the host. However, if these cancers are detected and treated surgically while they are still confined to the prostate, most can be cured (Fig. 14.1.3).[14,22,30] Serum PSA testing seems to be an excellent tool for the early detection of high-grade cancers while they are still confined to the prostate. In our own series of palpable (clinical stage T2 NX M0) cancers, 32% had a Gleason score of 7–10 in the prostate biopsy specimen, and only 28% of these were confined to the prostate (pathologic stage T2 N0 M0). In contrast, impalpable cancers detected by an elevated serum PSA (clinical stage T1c NX M0) were less likely to be poorly differentiated (24%) in the prostate biopsy specimen, but far more of these poorly differentiated cancers were confined to the prostate (49%). With early detection, more high-grade cancers are being diagnosed while still confined to the prostate. The prognosis for such cancers is excellent.

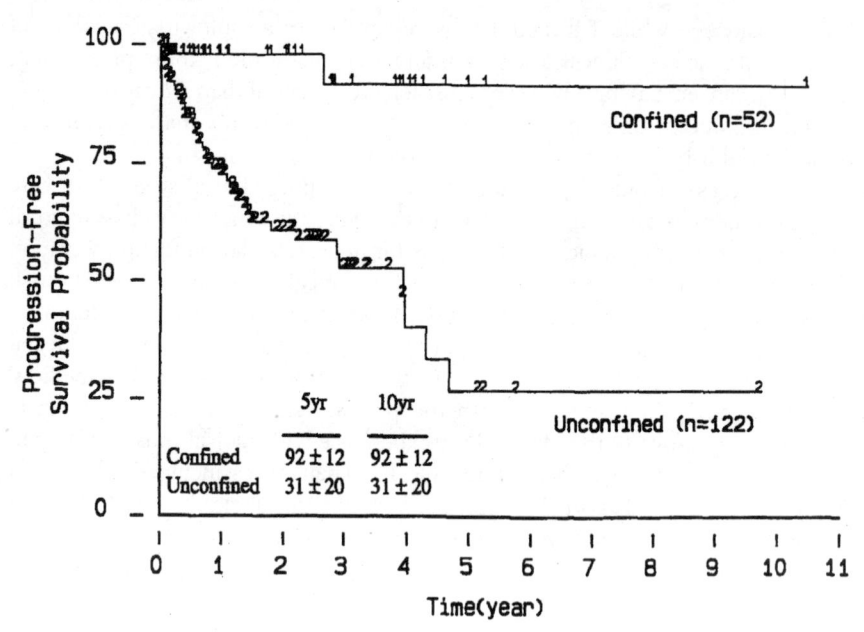

FIGURE 14.1.3 Progression-free rate by pathologic stage (confined vs. unconfined) after radical prostatectomy in 174 patients with clinically localized (clinical stage T1-T2 NxMo), poorly-differentiated (Gleason score 7-10) cancer on biopsy. (Reprinted with permission from Ref. 30).

Serum PSA Level PSA, a serine protease produced by both benign and malignant prostate epithelium, has been used for early diagnosis, staging, and monitoring treatment, and in immunohistochemical identification of malignant tumors of prostate origin. In prostate cancer, the level of serum PSA has been correlated with total tumor volume, clinical and pathological stage, and prognosis.[47] Freedom from PSA progression as a function of preoperative PSA is shown in Table 14.1.4.[21,44,45] Preoperative serum PSA levels are associated with the risk of progression after radical prostatectomy (Fig. 14.1.2D). As with clinical stage and biopsy Gleason score, increasing preoperative serum PSA levels are correlated with advanced pathologic stage but with considerable overlap. Higher preoperative serum PSA levels are not always associated with advanced pathologic features and lower valves do not necessarily suggest organ-confined disease. Therefore, the serum PSA level cannot definitely distinguish the stage of the cancer in an individual patient and cannot be used alone as a contraindication to definitive treatment.

Prognostic Models

By combining clinical prognostic factors, risk profiles have been developed to predict the outcome of patients with clinically localized prostate cancer who undergo radical prostatectomy. In a multicenter study, Partin et al[48] examined clinical and pathologic data from 4,133 men who underwent radical prostatectomy at the John Hopkins Hospital, Baylor College of Medicine, and the University of Michigan School of Medicine.[48] Serum PSA level, TNM clinical stage, and biopsy Gleason score were identified as significant predictors of pathologic stage. Nomograms were developed to predict the probability that a given tumor is a specific pathologic stage (Table 14.1.5).[48] Similarly, Kattan et al combined the serum PSA level, clinical stage, and biopsy Gleason score to develop a nomogram to predict the likelihood of recurrence of disease as detected by serum PSA level after radical prostatectomy (Fig. 14.1.4).[49,50] These prognostic models should enable patients and physicians to make more informed treatment decisions based on the patient's clinical situation.

CANCER CONTROL WITH RADICAL PROSTATECTOMY

Outcomes

Serum PSA level should decline to undetectable levels after radical prostatectomy. Although recurrence of prostate cancer after radical prostatectomy has been documented rarely in patients with an undetectable serum PSA level,[51–54] a detectable and rising serum PSA level will almost always precede clinical recurrence, usually by 3 to 5 years.[55,56] Therefore, after radical prostatectomy, treatment outcomes and cancer control should be based primarily on monitoring postoperative serum PSA levels.

Table 14.1.6 summarizes the actuarial probability of freedom from recurrence as detected by serum PSA level after radical prostatectomy from several recent series.[21,44,45,57] Remarkably similar 5-year, progression-free probabilities of 77%–80% of men undergoing surgery between 1966 and 1998 are noted. Our own data are based on 1000 patients with clinical stage T1–T2 prostate cancer who underwent radical prostatectomy between 1983 and 1998. No patient received postoperative irradiation or hormonal therapy prior to serum PSA recurrence. The actuarial 5- and 10-year nonprogression rates for these patients were 78% and 75%, respectively. Thus, data from modern surgical series clearly support the conclusion that cure is possible for many patients with prostate cancer that, if left alone or managed conservatively, would threaten the life and health of the host. Previously, palpation was the only method of early detection. Today, according to the results of a poll conducted with the aid of the George H. Gallup International Institute,[58] awareness of prostate cancer is widespread and routine testing is performed in over half of American men over the age of 50, increasing the capacity to detect those cancers that pose a threat to life and health while they are still curable with definitive local therapy.

Pathologic Prognostic Factors

In a multivariate analysis of clinical and pathologic prognostic factors, preoperative serum PSA level, pathologic stage, surgical margin status, and Gleason score in

TABLE 14.1.5 Predicted Probability of Each Pathologic Stage Based on Preoperative Serum Prostate-Specific Antigen (PSA) Level, Clinical Stage, and Gleason Grade in the Biopsy Specimen[a]

Gleason Score	PSA, 0.0–4.0 ng/mL T1c	T2a	T2b	PSA, 4.1–10.0 ng/mL T1c	T2a	T2b	PSA, 10.1–20.0 ng/mL T1c	T2a	T2b
Organ-confined Disease									
5	81 (76–84)	68 (63–72)	57 (50–62)	71 (67–75)	55 (51–60)	43 (38–49)	60 (54–65)	43 (38–49)	32 (26–37)
6	78 (74–81)	64 (59–68)	52 (46–57)	67 (64–70)	51 (47–54)	38 (34–43)	55 (51–59)	38 (34–43)	26 (23–31)
7	63 (58–68)	47 (41–52)	34 (29–39)	49 (45–54)	33 (29–38)	22 (18–26)	35 (31–40)	22 (18–26)	13 (11–16)
8–10	52 (41–62)	36 (27–45)	24 (17–32)	37 (28–46)	23 (16–31)	14 (9–19)	23 (16–32)	14 (9–19)	7 (5–11)
Established Capsular Penetration									
5	18 (15–22)	30 (26–35)	40 (34–46)	27 (23–30)	41 (36–46)	50 (45–55)	35 (30–40)	50 (45–56)	57 (51–63)
6	21 (18–25)	34 (30–38)	43 (38–48)	30 (27–33)	44 (41–48)	52 (48–56)	38 (34–42)	52 (48–57)	57 (51–62)
7	31 (26–36)	45 (40–50)	51 (46–57)	40 (35–44)	52 (48–57)	54 (49–59)	45 (40–50)	55 (50–60)	51 (45–57)
8–10	34 (27–44)	47 (38–56)	48 (40–57)	40 (33–49)	49 (42–57)	46 (39–53)	40 (33–49)	46 (38–55)	38 (30–47)
Seminal Vesicle Involvement									
5	1 (1–2)	2 (1–3)	3 (2–4)	2 (1–3)	3 (2–5)	5 (3–8)	3 (2–5)	5 (3–8)	8 (5–11)
6	1 (1–2)	2 (1–3)	3 (2–4)	2 (2–3)	3 (2–4)	5 (4–7)	4 (3–5)	5 (3–7)	7 (5–10)
7	4 (2–7)	6 (4–9)	10 (6–14)	8 (5–11)	10 (8–13)	15 (11–19)	12 (8–16)	14 (10–19)	18 (13–24)
8–10	9 (5–16)	12 (7–19)	17 (11–25)	15 (10–22)	19 (13–26)	24 (17–31)	20 (13–28)	22 (15–31)	25 (18–34)
Lymph Node Involvement									
5	0 (0–0)	0 (0–1)	1 (0–2)	0 (0–1)	1 (0–1)	2 (1–3)	1 (0–2)	2 (1–3)	4 (1–7)
6	0 (0–1)	1 (0–1)	2 (1–3)	1 (1–2)	2 (1–3)	4 (3–6)	3 (2–5)	4 (3–6)	10 (7–13)
7	1 (1–3)	2 (1–4)	5 (2–8)	3 (2–5)	4 (3–6)	9 (6–12)	8 (5–11)	9 (6–13)	17 (12–23)
8–10	4 (2–7)	5 (2–9)	10 (5–17)	8 (4–12)	9 (5–13)	16 (11–24)	16 (10–24)	17 (11–25)	29 (21–38)

PSA, prostate-specific antigen.
[a]Numbers represent percent predictive probability (95% confidence interval).
(Modified with permission, Partin et al.[48]).

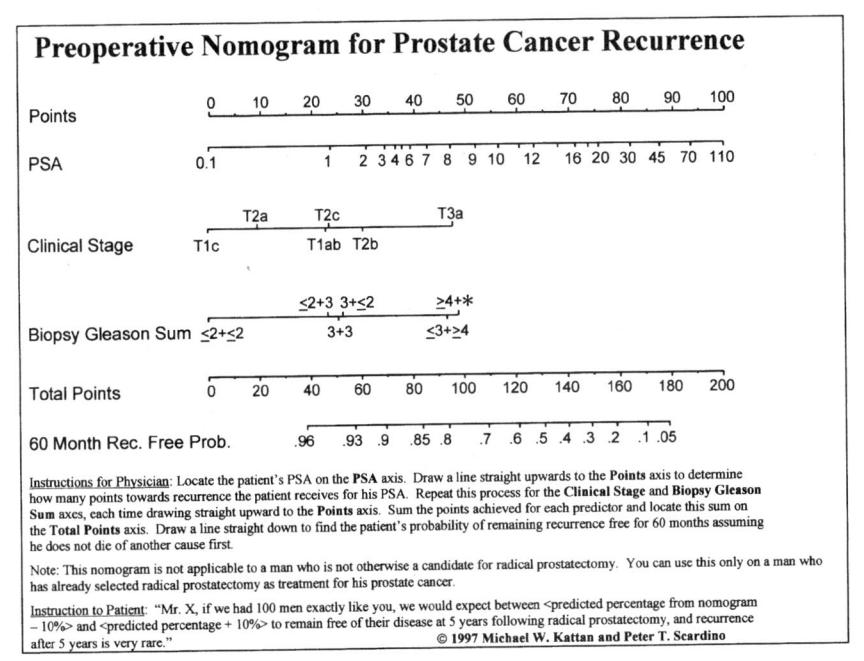

FIGURE 14.1.4 Nomogram that uses preoperative clinical factors (PSA level, biopsy, Gleason grade, and clinical stage) to predict the probability of freedom from progression (defined as a rising serum PSA level or the initiation of any other therapy for prostate cancer). (Modified from Ref. 49 and reprinted with permission).

the radical prostatectomy specimen were each independently associated with outcome after radical prostatectomy (Table 14.1.7). Several other indices have been considered in an attempt to improve the ability to describe the biologic potential of a given tumor. Some have considered tumor volume an important prognostic factor, but others have found no independent prognostic role for tumor volume.[29,59] Other parameters that have been reported to predict outcome include microvessel density, proliferative index, p53, E-cadherin, and measures of nuclear morphology. None, however, should be considered a necessary part of the evaluation of a patient with clinically localized prostate cancer at this time.

Pathologic Stage Considering all clinical and pathologic prognostic factors, the single most powerful prognostic factor is the pathologic stage of the cancer (Fig. 14.1.5).[50,60] For patients with prostate cancer pathologically confirmed to the prostate, 5-year disease-free recurrence determined with serum PSA measurements is excellent (> 90%). When the seminal vesicles or pelvic lymph nodes are involved with cancer, the prognosis is poor (Table 14.1.4).[21,44,45] A mistaken concept has arisen that prostate cancer can only be cured when it is confined to

TABLE 14.1.6 Actuarial 5-Year Progression-Free Probability Rates After Radical Retropubic Prostatectomy

Group	N	Years	PSA Nonprogression (%) 5 Yr	PSA Nonprogression (%) 10 Yr
Pound et al, 1997[44]	1623[a]	1982–95	80	68
Trapasso et al, 1994[57]	425[b]	1987–92	80	—
Zincke et al, 1994[21]	3170[b]	1966–91	77	54
Catalona and Smith, 1994[45]	925[c]	1983–93	78	—
Klein et al*	891[a]	—	80	—
Hull et al, 2000†	1000[b]	1983–98	78	75

Rates are for clinical stage T1 and T2 prostate cancers and are determined by PSA. (Modified from Ref. 30 with permission).
*Personal communication.
†Hull GW et al, unpublished data used with permission.
[a]Progression defined as a serum PSA > 0.2 ng/mL.
[b]Progression defined as a serum PSA > 0.4 ng/mL.
[c]Progression defined as a serum PSA > 0.6 ng/mL.

the prostate gland pathologically, lending further credence to the concept that the only curable cancers are those that do not need to be treated. On the contrary, data from our own series and from others clearly show that long-term cancer control is possible in 60%–70% of patients with microscopic extraprostatic extension without seminal vesicle invasion or lymph node metastases (pathologic stage T3a N0 M0 cancer).[14,24,30]

Patients can be classified as having an indolent, curable, or advanced prostate cancer depending on the pathologic features of the tumor on the radical prostatectomy specimen (see Table 14.1.1[14] for definitions). Overall risk of progression can be assigned to each of the three prognostic groups (Fig. 14.1.5).[14] This classification has implications for therapeutic decision making, such that indolent cancers, if recognized preoperatively, might be treated expectantly, whereas advanced cancers would be excellent candidates for adjuvant treatment when such therapy becomes available. In our series of 896 patients, 126 (14%) were considered to have indolent tumors, and none have progressed. A non-progression rate of 85% at 5 years was found for 592 (66%) men whose cancer had pathologic features consistent with a clinically important but curable tumor. Patients whose cancers had advanced pathologic features ($N = 178$, 20%) did poorly with only 28% disease free at 5 years (Hull GW et al, unpublished data used with permission).

Positive Surgical Margins Surgical technique certainly influences the long-term results after radical prostatectomy. Radical prostatectomy is curative only if the entire tumor is removed. If cancer extends to the margins of resection, the

TABLE 14.1.7 Multivariate Analysis of Risk of Progression[a]

Variable	Relative Risk (95% CI)	P Value
Preoperative Clinical Parameters		
Clinical stage		0.0071
T1a,b vs T1c		NS (0.60)
T1c vs T2a		NS (0.10)
T1c vs T2b	2.47 (1.52–4.03)	0.0003
T1c vs T2c	1.91 (1.06–3.42)	0.0304
Biopsy Gleason sum[a]		<0.0001
2–4 vs 5–6		NS (0.15)
5–6 vs 7	2.60 (1.75–3.87)	<0.0001
5–6 vs 8–10	3.21 (1.72–5.97)	0.0002
Log_2 (preoperative PSA)	1.80[b] (1.44–2.24)	<0.0001
Clinical and Pathologic Parameters		
Clinical stage		NS (0.15)
Biopsy Gleason sum		NS (0.12)
Log_2 (preoperative PSA)		NS (0.52)
Gleason sum in prostatectomy specimen		0.0008
2–4 vs 5–6		NS (0.97)
5–6 vs 7	2.48 (1.34–4.58)	0.0038
5–6 vs 8–10	4.55 (2.19–9.42)	<0.0001
Extracapsular extension		0.0019
Focal vs. none	2.17 (1.20–3.92)	0.011
Established vs. none	2.72 (1.56–4.74)	0.0004
Focal vs. established		NS (0.13)
Surgical margins		
Positive vs. negative	4.37 (2.90–6.58)	<0.0001
Seminal vesicle involvement		
Present vs. absent	2.61 (1.70–4.01)	<0.0001
Lymph node metastases		
Present vs. absent	3.31 (2.11–5.20)	<0.0001

CI, confidence interval; NS, not statistically significant ($P > 0.05$).
[a]Analysis of risk progression is based on preoperative clinical parameters alone and on clinical and pathologic parameters combined (Hull GW et al, unpublished data used with permission).
[b]Each doubling of the preoperative PSA level (one unit increase in log_2 preoperative PSA level) resulted in an increased relative risk of progression of 1.80.

probability of recurrence is 2 to 4 times greater per year of follow-up (Fig. 14.1.5).[24,50] With deliberate attention to surgical planning, we reduced our rate of positive margins from 24% before 1987 to 8% in 1993.[61] Consequently, we believe that while positive margins are common and that such margins reduce

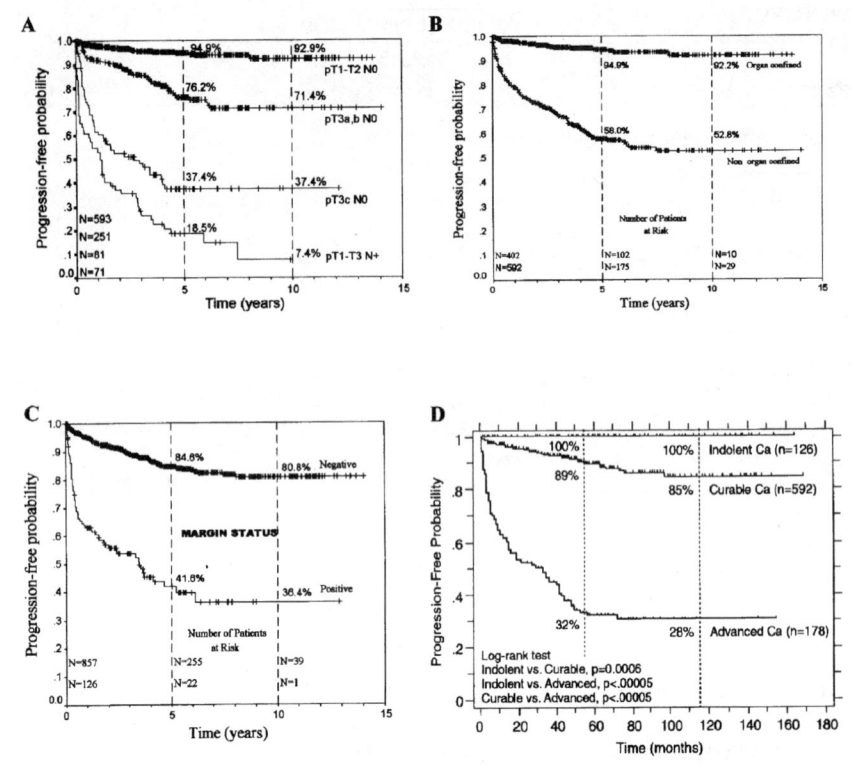

FIGURE 14.1.5 Progression-free probability curves based on the pathologic stage (A), whether or not the tumor is organ-confined (B), surgical margin status (C), and prognostic group (D). Abbreviations: ECE, extracapsular extension; SVI, seminal vesicle invasion; LN, positive lymph nodes; RRPGS, radical retropubic prostatectomy Gleason score. (Modified from Hull GW et al. unpublished data and reprinted with permission).

the chances that the cancer will be cured, most positive margins can be avoided with careful surgical planning.

Radical Prostatectomy Gleason Grade Perhaps the most convincing evidence that radical prostatectomy can interrupt the natural history of the disease is the long-term results of surgery for high-grade cancers.[22] We followed 174 patients with Gleason score 7–10 cancers. In 32% of cases, the cancer was confined to the prostate pathologically, and only one has had evidence of disease progression. However, if the cancer extends outside the prostate, progression occurs rapidly (Fig. 14.1.3).[14,30]

SURGICAL OUTCOMES DEPEND ON SURGICAL TECHNIQUES: TAILORING SURGERY TO THE INDIVIDUAL PATIENT

Urinary Incontinence

Urinary incontinence continues to be one of the most troubling side effects after radical prostatectomy. While an anatomic approach to the procedure has resulted in a diminished rate of this condition, incontinence rates vary widely (Table 14.1.8).[21,33–35,62–68] The National Cancer Institute-sponsored Prostate Cancer Outcomes Study recently reported longitudinal, community-based estimates of health outcomes in men diagnosed with prostate cancer.[67] Of 961 men who underwent radical prostatectomy and were continent preoperatively, 28% wore pads to stay dry and 9.6% had no urinary control or frequently leaked urine after surgery. Fowler et al reported that 31% of a sample Medicare population who underwent radical prostatectomy from 1988 to 1990 reported some degree of wetness.[66] In contrast, most medical centers whose physicians have a broad expertise in radical prostatectomy report that < 10% of patients are incontinent after surgery (Table 14.1.8).[21,33–35,62–68] Despite the relatively high rates of urinary incontinence reported in population surveys, most men were minimally bothered by incontinence and would make the same treatment decision again.[65,67]

TABLE 14.1.8 Incidence of Incontinence After Radical Prostatectomy

Series	No. of Patients	Incontinence (%)	Definition of Incontinence
Interview by Treating Physician at Center of Excellence			
Steiner et al, 1991[35]	593	8	Leaks with moderate activity
Leandri et al, 1992[62]	398	5	Leaks with moderate activity
Zincke et al, 1994[21]	1728	5	Requires 3 or more pads per day
Catalona et al, 1999[34]	1325	8	No pads
Geary et al, 1995[63]	458	20	Requires pads
Eastham et al, 1996[33]	581	9	Leaks with moderate activity
Series from Patient Surveys			
Murphy et al, 1994[64]	1796	19	Requires pads
Litwin et al, 1995[65]	98	25	"Bother" score
Population–Based Studies using Patient Surveys			
Fowler et al, 1993[66]	738	31	Pads or clamps
Potosky et al., 2000[67]	961	9.6	No control, leaks frequently
		28.1	Requires pads
Stanford et al, 2000[68]	1291	8.4	Severe incontinence
		21.6	Requires pads

(Modified from Eastham and Scardino[30] and reprinted with permission.)

The rate of incontinence is sensitive to surgical technique.[26,33,36] In 1990, we changed our technique to avoid retraction of the urethra during the prostatectomy, to place the anastomotic sutures through a small bite of urethra and a larger bite of lateral pelvic fascia surrounding the oversewn dorsal venous complex (Fig. 14.1.6 and Fig. 14.1.7),[50] and form a fully everted (stomatized) bladder neck (Fig. 14.1.8 and Fig. 14.1.9).[50] These changes improved the continence rates in our patients from 82% to 95% at 2 years and decreased the median time to recovery of continence from 5.6 to 1.5 months (Fig. 14.1.10).[33] Multivariate analysis has shown that factors independently associated with an increased chance of regaining continence were: (1) younger age, (2) preservation of both neurovascular bundles, (3) the absence of an anastomotic structure, and (4) the modifications in surgical technique outlined above.

Urodynamic evaluation of men who are incontinent after radical prostatectomy has not elucidated a predominant mechanism of incontinence. Most studies, however, have suggested that the functional urethral length is the most important factor in post-prostatectomy incontinence.[69-73] We believe a "no-touch" approach to the external sphincter tissues beyond the apex of the prostate and fixation of the urethra to the lateral pelvic fascia preserves the maximum amount of functional urethral length in the pelvis and contributes significantly to post-procedure continence.

Erectile Function

Return of erectile function after radical prostatectomy has been correlated with patient age, pathologic tumor stage, and the extent of preservation of the neurovascular bundles. Catalona and colleagues[34] evaluated 858 potent men between the ages of 44 and 77 years who underwent radical prostatectomy. For men younger than 50 years, 90% were potent if one or both neurovascular bundles were preserved. For men 50 years of age or older, potency was better if both neurovascular bundles were preserved: 67% of patients retained potency with bilateral neurovascular bundle preservation compared with 47% of men with unilateral nerve-sparing surgery.

Data on the recovery of potency after radical prostatectomy are quite different if one compares centers of excellence to population surveys.[34,62,64,66,68,73-75] Potosky et al initiated the Prostate Cancer Outcomes Study in 1994 to obtain community-based estimates of health outcomes in men undergoing treatment for prostate cancer.[67] These investigators reported that the prevalence of impotence following surgery, defined as erections insufficient for intercourse, was 80% in men who had undergone radical prostatectomy, although the degree of neurovascular bundle preservation was not documented. Litwin et al used a validated quality-of-life survey to assess sexual function in 214 men treated with watchful waiting, radiotherapy, or radical prostatectomy.[65] Potency status prior to treatment was not documented. In the patient group undergoing radical prostatectomy, nerve-

Treatment of Prostate Cancer: Surgery **297**

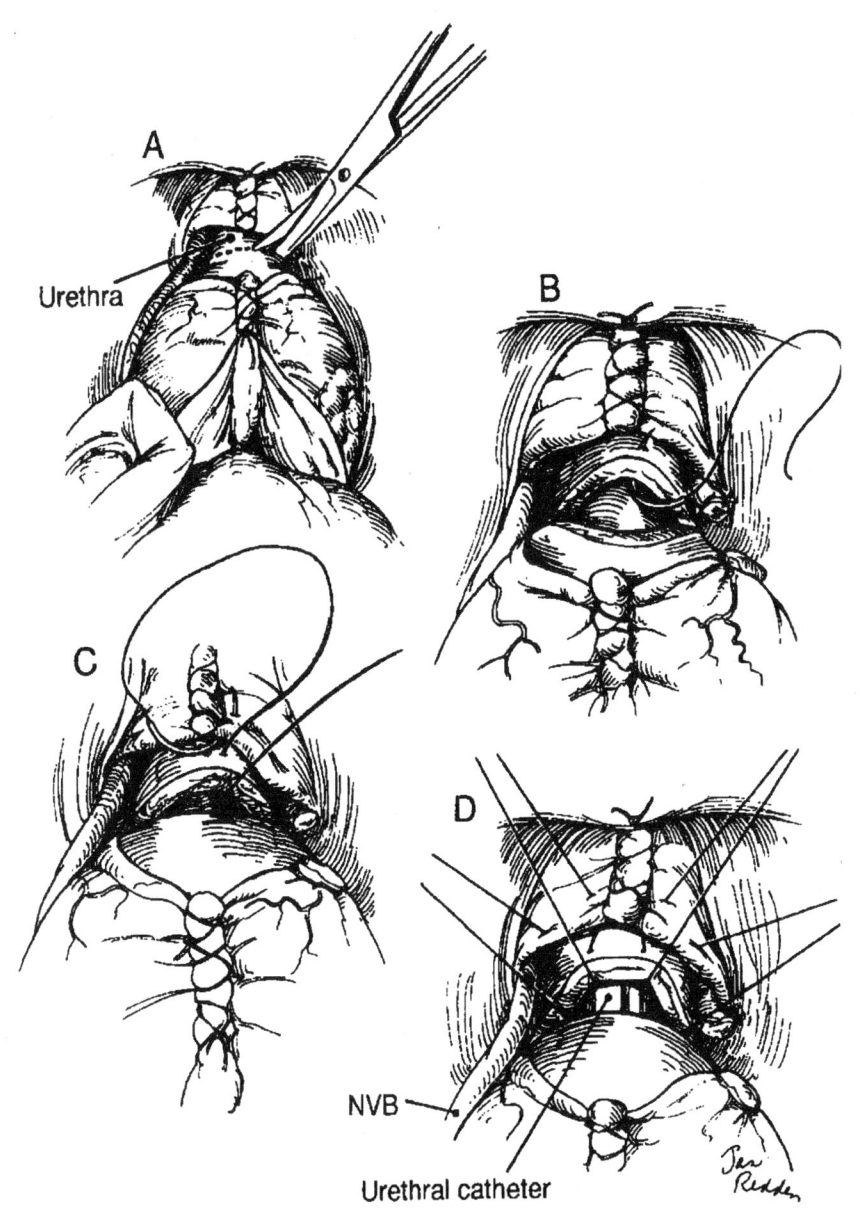

FIGURE 14.1.6 Close-up views of the urethra at the prostatic apex, illustrating the site of anterior division (A, B) and the placement of the anterior anastomotic sutures beneath the mucosa of the urethra and then separately through the thick layer of lateral pelvic fascia (C, D) that was oversewn to control the dorsal venous complex. Abbreviation: NVB, neurovascular bundle. (Reprinted with permission from Ref. 50).

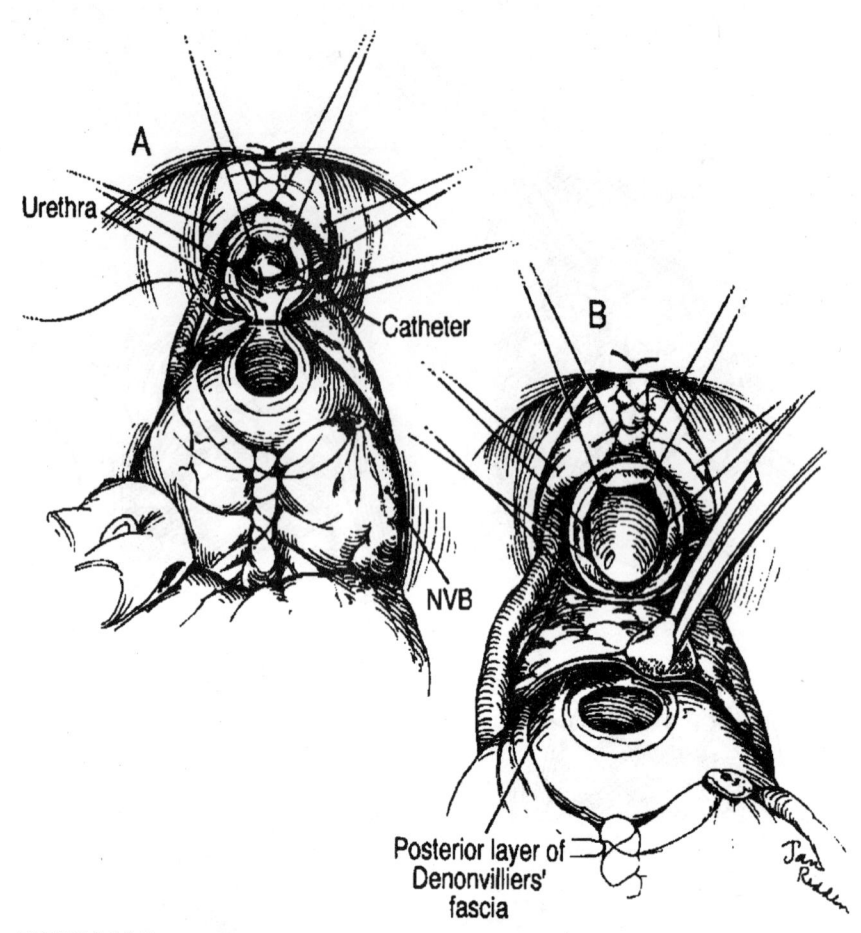

FIGURE 14.1.7 After the nerves have been dissected free (or divided), the remaining urethra and posterior layer of Denonvilliers' fascia beneath it are divided (A). Two posterior anastomotic sutures are placed at 5 or 7 o'clock through the fascia and urethra (A). The correct plane of dissection adjacent to the rectum is determined with the aid of a Kitner dissector (B). Abbreviation: NVB, neurovascular bundle. (Reprinted with permission from Ref. 50).

sparing techniques were used infrequently, yet 29% recovered erections satisfactory for sexual activity. These data and our own experience confirm that preservation of erectile function after radical prostatectomy is possible, but the probability of recovery depends on patient age, tumor stage, potency status before surgery, and the preservation of the neurovascular bundles.[37,74,76] The results are affected by subtle variations in surgical techniques.[38,75,76]

Because preservation of erectile function is a major concern for many men considering treatment for clinically localized prostate cancer, we analyzed various factors determined before and after radical prostatectomy to identify those associated with recovery of erections after surgery.[74] Between 1993 and 1996, 314

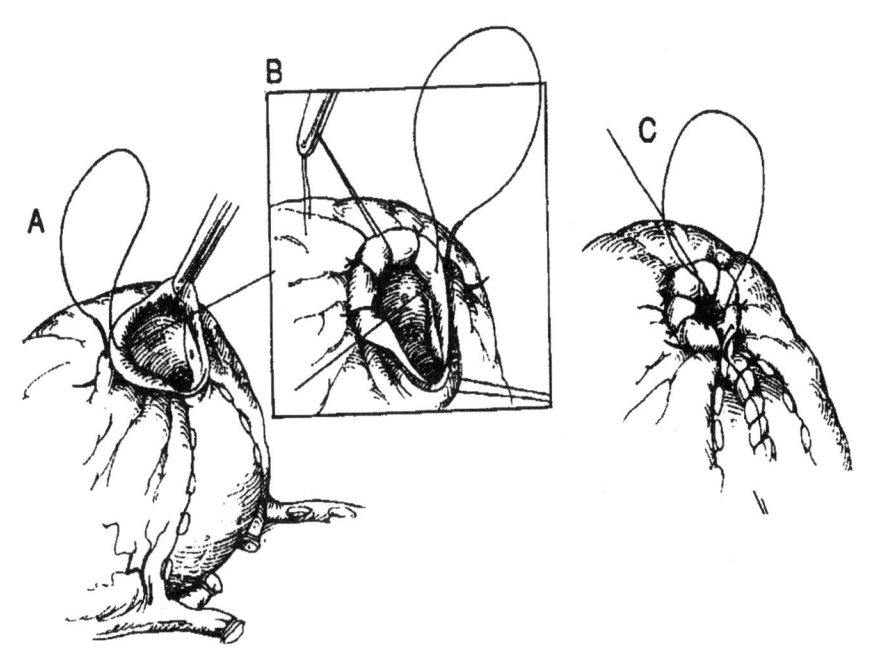

FIGURE 14.1.8 The bladder neck is reconstructed by everting the mucosa anteriorly (A, B) and closing the bladder neck posteriorly with a running suture, creating a "temo-racket" closure (C). The suture closest to the trigone should include muscle but little mucosa to avoid tethering the ureteral orifices. (Reprinted with permission from Ref. 50).

consecutive men with documentation of preoperative potency status underwent radical prostatectomy. Multivariate analysis determined that patient age, preoperative potency status, and the extent of neurovascular bundle preservation were predictive of the recovery of potency following surgery. Men under age 60 years with full erections before surgery who underwent bilateral neurovascular bundle preservation have a 76% likelihood of regaining erections sufficient for intercourse within 3 years of surgery (Table 14.1.9).[74] Partial damage to one or both neurovascular bundles reduced the chance of recovery to 67% compared to preserving both nerves, while unilateral nerve resection reduced the chance of recovery to 30% (Table 14.1.9).[74] Knowledge of preoperative erectile function, patient age, and the anticipated degree of preservation of the neurovascular bundles may aid in patient counseling regarding the recovery of erectile function after surgery (Fig. 14.1.11).[74]

Removal of the cancer and preserving the neurovascular bundle are often competing goals. Cancers most often penetrate the prostatic capsule posterolaterally, directly over the neurovascular bundles (Fig. 14.1.12).[50] A lateral approach to the neurovascular bundles allows wide exposure of the apex so that the apical tissue can be resected completely (Fig. 14.1.13).[50] The lateral pelvic fascia over

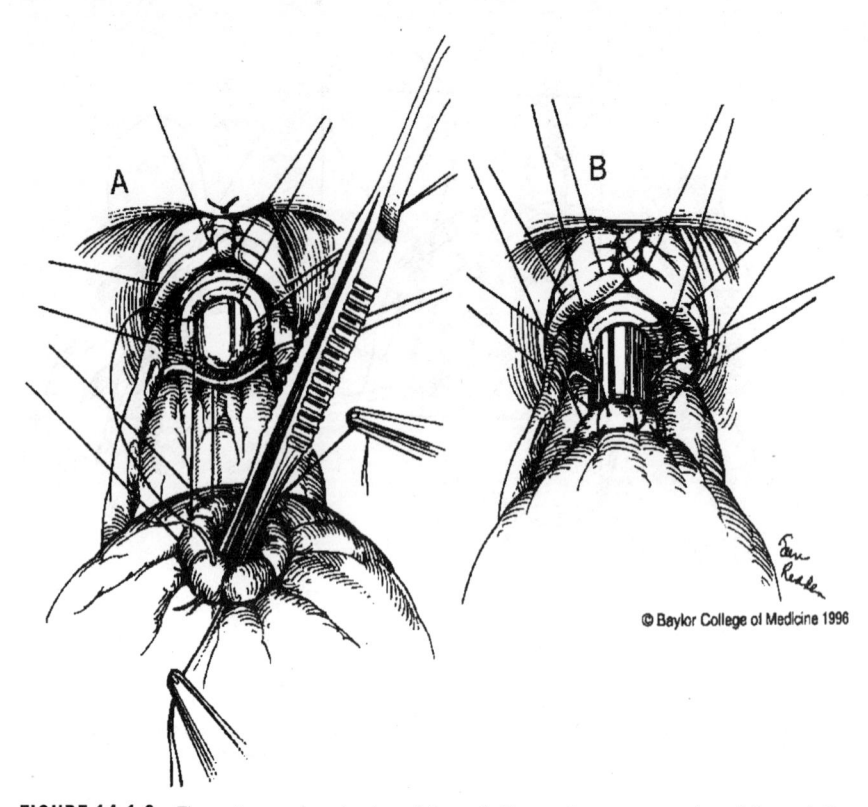

FIGURE 14.1.9 The sutures already placed through the urethra are now placed through the bladder neck (A) to provide a mucosa-to-mucosa anastomosis (B). (Reprinted with permission from Ref. 50).

the neurovascular bundle can be incised more medically or laterally to the nerve, depending on the location or extent of the tumor. Using this lateral approach, we have been successful in preserving most or all of both neurovascular bundles in the majority of patients, while still allowing a wider resection around the apex of the prostate, especially posteriorly.

When resection of one or both neurovascular bundles is necessary, we use a technique we developed for placing interposition grafts from the sural nerve to one or both neurovascular bundles (Fig. 14.1.14).[77] One-third of patients with bilateral nerve resection and placement of bilateral nerve grafts have had spontaneous, medically unassisted erections sufficient for sexual intercourse. The greatest return of function is observed 14–18 months after surgery.

Positive Surgical Margins

In a review of the literature from centers of excellence, reported rates of positive surgical margins vary from 14% to 41% with a mean of 25%.[61] Variations in

Treatment of Prostate Cancer: Surgery

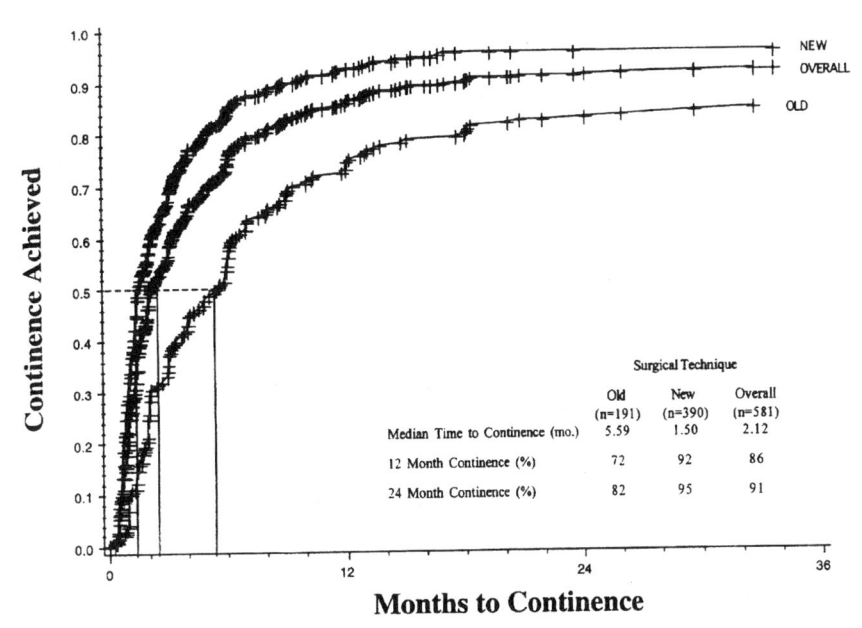

FIGURE 14.1.10 Time to recovery of continence for all 581 patients and for the old and new anastomotic techniques. For the 390 men who had the new technique (*see text for details*), median time to the recovery of continence was 1.5 months and 95% were continent by 24 months. (Reprinted with permission from Ref. 33).

	Surgical Technique		
	Old (n=191)	New (n=390)	Overall (n=581)
Median Time to Continence (mo.)	5.59	1.50	2.12
12 Month Continence (%)	72	92	86
24 Month Continence (%)	82	95	91

TABLE 14.1.9 Probability of Recovery of Potency by 24 and 36 Months Based on a Combination of Preoperative and Postoperative Parameters

Preoperative Potency	Probability (%) of Recovery of Potency by 24 Months (36 Months)		
	Age ≤ 60	Age = 60.1–65	Age > 65
Bilateral Nerve-Sparing			
Full Erection	70 (76)	49 (55)	43 (49)
Full Erection, Recently Diminished	53 (59)	34 (39)	30 (35)
Partial Erection	43 (49)	27 (31)	23 (27)
Unilateral or Bilateral Neurovascular Bundle Damage			
Full Erection	60 (67)	40 (46)	35 (41)
Full Erection, Recently Diminished	44 (50)	28 (32)	24 (28)
Partial Erection	35 (40)	21 (25)	18 (21)
Unilateral Neurovascular Bundle Resection			
Full Erection	26 (30)	15 (18)	13 (15)
Full Erection, Recently Diminished	17 (20)	10 (12)	8.5 (10)
Partial Erection	13 (15)	7.5 (8.8)	6.3 (7.5)

(Modified from Rabbani et al[74] with permission).

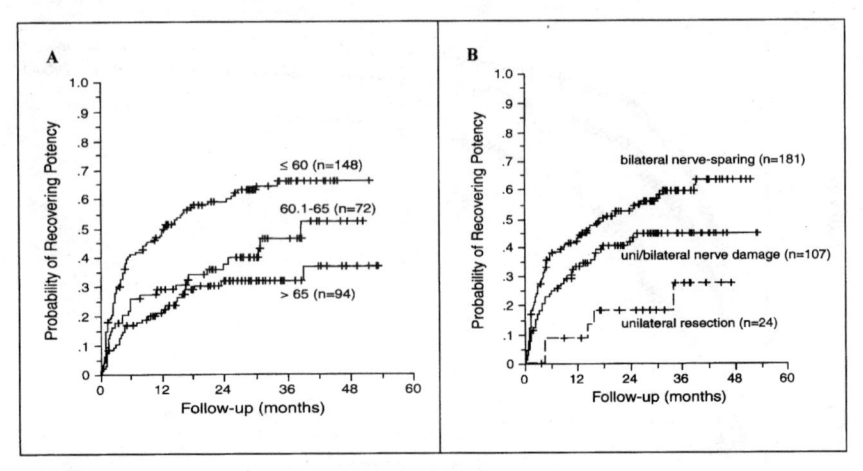

FIGURE 14.1.11 Probability of recovery of erections adequate for sexual activity as a function of time after radical prostatectomy among 322 potent men, according to patient age (A) and for all ages according to the extent of preservation of the neurovascular bundles (B). (Reprinted with permission from Ref. 74).

surgical margin rates are related not only to the extent of the tumor and to the processing of the specimen[61] but also to surgical technique. Key steps to reducing the frequency of positive margins include wide dissection around the apex of the prostate including dissection around the distal extension of the apex posteriorly, deep dissection beneath the posterior layer of Denonvilliers' fascia, selective resection of part or all of the neurovascular bundles posterolaterally, and division of the bladder neck proximately, away from the prostate and the prostatic urethra.[76] In each of the steps, the margin error is small: Only a few millimeters separates an incision into the cancer from an unnecessary resection of tissue vital to recovery of continence or erectile function.[63]

Because positive surgical margins are significantly associated with disease recurrence after radical prostatectomy (Table 14.1.4),[15-18] attempts have been made to reduce the rates with neoadjuvant androgen ablation. In a recent review of randomized, prospective trials, Scolieri et al determined that neoadjuvant hormonal therapy decreased the rate of positive margins in 6 of the 7 randomized prospective trials (Table 14.1.10).[78-85] No improvement was seen in the rate of seminal vesicle invasion or in the rate of lymph node metastases after neoadjuvant hormonal therapy compared to control subject. Similarly, there was no improvement in PSA-free survival (Table 14.1.11).[78,86-90] These investigators concluded that results from the available literature revealed no significant improvement in outcome to support the routine administration of neoadjuvant hormonal therapy before prostatectomy.

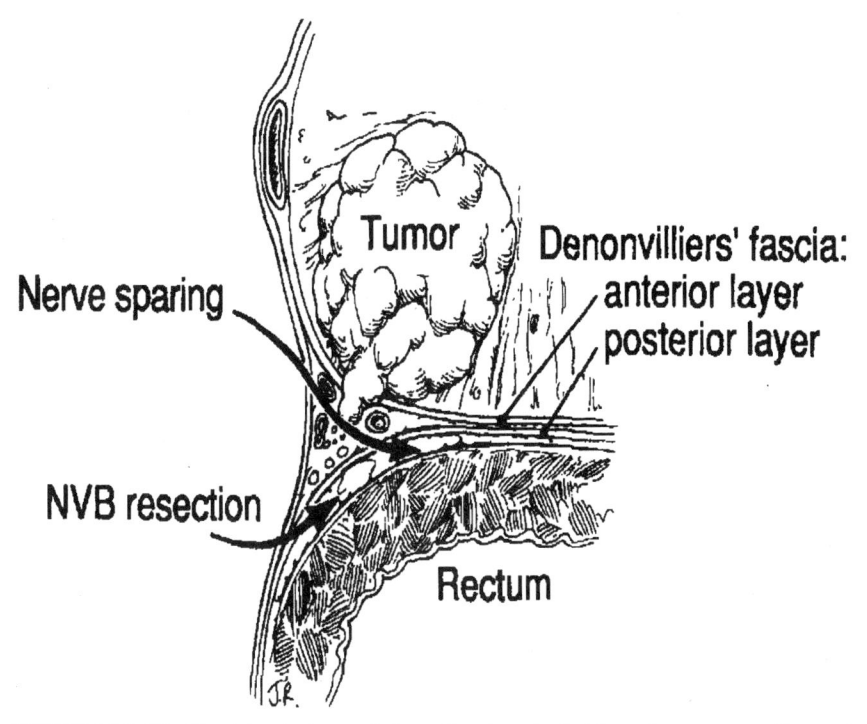

FIGURE 14.1.12 The lateral plane of dissection is selected based on preoperative and intraoperative assessment of the extent of the cancer. A wider resection, including resection of the entire neurovascular bundle, may be required to obtain adequate surgical margins. Abbreviation: NVB, neurovascular bundle. (Reprinted with permission from Ref. 50).

RATIONALE FOR SELECTING RADICAL PROSTATECTOMY AS THE TREATMENT OF CHOICE FOR CLINICALLY LOCALIZED PROSTATE CANCER

While randomized prospective clinical trials comparing different forms of therapy are lacking, reasonable comparisons can be made among different forms of local therapy when outcomes are reported for patients stratified by risk on the basis of the significant clinical prognostic factors of clinical stage, Gleason score, and serum PSA level. In several recent studies, biochemical outcome after radical prostatectomy, external beam radiation therapy, and/or interstitial radiation therapy for localized prostate have been compared.[91,92] Polascik et al compared biochemical progression rates in 76 men who underwent radical prostatectomy between 1988 and 1990 to 122 men treated with I^{125} brachytherapy without adjuvant treatment. The groups were carefully matched for Gleason score, serum PSA level, and clinical stage. Biochemical failure was defined as a serum PSA

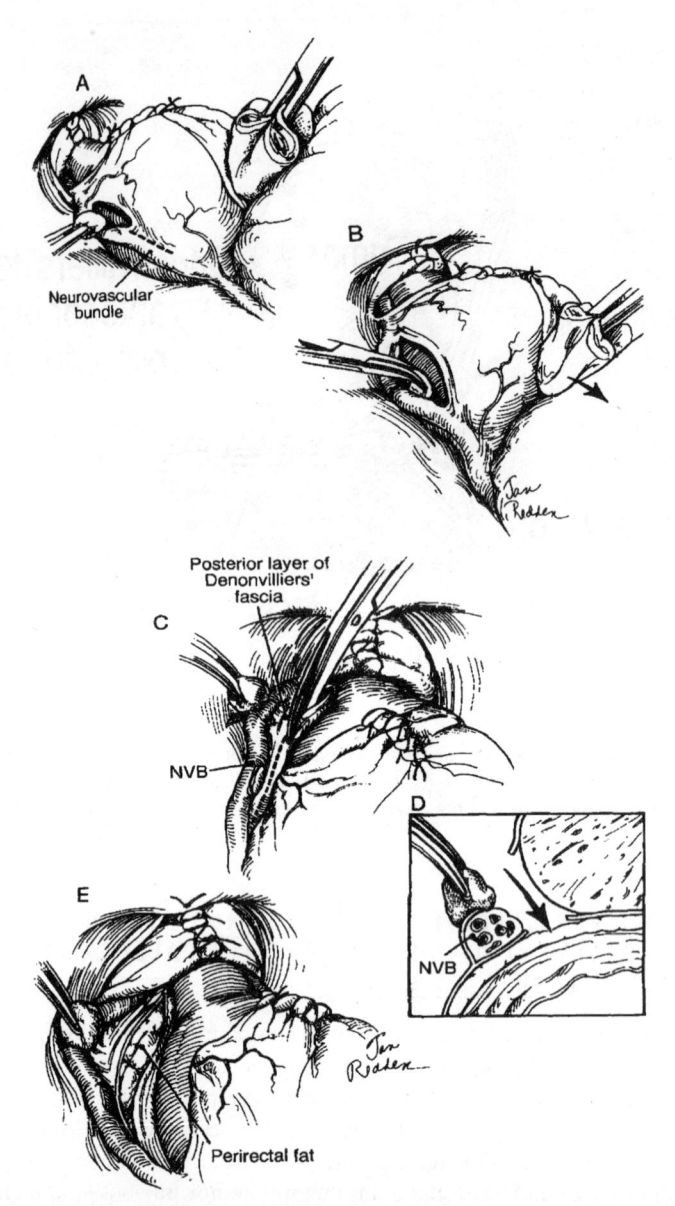

FIGURE 14.1.13 Preservation of the left neurovascular bundle (NVB). After the dorsal venous complex has been divided, the prostate is rotated to the right and the levator muscles are dissected away bluntly. The lateral pelvic fascia is incised in the groove between the prostate and the NVB. The NVB is most easily dissected away from the apical third of the prostate (A, B). The small branches of the vascular pedicle to the apex must be divided. The posterior layer of Denonvilliers' fascia is then incised, releasing the NVB from the prostate and urethra (C-E) so that the nerves will not be tethered when the anastomotic sutures are tied. (Reprinted with permission from Ref. 50).

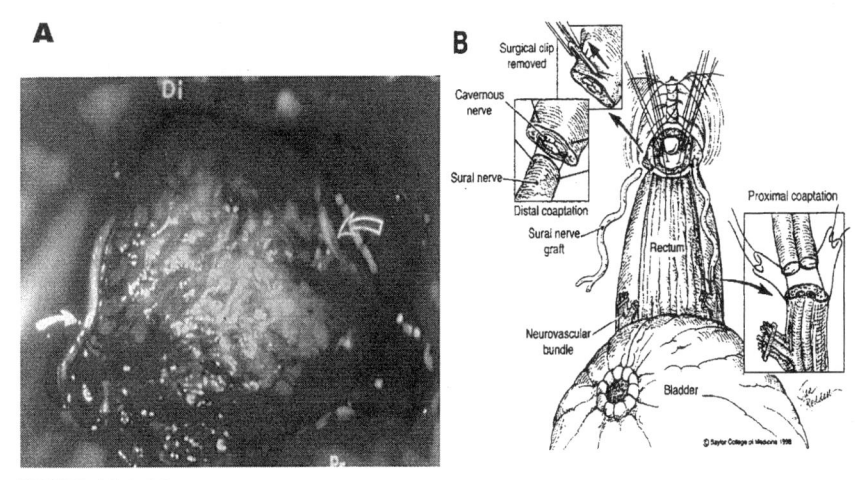

FIGURE 14.1.14 Sural nerve grafts can be interposed between the severed ends of the cavernous nerves when these nerves are resected to assure complete cancer excision. The nerve graft is reversed and digital branches are coapted to proximal ends of the cavernous nerves near the lateral vascular pedicle. (Reprinted with permission from Ref. 77).

level greater than 0.2 ng/mL and greater than 0.5 ng/mL for surgically and radiation managed patients, respectively. The 7-year actuarial PSA progression-free survival rate following radical prostatectomy was 98% [95% confidence interval (CI), 86%–99%] compared to 79% (95% CI, not published) for men treated with I^{125} brachytherapy. While the authors acknowledge that such comparisons have limitations, they conclude that such data provide a better comparison of biochemical progression than previously reported studies and emphasize the need for caution in interpreting the relative efficacy of brachytherapy in controlling localized prostate cancer.[80] D'Amico et al examined 1872 men treated between January 1989 and October 1997 with radical prostatectomy (N = 888), interstitial radiation therapy (N = 218), or external beam radiation therapy (N = 766).[92] Patients were assigned to one of three risk groups: low risk (stage T1c, T2a, and serum PSA level $\leq$ 10 ng/mL and Gleason score $\leq$ 6); intermediate risk (stage T2b or Gleason score 7 or serum PSA level > 10 and < 20 ng/mL); or high risk (stage T2c or serum PSA level $\geq$ 20 ng/mL or Gleason score $\geq$ 8). No difference was seen in the 5-year probability of freedom from progression for low-risk cancers treated with radical prostatectomy, three-dimensional (3D) conformal radiotherapy, and radioactive seed implants with or without neoadjuvant hormonal therapy (Fig. 14.1.15).[79,92] However, implants were significantly less effective for intermediate and high-risk cancers, and implants plus hormonal therapy were less effective for high-risk cancers (Fig. 14.1.15).[79,92] Comparing our own series of 1000 men undergoing radical prostatectomy for clinically localized prostate cancer (Hull GW et al, unpublished data used with permission) with

TABLE 14.1.10 Positive Margin Rates

References	Stage (No. Margins)	Neoadjuvant Hormonal Therapy	Radical Prostatectomy	Significant (P value)
Witjes et al[79]	T2 (92 vs 107)	14	36	Yes (< 0.01)
	T3 (72 vs 83)	43	59	No (0.14)
Overall (164 vs 190)		27	46	Yes (< 0.01)
Labrie et al[80]	B0	0	33	No
	B1	2.3	25.5	Yes
	B2	10.8	58.8	Yes
	C1	0	0	No
	C2	14.3	80	Yes
Overall		7.8	33.8	Yes
Soloway et al[81]	T2b (138 vs 144)	18	48	Yes
Hugosson et al[82]	T1b-c (10 vs 15)	30	33	
	T2a-b (vs 9)	22	11	
	T2c-T3a (37 vs 31)	22	61	Yes (0.0008)
Overall (56 vs 56)		23	41	Yes (0.013)
Dalkin et al[83]	T1c (17 vs 16)			
	T2a (8 vs 12)			
	T2b (3 vs 0)			
Overall (28 vs 28)[a]		17.9[a]	14.3[a]	No
Goldenberg et al[84]	T1b (5 vs 4)			
	T1c (5 vs 3)			
	T2a (30 vs 33)			
	T2b (19 vs 17)			
	T2c (42s vs 42)			
Overall (101 vs 91)		27.7	64.8	Yes
Van Poppel et al[85]	T2b (36 vs 37)	16.7	32.4	Yes
	T3 (29 vs 25)	41.3	44.0	No
Overall (65 vs 62)		27.7	37.1	

[a]Includes positive surgical margins and seminal vesicle invasion.
(Reprinted with permission from Ref. 78)

those published by D'Amico et al,[92] similar results are seen regardless of treatment modality for low-risk patients. For intermediate- and high-risk groups, patients in our series had significantly better 5-year cancer control rates (Fig. 14.1.15).[79,92] Despite the ease of risk group categorization, each group contains a heterogeneous population of cancers. This may account for the differences seen in Figure 14.1.15,[79,92] although surgical technique may also play a significant role.

CONCLUSION

Radical prostatectomy effectively eradicates prostate cancer in most men with clinically localized disease. Although technically complex, this procedure can generally

TABLE 14.1.11 PSA-Free Survival

References	N	Stage	Follow Up Months	% Neoadjuvant Hormonal Therapy	% No Neoadjuvant Hormonal Therapy
Witjes et al[86]	173	CT2	48	86	82
	320	CT2-3	48	81	77
Soloway et al[87]	256	CT2b	24	79	78.4
Aus et al[a88]	122	CT1b-3a	38	65.5	59.4
Goldenberg et al[89]	162	A2-B2	24	72	80.0
Fair et al[90]	194	cT1-2	29	84	89

[a]Includes lymph node metastasis and adjuvant therapy, considered treatment failure.
(Reprinted with permission from Ref. 78)

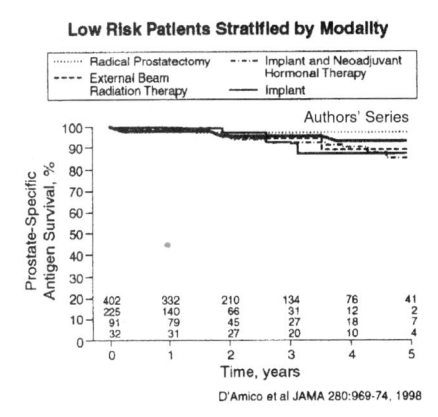

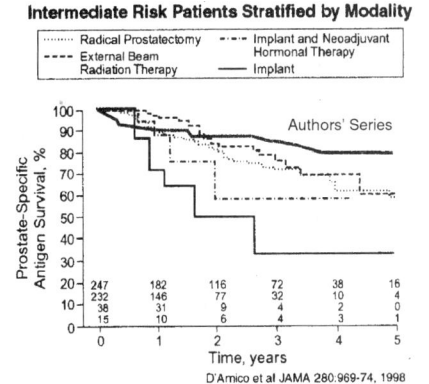

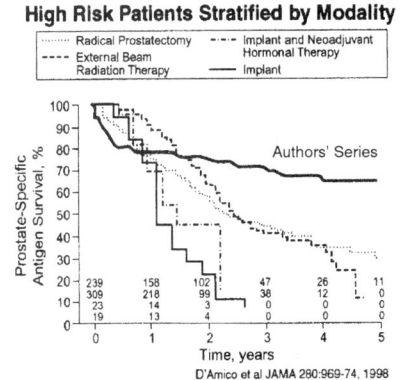

FIGURE 14.1.15 PSA progression-free survival for low-risk (A), intermediate-risk (B), and high-risk (C) patients, modified with permission from Ref. 79. The additional line "Authors' Series" indicates the results of radical prostatectomy in a separate group of 1,000 patients (Hull GW et al, unpublished data used with permission) not reported in the D'Amico article.[92]

be performed with a low level of acute and long-term morbidity, but the results are highly sensitive to fine details in surgical technique. Rates of urinary incontinence, erectile dysfunction, and positive surgical margins vary widely. With careful attention to surgical technique, cancer control rates will improve further and the effect of the operation on quality of life should continue to decrease.

ACKNOWLEDGMENT

We thank Brenna Nichols for expert editorial assistance.

REFERENCES

1. Greenlee RT, Murray T, Bolden S, Wingo PA. Cancer statistics, 2000. CA Cancer J Clin 2000;50: 7-33.
2. Fleming C, Wasson JH, Albertsen PC, Barry MJ, Wennberg JE. A decision analysis of alternative treatment strategies for clinically localized prostate cancer. Prostate Patient Outcomes Research Team [see comments]. JAMA 1993;269:2650-2658.
3. Beck JR, Kattan MW, Miles BJ. A critique of the decision analysis for clinically localized prostate cancer [see comments]. J Urol 1994;152:1894-1899.
4. Kattan MW, Miles BJ, Beck JR, Scardino PT. A reexamination of the decision analysis for clinically localized prostate cancer: Age and grade comparisons [abstract]. J Urol 1995;153:390A.
5. Gohagan JK, Prorok PC, Kramer BS, Cornett JE. Prostate cancer screening in the prostate, lung, colorectal and ovarian cancer screening trial of the National Cancer Institute [see comments]. J Urol 1994;152:1905-1909.
6. Wilt TJ, Brawer MK. The Prostate Cancer Intervention Versus Observation Trial (PIVOT). Oncology (Huntingt) 1997;11:1133-1139; discussion 1139-1140, 1143.
7. Catalona WJ, Smith DS, Ratliff TL et al. Measurement of prostate-specific antigen in serum as a screening test for prostate cancer [published erratum appears in N Engl J Med 1991;325:1324] [see comments]. N Engl J Med 1991;324:1156-1161.
8. Schmidt JD, Mettlin CJ, Natarajan N et al. Trends in patterns of care for prostatic cancer, 1974-1983: results of surveys by the American College of Surgeons. J Urol 1986;136:416-421.
9. Smith DS, Catalona WJ, Herschman JD. Longitudinal screening for prostate cancer with prostate-specific antigen [see comments]. JAMA 1996;276:1309-1315.
10. Soh S, Kattan MW, Berkman S et al. Has there been a recent shift in the pathological features and prognosis of patients treated with radical prostatectomy? [see comments]. J Urol 1997;157: 2212-2218.
11. Franks LM. Latent carcinoma of the prostate. J Pathol Bact 1954;68:603-616.
12. McNeal JE. Origin and development of carcinoma in the prostate. Cancer 1969;23:24-34.
13. Sakr WA, Grignon DJ, Crissman JD et al. High grade prostatic intraepithelial neoplasia (HGPIN) and prostatic adenocarcinoma between the ages of 20-69: an autopsy study of 249 cases. In Vivo 1994;8:439-443.
14. Ohori M, Wheeler TM, Dunn JK et al. The pathological features and prognosis of prostate cancer detectable with current diagnostic tests [see comments]. J Urol 1994;152:1714-1720.
15. Chodak GW, Thisted RA, Gerber GS et al. Results of conservative management of clinically localized prostate cancer [see comments]. N Engl J Med 1994;330:242-248.
16. Albertsen PC, Fryback DG, Storer BE et al. Long-term survival among men with conservatively treated localized prostate cancer [see comments]. JAMA 1995;274:626-631.

17. Albertsen PC, Hanley JA, Gleason DF, Barry MJ. Competing risk analysis of men aged 55 to 74 years at diagnosis managed conservatively for clinically localized prostate cancer [see comments]. JAMA 1998;280:975–980.
18. Johansson JE, Holmberg L, Johansson S et al. Fifteen-year survival in prostate cancer. A prospective, population-based study in Sweden [see comments] [published erratum appears in JAMA 1997; 278:206]. JAMA 1997;277:467–471.
19. Dillioglugil O, Leibman BD, Kattan MW et al. Hazard rates for progression after radical prostatectomy for clinically localized prostate cancer. Urology 1997;50:93–99.
20. Partin AW, Pound CR, Clemens JQ et al. Serum PSA after anatomic radical prostatectomy. The Johns Hopkins experience after 10 years. Urol Clin North Am 1993;20:713–725.
21. Zincke H, Oesterling JE, Blute ML et al. Long-term (15 years) results after radical prostatectomy for clinically localized (stage T2c or lower) prostate cancer [see comments]. J Urol 1994;152: 1850–1857.
22. Ohori M, Goad JR, Wheeler TM et al. Can radical prostatectomy alter the progression of poorly differentiated prostate cancer? [see comments]. J Urol 1994;152:1843–1849.
23. Gerber GS, Thisted RA, Scardino PT et al. Results of radical prostatectomy in men with clinically localized prostate cancer [see comments]. JAMA 1996;276:615–619.
24. Wheeler TM, Dillioglugil O, Kattan MW et al. Clinical and pathological significance of the level and extent of capsular invasion in clinical stage T1–2 prostate cancer. Hum Pathol 1998;29: 856–862.
25. Scardino PT, Wheeler TM, Kattan MW. Is cure of prostate cancer possible in those for whom it is necessary? In: Kurth KH, Mickisch GH, Schroder FH, eds. Renal, Bladder and Prostate Cancer: An Update. London:The Parthenon Publishing Group 1999:131–137.
26. Goad JR, Scardino PT. Modifications in the technique of radical retropubic prostatectomy to minimize blood loss. Atlas Urol Clin North Am 1994;2:65–80.
27. Smith JA, Bray WL, Koch NO. Cost efficient management of the patient with localized prostate cancer. AUA Update Series 1997;16:122–131.
28. Leibman BD, Dillioglugil O, Abbas F et al. Impact of a clinical pathway for radical retropubic prostatectomy. Urology 1998;52:94–99.
29. Ohori M, Wheeler TM, Scardino PT. The New American Joint Committee on Cancer and International Union Against Cancer TNM classification of prostate cancer. Clinicopathologic correlations. Cancer 1994;74:104–114.
30. Eastham JA, Scardino PT. Radical prostatectomy. In: Walsh PC, Retik AB, Vaughan ED Jr, Wein AJ, eds. Campbell's Urology, 7th edn. Philadelphia:W.B. Saunders Company, 1998:2547–2564.
31. Klein EA, Kupelian PA, Tuason L, Levin HS. Initial dissection of the lateral fascia reduces the positive margin rate in radical prostatectomy. Urology 1998;51:766–773.
32. Wieder JA, Soloway MS. Incidence, etiology, location, prevention and treatment of positive surgical margins after radical prostatectomy for prostate cancer. J Urol 1998;160:299–315.
33. Eastham JA, Kattan MW, Rogers E et al. Risk factors for urinary incontinence after radical prostatectomy [see comments]. J Urol 1996;156:1707–1713.
34. Catalona WJ, Carvalhal GF, Mager DE, Smith DS. Potency, continence and complication rates in 1,870 consecutive radical retropubic prostatectomies. J Urol 1999;162:433–438.
35. Steiner MS, Morton RA, Walsh PC. Impact of anatomical radical prostatectomy on urinary continence. J Urol 1991;145:512–514; discussion 514–515.
36. Steiner MS. Continence-preserving anatomic radical retropubic prostatectomy. Urology 2000;55: 427–435.
37. Walsh PC, Marschke P, Ricker D, Burnett AL. Patient-reported urinary continence and sexual function after anatomic radical prostatectomy. Urology 2000;55:58–61.

38. Walsh PC, Marschke P, Ricker D, Burnett AL. Use of intraoperative video documentation to improve sexual function after radical retropubic prostatectomy [see comments]. Urology 2000; 55:62–67.
39. Aus G, Hugosson J, Norlen L. Long-term survival and mortality in prostate cancer treated with noncurative intent [see comments]. J Urol 1995;154:460–465.
40. Dillioglugil O, Leibman BD, Leibman NS et al. Risk factors for complications and morbidity after radical retropubic prostatectomy. J Urol 1997;157:1760–1767.
41. Chodak GW. The role of watchful waiting in the management of localized prostate cancer [see comments]. J Urol 1994;152:1766–1768.
42. Brasso K, Friis S, Juel K, Jorgensen T, Iversen P. The need for hospital care of patients with clinically localized prostate cancer managed by noncurative intent: a population based registry study. J Urol 2000;163:1150–1154.
43. Martin JA, Smith BL, Mathews TJ, Ventura SJ. Births and deaths: Preliminary data for 1998. Natl Vital Stat Rep 1999;47:1–45.
44. Pound CR, Partin AW, Epstein JI, Walsh PC. Prostate-specific antigen after anatomic radical retropubic prostatectomy. Patterns of recurrence and cancer control. Urol Clin North Am 1997;24:395–406.
45. Catalona WJ, Smith DS. 5-year tumor recurrence rates after anatomical radical retropubic prostatectomy for prostate cancer [see comments]. J Urol 1994;152:1837–1842.
46. Lerner SE, Blute ML, Iocca AJ, Zincke H. Primary surgery for clinical stage T3 adenocarcinoma of the prostate. In: Vogelzang NJ, Scardino PT, Shipley WU, Coffey DS, eds. Comprehensive Textbook of Genitourinary Oncology, 2nd edn. Philadelphia: Lippincott William & Wilkins, 2000:789–799.
47. Oesterling JE. Prostate specific antigen: a critical assessment of the most useful tumor marker for adenocarcinoma of the prostate. J Urol 1991;145:907–923.
48. Partin AW, Kattan MW, Subong EN et al. Combination of prostate-specific antigen, clinical stage, and Gleason score to predict pathological stage of localized prostate cancer. A multi-institutional update [see comments] [published erratum appears in JAMA 1997;278:118]. JAMA 1997;277: 1445–1451.
49. Kattan MW, Eastham JA, Stapleton AM et al. A preoperative nomogram for disease recurrence following radical prostatectomy for prostate cancer. J Natl Cancer Inst 1998;90:766–771.
50. Eastham JA, Scardino PT. Radical prostatectomy for clinical stage T1 and T2 prostate cancer. In: Vogelzang NJ, Scardino PT, Shipley WU, Coffey DS, eds. Comprehensive Textbook of Genitourinary Oncology, 2nd ed. Philadelphia: Lippincott, Williams & Wilkins, 2000:722–738.
51. Goldrath DE, Messing EM. Prostate specific antigen: not detectable despite tumor progression after radical prostatectomy. J Urol 1989;142:1082–1084.
52. Takayama TK, Krieger JN, True LD, Lange PH. Recurrent prostate cancer despite undetectable prostate specific antigen. J Urol 1992;148:1541–1542.
53. Leibman BD, Dillioglugil O, Wheeler TM, Scardino PT. Distant metastasis after radical prostatectomy in patients without an elevated serum prostate specific antigen level. Cancer 1995;76: 2530–2534.
54. Oefelein MG, Smith N, Carter M et al. The incidence of prostate cancer progression with undetectable serum prostate specific antigen in a series of 394 radical prostatectomies. J Urol 1995;154: 2128–2131.
55. Abi-Aad AS, Macfarlane MT, Stein A, deKernion JB. Detection of local recurrence after radical prostatectomy by prostate specific antigen and transrectal ultrasound. J Urol 1992;147:952–955.
56. Paulson DF. Impact of radical prostatectomy in the management of clinically localized disease. J Urol 1994;152:1826–1830.
57. Trapasso JG, deKernion JB, Smith RB, Dorey F. The incidence and significance of detectable levels of serum prostate specific antigen after radical prostatectomy [see comments]. J Urol 1994;152: 1821–1825.

58. Cowen ME, Kattan MW, Miles BJ. A national survey of attitudes regarding participation in prostate carcinoma testing. Cancer 1996;78:1952–1957.
59. McNeal JE, Villers AA, Redwine EA et al. Histologic differentiation, cancer volume, and pelvic lymph node metastasis in adenocarcinoma of the prostate. Cancer 1990;66:1225–1233.
60. Epstein JI, Pizov G, Walsh PC. Correlation of pathologic findings with progression after radical retropubic prostatectomy. Cancer 1993;71:3582–3593.
61. Abbas F, Scardino PT. Why neoadjuvant androgen deprivation prior to radical prostatectomy is unnecessary. Urol Clin North Am 1996;23:587–604.
62. Leandri P, Rossignol G, Gautier JR, Ramon J. Radical retropubic prostatectomy: morbidity and quality of life. Experience with 620 consecutive cases. J Urol 1992;147:883–887.
63. Geary ES, Dendinger TE, Freiha FS, Stamey TA. Incontinence and vesical neck strictures following radical retropubic prostatectomy. Urology 1995;45:1000–1006.
64. Murphy GP, Mettlin C, Menck H et al. National patterns of prostate cancer treatment by radical prostatectomy: results of a survey by the American College of Surgeons Commission on Cancer [see comments]. J Urol 1994;152:1817–1819.
65. Litwin MS, Hays RD, Fink A et al. Quality-of-life outcomes in men treated for localized prostate cancer [see comments]. JAMA 1995;273:129–135.
66. Fowler FJ Jr, Barry MJ, Lu-Yao G et al. Patient-reported complications and follow-up treatment after radical prostatectomy. The National Medicare Experience: 1988–1990 (updated June 1993). Urology 1993;42:622–629.
67. Potosky AL, Legler J, Albertsen PC et al. Health outcomes after prostatectomy or radiotherapy for prostate cancer: Results from the Prostate Cancer Outcomes Study. J Natl Cancer Inst 2000; 92:1582–1592.
68. Stanford JL, Feng Z, Hamilton AS et al. Urinary and sexual function after radical prostatectomy for clinically localized prostate cancer: the Prostate Cancer Outcomes Study [see comments]. JAMA 2000;283:354–360.
69. Hutch JA, Fisher R. Continence after radical prostatectomy. Br J Urol 1968;40:62–67.
70. Rudy DC, Woodside JR, Crawford ED. Urodynamic evaluation of incontinence in patients undergoing modified Campbell radical retropubic prostatectomy: a prospective study. J Urol 1984;132: 708–712.
71. Presti JC Jr, Schmidt RA, Narayan PA et al. Pathophysiology of urinary incontinence after radical prostatectomy. J Urol 1990;143:975–978.
72. Krane RJ. Urinary incontinence after treatment for localized prostate cancer. Mol Urol 2000;4: 279–286.
73. Quinlan DM, Epstein JI, Carter BS, Walsh PC. Sexual function following radical prostatectomy: influence of preservation of neurovascular bundles. J Urol 1991;145:998–1002.
74. Rabbani F, Stapleton AM, Kattan MW et al. Factors predicting recovery of erections after radical prostatectomy. J Urol 2000;164:1929–1934.
75. Walsh PC. Technique of vesicourethral anastomosis may influence recovery of sexual function following radical prostatectomy. Atlas Urol Clin North Am 1994;2:59–64.
76. Stapleton AMF, Scardino PT. Nerve-sparing radical retropubic prostatectomy. In: Vaughan ED, Jr., Perlmutter AP, eds. Atlas of Clinical Urology, Vol 2. Philadelphia: Current Medicine, 1999: 11.1–11.11.
77. Kim ED, Scardino PT, Hampel O et al. Interposition of sural nerve restores function of cavernous nerves resected during radical prostatectomy. J Urol 1999;161:188–192.
78. Scolieri MJ, Altman A, Resnick MI. Neoadjuvant hormonal ablative therapy before radical prostatectomy: A review. Is it indicated? J Urol 2000;164:1465–1472.

79. Witjes WP, Schulman CC, Debruyne FM. Preliminary results of a prospective randomized study comparing radical prostatectomy versus radical prostatectomy associated with neoadjuvant hormonal combination therapy in T2–3 N0 M0 prostatic carcinoma. The European Study Group on Neoadjuvant Treatment of Prostate Cancer. Urology 1997;49:65–69.
80. Labrie F, Cusan L, Gomez JL et al. Neoadjuvant hormonal therapy: the Canadian experience. Urology 1997;49:56–64.
81. Soloway MS, Sharifi R, Wajsman Z et al. Randomized prospective study comparing radical prostatectomy alone versus radical prostatectomy preceded by androgen blockade in clinical stage B2 (T2bNxM0) prostate cancer. The Lupron Depot Neoadjuvant Prostate Cancer Study Group. J Urol 1995;154:424–428.
82. Hugosson J, Abrahamsson PA, Ahlgren G et al. The risk of malignancy in the surgical margin at radical prostatectomy reduced almost three-fold in patients given neo-adjuvant hormone treatment. Eur Urol 1996;29:413–419.
83. Dalkin BL, Ahmann FR, Nagle R, Johnson CS. Randomized study of neoadjuvant testicular androgen ablation therapy before radical prostatectomy in men with clinically localized prostate cancer. J Urol 1996;155:1357–1360.
84. Goldenberg SL, Klotz LH, Srigley J et al. Randomized, prospective, controlled study comparing radical prostatectomy alone and neoadjuvant androgen withdrawal in the treatment of localized prostate cancer. Canadian Urologic Oncology Group [see comments]. J Urol 1996;156:873–877.
85. Van Poppel H, De Ridder D, Elgamal AA et al. Neoadjuvant hormonal therapy before radical prostatectomy decreases the number of positive surgical margins in stage T2 prostate cancer: interim results of a prospective randomized trial. The Belgian Uro-Oncological Study Group. J Urol 1995;154:429–434.
86. Witjes WPJ, Schulman CC, Debruyne FMJ et al. Neoadjuvant combined androgen deprivation therapy in locally confined prostatic carcinoma: 3–4 years of followup of a European randomized study [abstract]. J Urol 1998;159:254.
87. Soloway M, Shaaifi R, Wajsman Z, et al. Radical prostatectomy alone vs. radical prostatectomy preceded by androgen blockade in cT2b prostate cancer: 24 month results [abstract]. J Urol 1997; 157:160.
88. Aus G, Abrahamsson PA, Ahlgren G et al. Hormonal treatment before radical prostatectomy: a 3-year followup. J Urol 1998;159:2013–2016; discussion 2016–2017.
89. Goldenberg SL, Klotz L, Jewett MA et al. A randomized trial of neoadjuvant androgen withdrawal therapy prior to radical prostatectomy: 24 months post-treatment PSA results [abstract]. J Urol 1997;157:92.
90. Fair WR, Cookson MS, Stroumbakis N et al. The indications, rationale, and results of neoadjuvant androgen deprivation in the treatment of prostatic cancer: Memorial Sloan-Kettering Cancer Center results. Urology 1997;49:46–55.
91. Polascik TJ, Pound CR, DeWeese TL, Walsh PC. Comparison of radical prostatectomy and iodine 125 interstitial radiotherapy for the treatment of clinically localized prostate cancer: a 7-year biochemical (PSA) progression analysis [see comments]. Urology 1998;51:884–889; discussion 889–890.
92. D'Amico AV, Whittington R, Malkowicz SB et al. Biochemical outcome after radical prostatectomy, external beam radiation therapy, or interstitial radiation therapy for clinically localized prostate cancer [see comments]. JAMA 1998;280:969–974.
93. Gerber GS, Thisted RA, Chodak GW et al. Results of radical prostatectomy in men with locally advanced prostate cancer: multi-institutional pooled analysis. Eur Urol 1997;32:385–390.

Treatment of Prostate Cancer: External-Beam Radiotherapy

Steven A. Leibel

Zvi Fuks

Michael J. Zelefsky

C. Clifton Ling

Curative approaches of external-beam irradiation for prostate cancer became available in the 1950s with the emergence of megavoltage ^{60}Co teletherapy units[1] and linear accelerators.[2] This technology provided for the first time the opportunity to deliver tumoricidal doses to the prostate without excessive damage to the skin and normal tissues.[3] Incremental advances in radiation dosimetry, treatment planning, and delivery have since evolved to enhance precision, increase the dose, and reduce the toxicity of radiation therapy. Despite these improvements, the conventional radiation dose levels of 65–70 Gy, the maximum feasible with traditional techniques, have limited the ability of conventional external-beam radiation therapy to achieve maximal levels of tumor control in localized prostate cancer. Dose escalation with three-dimensional conformal radiation therapy (3D-CRT) and intensity-modulated radiation therapy (IMRT) and the use of concomitant androgen deprivation are being investigated as approaches to overcome the resistance of tumor clonogens to the dose levels administered with conventional radiotherapeutic techniques.

Three-dimensional treatment planning systems use advanced imaging technology and sophisticated radiation dose calculation algorithms to generate plans that conform the prescribed dose to the tumor target. At the same time, the volume of surrounding normal tissues carried to high dose levels is reduced, permitting an increase in tumor dose without a concomitant increase in normal tissue toxicity. The development of computer-automated optimization for treatment planning and the introduction of delivery systems for intensity-modulated radiation fields have significantly enhanced the precision of tumor targeting and escalation of the tumor dose to previously unattainable levels. Recent experience demonstrates that the 3D approach represents a breakthrough in the ability to improve the local cure of prostate cancer.[4-6]

Combining androgen deprivation with radiation therapy is another therapeutic strategy being tested. Both normal and neoplastic prostate cells are sensitive to androgen withdrawal. The availability of new, less toxic agents has led to their use as neoadjuvant or adjuvant treatments in combination with radiation therapy. Data from several randomized trials have indicated significantly reduced local failures in locally advanced, unfavorable-risk prostate cancer.[6,7]

LIMITS OF CONVENTIONAL RADIATION THERAPY

Much of the available long-term outcome data for irradiation in prostatic carcinoma is derived from patients who were treated in the 1970s, before the era of computed tomography (CT) and magnetic resonance imaging. The anatomical boundaries of the prostate and the design of treatment fields were determined by plain-film radiographic simulator techniques,[8] and large safety margins were required to address uncertainties of tumor target definition. Early conventional delivery methods used 6 × 6 cm to 8 × 8 cm fields delivered with rotational arc techniques.[2,8] Although this was acceptable for many T1 and T2a tumors,[9] reconstruction of such fields using CT imaging clearly indicated that this approach would be insufficient to cover most locally advanced tumors, especially when it was necessary to encompass the seminal vesicles.[10,11]

More contemporary conventional treatment techniques have been based on CT-assisted planning. A four-field whole-pelvis approach is used to treat the prostate, seminal vesicles, and regional lymph nodes.[12] The cross section of each beam is shaped with individualized Cerrobend (low-melting-point alloy) blocks to shield the small bowel, the posterior wall of the rectum, the anal canal and sphincter, and the uninvolved bladder and urethra. Treatment is delivered in daily fractions of 1.8–2 Gy, given five sessions per week, to a cumulative dose of 45–50 Gy. An additional "boost" to the prostate and seminal vesicles encompassed by 1–2 cm of normal tissue subsequently is administered with either a bilateral 120-degree-arc rotational technique[3,8] or with a four-field arrangement.[12] The standard boost dose is 20 Gy, delivered by the same fractionation scheme as is used in the pelvic fields, for a total dose to the prostate of 65–70 Gy. For

T1 and small T2 tumors with a low Gleason score, treatment is confined to the prostate only (carried to 65–70 Gy), because the probability of seminal vesicle involvement and metastatic spread to the pelvic lymph nodes in such patients is very small.[12]

Data collected over the last three decades for patients treated with conventional (non-3D) techniques demonstrated that 10-year rates of clinically assessed [without prostate-specific antigen (PSA) measurements] local control were 85%–96% for stages T1b–T2 tumors and 58%–65% for T3–T4 tumors.[13] These estimates, however, appear to be high, inasmuch as more recent PSA relapse-free survival rates were reported to be 65% in patients with stages T1–T2 disease[14] and 24% in more locally advanced T3 tumors.[15] Moreover, biopsy-proven local recurrence rates range from 23% to 65% in patients with T1–T3 tumors treated to dose levels of 65–70 Gy.[16,17] These data indicate a need to improve local tumor control in prostate cancer, particularly in patients with locally advanced disease whose only curative treatment option is external-beam irradiation.[18]

The relative inability of conventional techniques to eradicate localized prostate cancer results, in part, from resistance of subpopulations of tumor clonogens to the traditional dose levels of 65–70 Gy. Several studies provide evidence for a direct relationship between local tumor control and dose and suggest that the dose levels necessary for controlling prostate cancer exceed 70 Gy. In an analysis of 624 stage T3 prostate cancer patients, the actuarial 7-year clinical local recurrence rates were 36% for those receiving 60–64.9 Gy, 32% for 65–69.9 Gy, and 24% for patients treated to at least 70 Gy.[19] Zagars et al[15] concluded that for T3 tumors, a dose of less than 68 Gy was essentially ineffective. A recent study from the Radiation Therapy Oncology Group (RTOG) indicated that patients with Gleason scores of 8–10 who received more than 66 Gy (median, 69 Gy) had significant improvements in disease-specific and overall survival rates as compared with those treated to no more than 66 Gy (median, 64 Gy).[20] The ability to administer high doses with conventional techniques has been limited by rectal and bladder complications, resulting from the use of wide safety margins around the prostate. The American College of Radiology Patterns of Care study found that the likelihood of severe (grade 3–4) rectal and bladder complications almost doubled (from 3.5% to 6.9%) when doses of more than 70 Gy were administered with conventional treatment methods.[21] Moreover, in a dose-escalation study using such techniques, the 2-year rate of moderate to severe proctitis increased from 20% for patients receiving not more than 75 Gy to 60% for those treated to higher dose levels.[22]

The lack of sophisticated treatment planning tools to delineate between the prostate and its surrounding pelvic organs and to calculate the dose at each pixel of the irradiated tissue volume has limited the ability of conventional radiation therapy to increase the tumor dose safely to more than 70 Gy. Because dose computations are labor-intensive, conventional dose calculation methods until recently provided limited information on dose distributions, restricted mainly to the midaxial tissue plane. The dose to the remainder of the tumor was assumed based on reasonable, albeit imprecise, projections.

THREE-DIMENSIONAL CONFORMAL RADIATION THERAPY

Advances in computer technology and engineering have enabled the implementation of 3D-CRT as an approach to overcome many of these obstacles. The availability of high-performance workstations and sophisticated algorithms capable of rapid dose computations and the design of new computer-aided treatment delivery systems with multileaf collimation (MLC) and on-line real-time portal imaging have made 3D-CRT feasible for prostate cancer and several other human tumors. Three-dimensional treatment planning is predicated on the ability to define anatomically each critical subvolume within the entire 3D space of irradiated tissues and to calculate precisely the dose delivered at each point. It uses advanced imaging technology for tumor and normal organ segmentation and computer-aided optimization to generate treatment plans that conform the prescribed dose to the entire 3D configuration of the prostatic target volume's anatomical boundaries while maximally excluding the adjacent normal organs.[23,24]

Biological Basis of 3D-CRT

The ability to reduce the volume of normal tissues receiving high radiation dose levels is a critical attribute of the 3D-CRT paradigm. The biological effects of radiation on both the tumor and the normal tissues result in sigmoid-shaped dose-response patterns.[25,26] The observation that dose-response curves for tumor control are at a lower dose range than the corresponding toxicity curves for adjacent normal tissues provides the underlying foundation of curative radiation therapy. When tumor control and normal tissue complication curves are approximately parallel in shape and sufficiently well separated, the dose levels necessary to cure disease in a high percentage of patients can be administered without producing excessive damage to normal tissue. However, clinical data indicate that human tumor control probability curves represent population averages of patients with a spectrum of tumor radiosensitivity, whereas the range of variations in normal tissue sensitivity appear to be considerably smaller. Therefore, the slopes of tumor control curves are typically less steep than those for normal tissue injury,[27,28] limiting the ability to deliver high radiation doses, as are frequently required for tumor cure. However, recent clinical data of prostate cancer treated with radiation therapy have indicated that reduction in the rectal volume exposed to radiation shifts the effective normal tissue complication curve to the higher dose region (the so-called volume effect).[29] This finding suggests that the reduction of rectal volume by the 3D-CRT approach should permit a safe escalation in tumor dose. Several recent reports have validated this concept, demonstrating the effectiveness of 3D-CRT in dose-escalation schemes in prostate cancer, thus defining new standards for curative radiation therapy in this disease.[4–6,30–34]

3D-CRT Planning and Delivery

Currently available 3D treatment–planning systems vary in several features but are based on common principles.[24,35] All systems use CT-guided simulation to delineate the prostate and normal organs and to generate high-resolution 3D reconstructions. Patients are immobilized within individually fabricated thermoplastic casts to minimize setup uncertainties and to ensure daily reproducibility of positioning on the treatment couch.[36] The planning target volume (PTV)[37] is delineated on each CT slice by encompassing the prostate and seminal vesicle tissue with a 1-cm margin around the clinical target volume. In some systems, the safety margin at the interface with the rectum is reduced to 0.6 cm. The walls of the rectum and bladder, the pelvic bones, and the skin surface also are identified on each CT slice. Portions of the small bowel or sigmoid colon within or adjacent to the PTV also are contoured and taken into consideration, if necessary, in designing the treatment plan. The PTV and normal organs are reconstructed in 3D and displayed with the beam's-eye view technique, using wire-frame or solid graphics to delineate surfaces and color to distinguish each structure.[24,35] Early in the 3D-CRT experience, patients were treated with a coplanar six-field 3D-CRT approach (two lateral opposed fields and two pair of oblique fields)[11] using computer-driven MLC to shape the aperture of each field.[38] The target dose was prescribed to the maximum isodose surface distribution that completely encompassed the PTV. This technique was used to administer prescription doses of at least 75.6 Gy.

INTENSITY MODULATED RADIATION THERAPY

More recently, IMRT was developed as an advanced form of 3D-CRT.[5,39,40] IMRT uses the inverse treatment-planning approach to generate beam profiles with changing intensities across the treatment field and treatment delivery using a variety of methods to apply nonuniform beam intensities. This technique thus is different from conventional and first-generation 3D treatment planning for prostate cancer, both of which use a "forward" approach and beams with uniform intensities. Multiple IMRT beams with different profiles are used to achieve a composite with a homogeneous dose distribution within the PTV. The resultant plan typically conforms tightly to the PTV and exhibits a rapid fall-off of the dose within the surrounding tissue.

The process of inverse treatment planning for IMRT is initiated with definition of the desired dose distribution to the target volume and normal organs. Using a computer-aided optimization algorithm, the intensity profile of each beam is iteratively adjusted to satisfy the predefined dose specifications to the tumor and normal tissue structures.[41] The output of the inverse planning process is a series of beam intensity profiles that serve as a template for treatment delivery. Unlike the first-generation 3D-CRT in which MLC is used for beam shaping, the Memorial Sloan-Kettering Cancer Center (MSKCC) system for IMRT delivery uses MLC in a dynamic mode (dynamic multileaf collimation).[42] Each pair of opposing leaves forms an individual "sliding window" that travels across the target under computer control during radiation delivery. The width of the window and the speed of the leaves are adjusted continuously, according to a prescribed scheme, to produce the required intensity pattern. A computer program directs the function of the MLC during treatment. Other methods for delivering intensity-modulated beams include the multisegment static multileaf collimation (step-and-shoot) approach and the slit-beam technique, in which leaf shutters are driven in and out of the beam path.[43] At MSKCC, a coplanar five-field IMRT technique is used to treat patients to dose levels of 81 Gy or more.[44]

The MSKCC Dose-Escalation Study

The validity of the 3D-CRT concept in prostate cancer was confirmed at MSKCC in an institutional review board–approved dose-escalation study.[4,5,36,45] The study was designed to assess the morbidity of high-dose 3D-CRT, to establish the highest feasible dose with the 3D-CRT approach, and to evaluate the impact of dose on the rates of local tumor control. The radiation dose was systematically increased from 64.8 to 86.4 Gy by increments of 5.4 Gy in consecutive groups of patients. Treatment was given in daily fractions of 1.8 Gy with 15 MV x-rays. A total of 1100 patients were treated in a 10-year period through October 1998, and their characteristics are shown in Table 14.2.1.

The treatment volume included the entire prostate and seminal vesicles but did not encompass the regional pelvic lymph nodes.[36] A 3-month course of neoadjuvant androgen deprivation (NAAD) therapy was administered to 427 patients (39%) having large-volume prostate glands to decrease the target volume for irradiation and, hence, to reduce the risk of treatment-related complications.[46] In all such cases, NAAD was discontinued at the completion of irradiation. In other patients, hormonal therapy was given only when indicated for relapsing disease. Disease status and late toxicity (using the RTOG morbidity grading system[47]) end points were analyzed in November 2000. The median follow-up time was 60 months, with a range of 24–142 months.

Toxicity of 3D-CRT and IMRT

An important component of the 3D paradigm is the ability to deliver high radiation doses with a minimal risk of normal tissue toxicity. The rates of long-term rectal and urinary complications observed in the 1100 patients treated with 3D-CRT and IMRT are shown in Figure 14.2.1.[45] The 5-year actuarial rate of grade 3 or higher rectal toxicity was 1.2%, and no correlation between dose and the rates

TABLE 14.2.1 Characteristics of 1100 Stage T1c-T3 Prostate Cancer Patients Treated with 3D-CRT and IMRT

Characteristic	No. of Patients (%)
Clinical stage	
T1c	284 (26)
T2a	354 (32)
T2b	200 (18)
T3	262 (24)
Gleason score	
≤ 6	572 (52)
≥ 7	528 (48)
Pretreatment PSA	
≤ 10 ng/mL	522 (47)
> 10 ng/mL	578 (53)
Tumor dose (Gy)	
64.8	96 (9)
70.2	269 (24)
75.6	445 (40)
81.0	250 (23)
86.4	40 (4)
Prognostic group	
Favorable[a]	279 (25)
Intermediate	405 (37)
Unfavorable	416 (38)
3D technique	
6-Field 3D-CRT to 64.8–75.6 Gy	810 (74)
Two-phase 3D-CRT to 81 Gy	61 (5)
5-Field IMRT to 81–86.4 Gy	229 (21)
Neoadjuvant androgen deprivation	
No	673 (61)
Yes	427 (39)

3D-CRT, three-dimensional conformal radiation therapy; IMRT, intensity-modulated radiation therapy; PSA, prostate-specific antigen.
[a]See text.[4,24]

of complications was found within the range of 64.8–81 Gy.[5] For 3D-CRT, there was, however, a dose-related increase in late grade 2 rectal bleeding. The 5-year actuarial rate of grade 2 rectal bleeding for patients receiving 64.8–70.2 Gy was 5% as compared to 17% for those treated to 75.6 Gy ($P < 0.001$).[45]

When the dose was escalated to 81 Gy, a safety constraint was imposed during planning to restrict to 30% or less the volume of the rectal wall receiving 75.6 Gy. To meet this requirement, a two-phase approach was used with the 3D-CRT technique in which the first 72 Gy was administered with the coplanar six-field

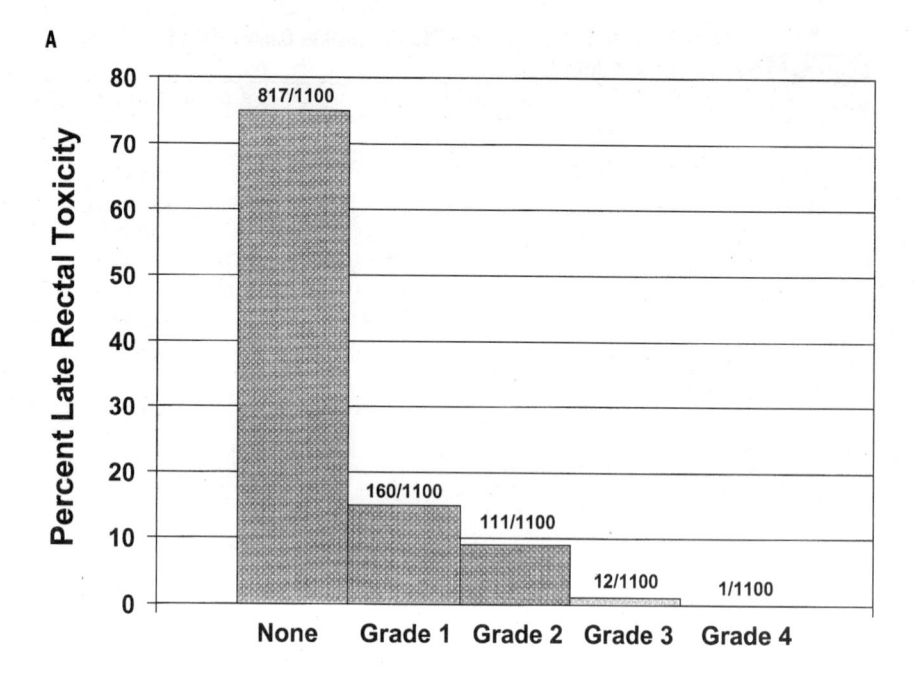

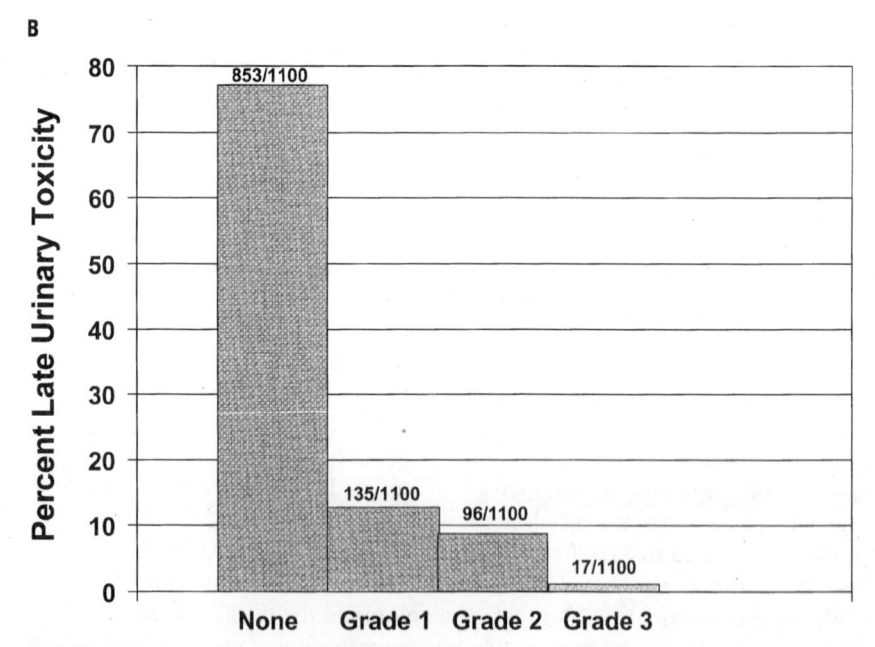

FIGURE 14.2.1 Incidence of late rectal (A) and late urinary (B) complications by grade according to the RTOG morbidity grading system.[47]

design, followed by a separate multifield plan for the remaining 9 Gy (five treatment fractions). The boost phase assured that the rectum was completely blocked in each field.[36] With this approach, the 5-year actuarial rate of late grade 2 rectal bleeding was 15%.[44,45] Because this technique did not substantially decrease the rate of grade 2 toxicity, an IMRT approach was introduced to improve the conformality of treatment to 81 Gy.[5,39,40,44]

Figure 14.2.2 depicts the rectal toxicity in the first 189 patients treated with IMRT to 81 Gy as compared with 61 patients treated with the two-phase 3D-CRT approach to the same dose level. The 3-year actuarial rate of late grade 2–3 rectal bleeding was 3% for IMRT as compared to 17% for the two-phase technique ($P < 0.001$). Only one case of grade 3 rectal bleeding was observed in each treatment group. Of 560 patients now treated with IMRT (median follow-up, 30 months; range, 6–56 months), only 8 (1.4%) have thus far developed grade 2 rectal bleeding, and 3 patients (0.5%) have experienced grade 3 toxicity. These findings demonstrate that the improved conformality and reduction of irradiated rectal tissue with IMRT translated into a decrease in rectal toxicity, providing an opportunity for further dose escalation. Indeed, 41 patients were accrued to the 86.4 level of the dose-escalation study and, with a median follow-up time of 31

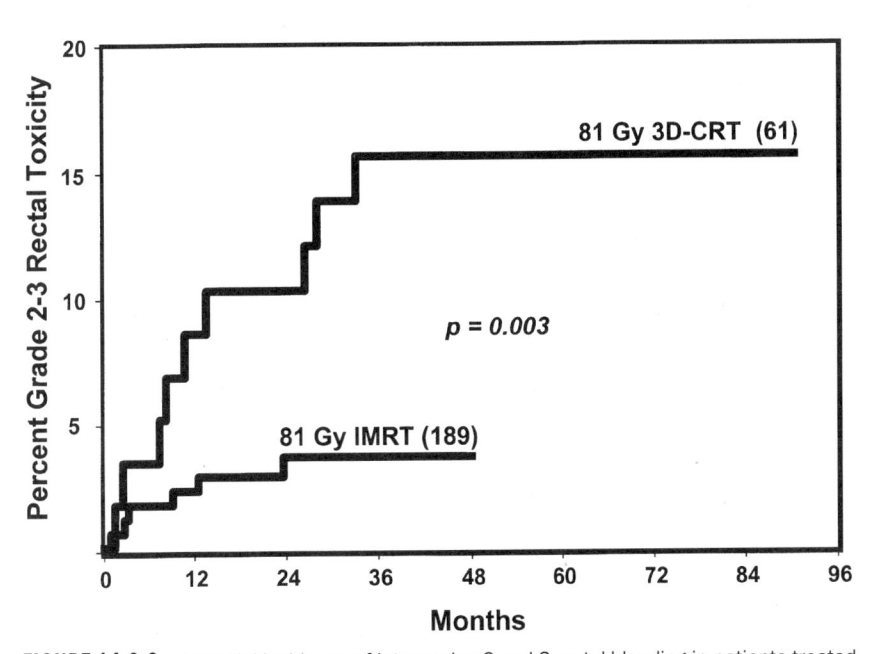

FIGURE 14.2.2 Actuarial incidence of late grades 2 and 3 rectal bleeding in patients treated with 81 Gy by intensity-modulated radiation therapy (IMRT) as compared with 81 Gy delivered by the two-phase three-dimensional conformal radiation therapy (3D-CRT) technique. Only one case of grade 3 rectal bleeding was noted in each treatment group.

months (range, 24–40 months), no grade 3 or higher toxicities have been observed. Only two patients (5%) have developed grade 2 rectal bleeding.[45]

Does Dose Escalation Improve the Outcome?

The MSKCC study has generated extensive information on the efficacy of dose escalation both on long-term disease-free survival and local control. High radiation dose levels (≥ 75.6 Gy) had a significant impact on PSA relapse-free survival. PSA relapse was defined as three successive increases in the PSA value after a posttreatment nadir level was achieved.[48] The date of failure was the midpoint in time between the last nonrising and the first rising PSA value.[14] For this analysis, patients were categorized into three prognostic groups according to pretreatment variables that independently affected the PSA outcome.[4,24] Patients with stages T1–T2 disease, a pretreatment PSA level of 10 ng/mL or less, and a Gleason score no higher than 6 were classified as a favorable prognosis group. An increase in one of the variables classified the patient in an intermediate prognosis group, and an increase in two or more variables in an unfavorable prognosis group. The 7-year actuarial PSA relapse-free survival for favorable-risk patients who received at least 75.6 Gy was 90%, as compared to 77% for those treated to 64.8–70.2 Gy ($P = 0.05$) (Fig. 14.2.3A). The corresponding rates for patients in the intermediate-risk group were 70% and 50%, respectively ($P = 0.001$) (see Fig. 14.2.3B). The 7-year actuarial PSA relapse-free survival for unfavorable-risk patients who received at least 75.6 Gy was 47%, as compared to 21% for those treated to 64.8–70.2 Gy ($P = 0.002$). Moreover, unfavorable-risk patients who received 81 Gy had a better outcome than those who were treated with lower doses. Figure 14.2.4 shows that the 7-year PSA relapse-free survival rate for patients who received 81 Gy was 67%, as compared to 43% for those treated to 75.6 Gy ($P = 0.05$).[45]

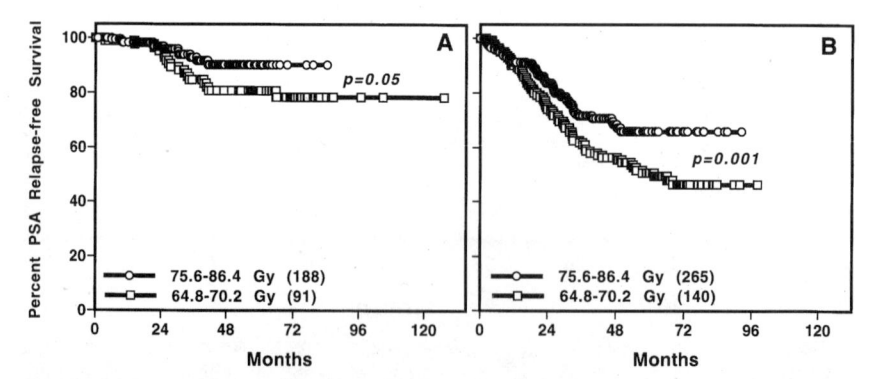

FIGURE 14.2.3 Actuarial prostate-specific antigen (PSA) relapse-free survival according to dose for patients in the favorable (A) and intermediate (B) prognostic groups.

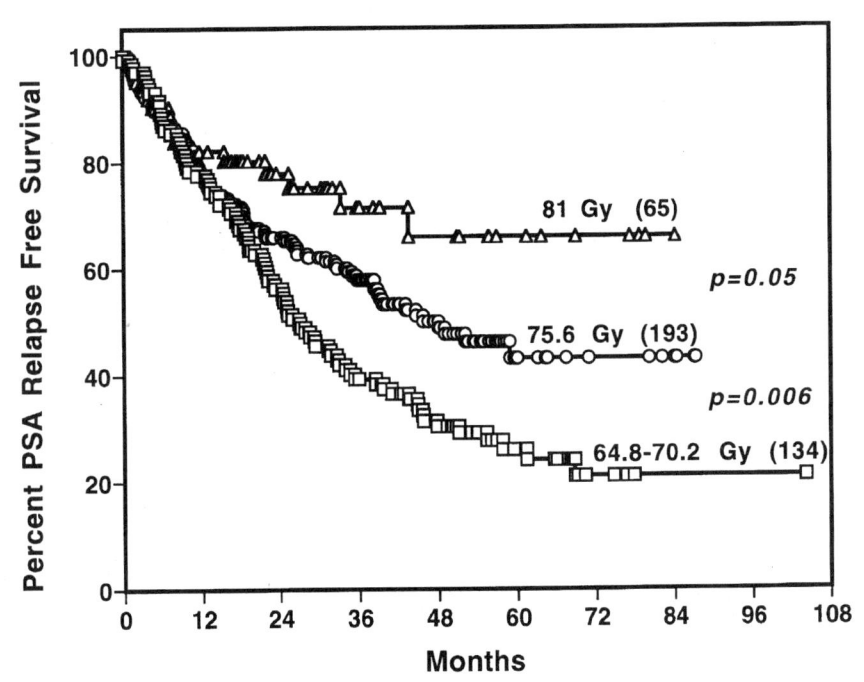

FIGURE 14.2.4 Actuarial prostate-specific antigen (PSA) relapse-free survival according to dose for patients in the unfavorable prognostic group.

Because radiation was confined to the prostate alone, it is reasonable to assume that the improvement in PSA relapse-free survival with increasing dose could be attributed, for the most part, to improved local control. To explore this notion further, sextant prostate biopsies were performed at 2.5 years (median, 35 months) after 3D-CRT or IMRT or later in 252 patients. Of the patients receiving 81 Gy, 37 of 41 (90%) had negative biopsies, indicating local tumor control, as compared with 92 of 119 (77%) after 75.6 Gy, 45 or 68 (66%) after 70.2 Gy, and 11 of 24 (46%) after 64.8 Gy (81 Gy vs 75.6 Gy; $P = 0.22$; 81 Gy vs 70.2 Gy, $P = 0.01$).[45] Table 14.2.2 summarizes the biopsy findings according to prognostic risk groups and dose levels. Within each risk group, the incidence of positive biopsies decreased with increasing dose. In addition, the rate of positive biopsies within each dose bin increased as the prognostic group became less favorable, except for the group of patients receiving 81 Gy, for which the number of patients who have undergone biopsy thus far is too small to permit a pattern analysis.

When fitted to a tumor control probability model, the mean dose to the PTV was found, within each prognostic risk group, to be directly related to the biopsy outcome. The median tumor control dose (TCD_{50}), or the dose required to achieve a tumor control probability of 50%, for the favorable-risk patients was 68.3 Gy,

TABLE 14.2.2 Local Failure According to Prognostic Risk Group and Dose Assessed by Biopsies in 252 Patients at ≥ 2.5 Years After 3D-CRT and IMRT

Dose (Gy)	Positive Biopsy Specimens/Total Biopsies (%)		
	Favorable	Intermediate	Unfavorable
81	0/7 (0)	3/18 (17)	1/16 (6)
75.6	2/18 (11)	8/44 (19)	17/57 (30)
70.2	3/20 (15)	5/21 (24)	15/27 (56)
64.8	1/3 (33)	6/13 (46)	6/8 (75)
Total	6/48 (13)	22/96 (23)	39/108 (37)

3D-CRT, three-dimensional conformal radiation therapy; IMRT, intensity-modulated radiation therapy.

as compared with 72.8 Gy for the intermediate-risk and 77.3 Gy for the unfavorable-risk groups (unpublished data). These data indicate that the more aggressive biological phenotypes of prostate tumor cells are more radioresistant. However, the data indicate that even for more favorable phenotypes, conventional doses of 65–70 Gy appear insufficient and that doses of 81 Gy or more are necessary for a maximal local cure. Based on these data, patients at MSKCC with intermediate- and unfavorable-risk features now are being treated to 86.4 Gy. Whether this or higher doses will decrease the risk of local relapse will require further investigation. Nonetheless, it is clear that such high dose levels can be delivered only with advanced IMRT techniques.

Similar conclusions regarding a need for increased radiation doses to achieve a maximal local cure can be derived from other studies. Investigators from the Fox Chase Cancer Center reported the results of a matched-pair analysis in which 357 patients who received at least 74 Gy with 3D-CRT were compared to the same number of patients treated with less than 74 Gy with either conventional or conformal techniques. The 5-year PSA relapse-free survival rates were 71% and 56% for the high- and low-dose groups, respectively ($P = 0.003$). Dose also had a significant impact on the 5-year freedom from distant metastasis (97% vs 88%; $P = 0.0004$), cause-specific survival (99% vs 94%; $P = 0.007$) and overall survival (88% vs 79%; $P = 0.01$).[49] Pollack and Zagars[50] observed a dose effect in a retrospective analysis of 94 patients with localized prostate cancer treated with high-dose 3D-CRT (74–78 Gy) and 844 patients treated with conventional-dose irradiation (60–70 Gy). Patients were divided into low-dose (< 67 Gy), intermediate-dose (67–77 Gy), and high-dose (> 77 Gy) groups. The 3-year PSA relapse-free survival rates were 61%, 74%, and 96% for the low-, intermediate- and high-dose groups, respectively ($P < 0.01$). When patients were stratified by the pretreatment PSA (≤ 4 vs > 4–10 vs > 10–20 vs > 20 ng/mL), clinical stage (T1–T2 vs T3–T4), or Gleason score (2–6 vs 7–10), a significantly improved biochemical outcome was observed in all subgroups except for those with pretreatment PSA levels of not more than 4.0 ng/mL.

To prove further the impact of dose on the outcome, these investigators randomized 301 patients to receive either 70 Gy using a four-field conventional technique or the same treatment plus a six-field conformal boost to a total of 78 Gy.[50] The overall 5-year PSA relapse-free survival rates were 69% for patients treated with 70 Gy and 79% for those who received 78 Gy ($P = 0.058$). A significant difference in biochemical outcome was observed in a subgroup of these patients whose pretreatment PSA level was greater than 10 ng/mL (48% for 70 Gy vs 75% for 78 Gy; $P = 0.011$), with the most striking effect observed in T1–T2 patients in this subgroup (60% for 70 Gy vs 90% for 78 Gy; $P = 0.011$). The difference in the PSA outcome for patients with a pretreatment PSA level of not more than 10 ng/mL was not significant.[31]

ANDROGEN DEPRIVATION AND RADIATION THERAPY

Biological Basis of Combining Androgen Deprivation with Radiation Therapy

In contrast to 3D-CRT and IMRT, the goal of androgen deprivation is to shift the tumor control curve of prostate cancer to the lower dose region to enhance the probability of cure at the conventional dose levels of 65–70 Gy. Androgen withdrawal leads to inhibition of DNA synthesis and cell proliferation and induces apoptotic cell death in both normal and malignant prostate tissues.[51] The rationale for using NAAD is to reduce the volume of the prostate and to decrease the number of tumor clonogens prior to irradiation. Whether NAAD also sensitizes tumor clonogens to the effects of radiation is not entirely clear. The aim of adjuvant androgen deprivation is to eradicate residual tumor clones remaining after radiation therapy, either within the prostate or at distant metastatic sites.

Experimental studies using the androgen-sensitive Dunning R3327-G rat prostate tumor and Shionogi mouse mammary carcinoma model systems have provided information on the impact of timing and sequencing on the outcome of androgen deprivation and radiation. Zeitman et al[52,53] found an approximately twofold reduction in the TCD_{50} when radiation was administered after a maximal tumor regression from androgen deprivation was achieved. This effect was less striking when radiation was given before maximal tumor reduction, indicating that androgen deprivation provided at least an additive effect on cell killing. A smaller decrease in TCD_{50} was observed when androgen deprivation was induced after radiation therapy. Pollack et al[54] demonstrated that the combination of androgen deprivation and subsequent fractionated irradiation resulted in a greater delay of tumor growth than the sum of the individual effects of the two treatments, consistent with a supraadditive enhancement of tumor growth inhibition.

Has Combined Androgen Deprivation and Radiation Therapy Achieved Its Goals?

Considerable evidence supports the use of androgen deprivation with radiation therapy in selected prostate cancer patients, especially those with locally advanced, unfavorable-risk disease. Several groups have demonstrated the effectiveness of NAAD in decreasing the size of the prostate before radiation therapy, thus improving the ability to deliver maximal radiation doses without exceeding normal tissue tolerance.[46,55,56] For example, Zelefsky et al[46] demonstrated that 3 months of leuprolide acetate and flutamide or bicalutamide reduced the prostate PTV by a mean of 25% (range, 3%–52%).

Table 14.2.3 summarizes the results of four multiinstitutional randomized trials that tested the impact of neoadjuvant or adjuvant androgen deprivation on the outcome of radiation therapy. In each trial, the pelvic lymph nodes received 45–50 Gy and the prostate was treated with 65–70 Gy using conventional tech-

TABLE 14.2.3 Five-Year Outcomes of Randomized Trials Testing the Effect of Androgen Deprivation Combined with Radiation Therapy

	RTOG 86–10[57–59]	RTOG 85–31[59–61]	RTOG 92–02[62]	EORTC 22863[63,64]
Study arm[a]	Neo Gos/Flu	Adj Gos	Neo Gos/Flu Adj Gos	Adj Gos
Control arm	RT alone	RT alone	Neo Gos/Flu	RT alone
No. of patients	471	977	1554	415
Median follow-up (yr)	6	5.6	4.8	3.7
Local failure				
Study	22%	15%	6.2%	3%
Control	35%	31%	13%	23%
Distant metastases				
Study	29%	15%	11%	2%
Control	39%	29%	17%	44%
PSA RFS				
Study	39%	54%	46%	81%
Control	20%	21%	21%	43%
Overall survival				
Study	72%[b]	75%[b]	78%[b]	79%
Control	68%	71%	79%	62%

Adj, adjuvant; EORTC, European Organization for Research and Treatment of Cancer; Flu, flutamide; Gos, goserelin; Neo, neoadjuvant; PSA, prostate-specific antigen; RFS, relapse-free survival; RT, radiation therapy; RTOG, Radiation Therapy Oncology Group.
[a]See text.
[b]Differences not significant.

niques. The clinical value of the neoadjuvant approach was tested in RTOG trial 86-10, in which patients with large (at least 5 × 5 cm) T2–T4 prostate tumors were randomized to receive goserelin acetate and flutamide for 2 months before and during radiation therapy or radiation alone.[57–59] The adjuvant approach was tested in three studies. RTOG trial 85-31 randomized patients with stages T3–T4 disease (smaller than 5 × 5 cm) or those with T1–T2 tumors and lymph node involvement to receive goserelin either beginning during the last week of radiation and continued indefinitely or being initiated on evidence of postirradiation relapse.[59–61] In RTOG trial 92-02, patients with stages T2c–T4 tumors were administered neoadjuvant goserelin and flutamide for 2 months before and 2 months during radiation treatment and then were randomized either to receive adjuvant goserelin for 2 years or to receive no additional treatment.[62] The European Organization for Research and Treatment of Cancer trial 22863 randomly assigned patients with high-grade T1–T2 or T3–T4 prostate cancer to receive radiation therapy alone or radiation therapy plus goserelin, initiated at the beginning of radiation therapy and continued after irradiation for 3 years. Cyproterone acetate also was administered during the first month of treatment.[63,64]

These studies have uniformly demonstrated significant improvements in local control, freedom from distant metastases, and PSA relapse-free survival for patients receiving combined-modality therapy. The European Organization for Research and Treatment of Cancer trial has drawn considerable attention as it showed a significant overall survival advantage for patients receiving adjuvant androgen deprivation.[63,64] However, the validity of this observation has been questioned, because the survival of the radiation-alone group (62%) appears noticeably lower than published rates for similar patients as well as those in other trials testing androgen deprivation.[7] Survival improvements in the RTOG adjuvant therapy trials (85-31 and 92-02) have thus far been observed only in patients with Gleason scores of 8–10.[59–62] In contrast, subset analysis of the RTOG NAAD trial (86-10) indicated that outcome improvements, including overall survival, occurred primarily in patients with Gleason scores of 2–6.[58,59] Longer follow-up of patients in these trials will be needed to determine whether adjuvant androgen deprivation prevents or only delays the appearance of distant metastases and whether a survival benefit will be observed for all patients.

The effect of androgen deprivation on local tumor control has been demonstrated also in posttreatment biopsy studies. Laverdière et al[17] reported preliminary results of a three-arm randomized trial of stages T2–T3 prostate cancer patients from whom biopsies were obtained at 24 months after radiation therapy. Patients treated for 3 months with NAAD (leuprolide and flutamide) followed by 64 Gy had a 28% rate of tumor-positive biopsies as compared with a 65% rate for those receiving radiation alone. However, androgen deprivation given for 3 months before and 6 months after radiation therapy to 64 Gy was associated with only a 5% rate of positive biopsies, consistent with an additive rather than a radiation-sensitizing effect.

Effect of Androgen Deprivation on the Outcome After High-Dose 3D-CRT and IMRT

Whereas the randomized trials demonstrating improved outcome with androgen deprivation have used exclusively conventional dose levels of 65–70 Gy, the question remains as to whether androgen deprivation would lead to similar improvements in patients receiving high-dose conformal radiation therapy. The MSKCC study demonstrated improvements in local tumor control for patients receiving NAAD. Table 14.2.4 shows that for patients treated with NAAD and 3D-CRT or IMRT, 9% (8 of 84) had positive biopsies at 2.5 years or more beyond completion of treatment, as compared to 35% (59 of 168) in those who received radiation therapy alone ($P < 0.001$).[45] Although androgen deprivation significantly affected the rate of tumor-positive biopsies for patients receiving 70.2 and 75.6 Gy, no benefit has thus far been observed in those treated with 81 Gy. Furthermore, androgen deprivation did not improve PSA relapse-free survival of patients in any of the risk groups.[45,65]

These findings suggest that while affecting the radiation response of prostate tumor cells, this short-term androgen deprivation regimen may not have influenced the development of metastatic disease. Indeed, in unfavorable-risk patients, the 5-year rates of distant metastases were 20%, regardless of whether NAAD therapy was given. The 5-year disease-free survival rates were 76% for unfavorable-risk patients receiving NAAD and 62% for patients treated with radiation alone ($P = 0.06$). The corresponding overall 5-year survival rates were 84% and 86%, respectively ($P = 0.58$). The 5-year PSA relapse-free survival for patients receiving androgen deprivation was 50%, as compared to 32% for those treated with radiation therapy alone ($P = 0.29$). Figure 14.2.5 shows that when the biochemical outcome was examined according to dose, patients who received 81 Gy with androgen deprivation had a 5-year PSA relapse-free survival of 68%, as compared to 62% for those treated with radiation therapy alone. In contrast, the

TABLE 14.2.4 Impact of Neoadjuvant Androgen Deprivation on Local Control Assessed by Biopsies in 252 Patients at ≥ 2.5 Years After 3D-CRT and IMRT

Dose (Gy)	Positive Biopsy Specimens/ Total Biopsies (%) No NAAD	NAAD	P value
64.8	13/24 (54)	ND	
70.2	21/52 (40)	2/16 (12)	0.03
75.6	22/68 (32)	5/51 (10)	0.001
81	3/24 (12)	1/17 (6)	0.8
Total	59/198 (35)	8/84 (9)	<0.001

3D-CRT, three-dimensional conformal radiation therapy; IMRT, intensity-modulated radiation therapy; NAAD, neoadjuvant androgen deprivation; ND, no data.

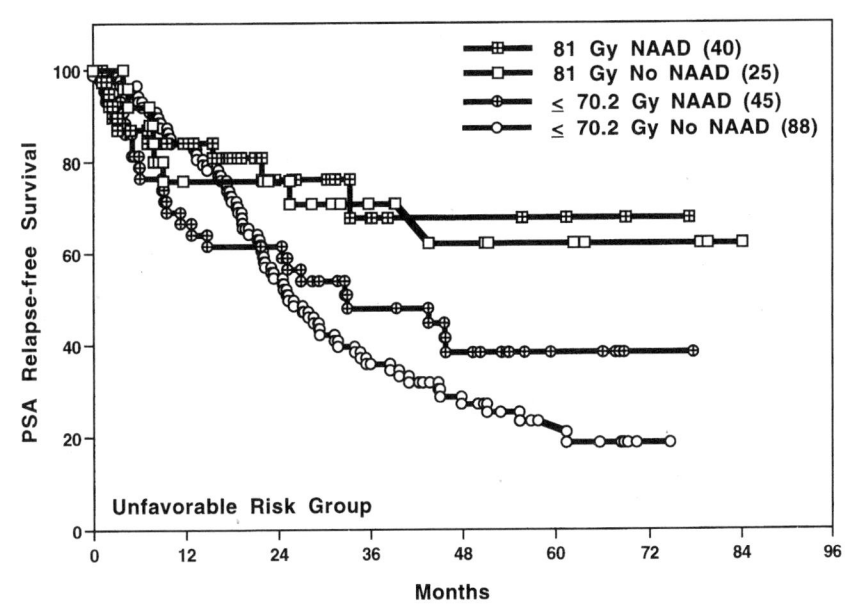

FIGURE 14.2.5 Actuarial prostate-specific antigen (PSA) relapse-free survival for unfavorable-risk patients treated with 81 Gy alone or with neoadjuvant androgen deprivation (NAAD), as compared with those treated with no more than 70 Gy alone or in combination with NAAD. Within each dose level, the differences were not statistically significant.

corresponding rates for those treated with not more than 70 Gy were 38% and 21%, respectively. These data indicate that higher doses significantly improve the PSA outcome over conventional dose levels ($P = 0.009$), regardless of whether NAAD is administered, and that neoadjuvant therapy may not provide an additional improvement at higher dose levels.

CONCLUSION

The last decade has witnessed dramatic advances in external-beam irradiation for the treatment of patients with prostate cancer. 3D-CRT and IMRT have greatly enhanced the precision of radiation therapy. The results of the MSKCC dose-escalation study confirm the validity of the 3D-CRT paradigm both in terms of reducing late radiation-induced morbidity and in improving local tumor control and disease-free survival. The 3D-CRT/IMRT approach thus represents a significant advancement in the use of radiation for the cure of prostate cancer. As the safety of an 86.4 Gy radiation dose has now been established, it remains to be demonstrated whether this dose would further improve the outcome, especially for patients with unfavorable risk factors.

Androgen deprivation combined with conventional-dose radiation therapy has also produced noteworthy improvements in outcome. Issues regarding patient selection for combined treatment, the sequencing of androgen deprivation and radiation therapy, and the optimal length of time that androgen deprivation therapy should be administered have yet to be resolved.[7,66] It is not clear whether patients with favorable and intermediate disease characteristics benefit from androgen deprivation.[67] The use of NAAD for patients with stages T1–T2, good-prognosis tumors is currently being tested in RTOG trial 94-08. Combined adjuvant chemotherapy and conventional radiation therapy also is being evaluated in high-risk prostate cancer patients.[68] For example, in RTOG trial 99-02 patients receive NAAD for 2 months before and during radiation therapy and are randomized to receive an additional 2 years of androgen deprivation or four cycles of chemotherapy in the form of estramustine, etoposide, and paclitaxel.

The ongoing dose-escalation studies soon will establish the maximal tolerable dose with 3D-CRT and IMRT. Whether androgen deprivation will obviate the need for dose escalation or whether androgen deprivation may be unnecessary when higher dose levels are administered remains unknown. Indeed, in some patients, both approaches combined may further improve the outcome. It should be emphasized, however, that androgen deprivation is associated with several side effects, such as hot flashes, loss of libido, impotence, decreased muscle tone, osteoporosis, and anemia, which can significantly impair the quality of life in treated patients. In RTOG trial 92-02, adjuvant androgen deprivation was associated, for reasons that are not clear, with a significant increase in late grade 3 and 4 bowel complications.[62] In view of the apparent favorable benefit-risk ratio of high-dose IMRT when administered as a single modality, the conduct of clinical trials to reconcile these important questions will be essential.

ACKNOWLEDGMENT

This work was supported in part by grant CA 59017 from the National Cancer Institute, Department of Health and Human Services, Bethesda, Maryland.

REFERENCES

1. Del Regato J. Radiotherapy in the conservative treatment of operable and locally inoperable carcinoma of the prostate. Radiology 1967;88:761–766.
2. Bagshaw MA, Kaplan HS, Sagerman RH. Linear accelerator supervoltage therapy: VII. Carcinoma of the prostate. Radiology 1965;85:121–129.
3. Ray GR, Cassady JR, Bagshaw MA. Definitive radiation therapy of carcinoma of the prostate. Radiology 1973;106:407–418.
4. Zelefsky MJ, Leibel SA, Gaudin PB et al. Dose escalation with three-dimensional conformal radiation therapy affects the outcome in prostate cancer. Int J Radiat Oncol Biol Phys 1998;41:491–500.

5. Leibel SA, Fuks Z, Zelefsky MJ, Ling CC. Prostate cancer: three-dimensional conformal and intensity modulated radiation therapy. PPO Updates 2000;14:1–9.
6. Horowitz EM, Hanks GE. External beam radiation for prostate cancer. CA Cancer J Clin 2000; 50:349–375.
7. Pollack A, Zagars GK. Androgen ablation in addition to radiation therapy for prostate cancer: Is there a true benefit? Semin Radiat Oncol 1998;8:95–106.
8. Bagshaw MA. Definitive megavoltage radiation therapy in carcinoma of the prostate. In: Fletcher GH, ed. Textbook of Radiotherapy (2nd ed). Philadelphia: Lea & Febiger, 1973:752–767.
9. Bagshaw MA. External radiation therapy of carcinoma of the prostate. Cancer 1980;45:1912–1921.
10. Lee D-J, Leibel S, Shiels R et al. The value of ultrasonic imaging and CT scanning in planning the radiotherapy of prostatic carcinoma. Cancer 1980;45:724–727.
11. Ten Haken RK, Perez-Tamayo C, Tesser RJ et al. Boost treatment of the prostate using shaped fixed beams. Int J Radiat Oncol Biol Phys 1989;16:193–200.
12. Epstein BE, Hanks GE. Radiation therapy techniques and dose selection in the treatment of prostate cancer. Semin Radiat Oncol 1993;3:179–186.
13. Hanks GE, Krall JM, Hanlon AL et al. Patterns of care and RTOG studies in prostate cancer: long-term survival, hazard rate observations, and possibilities of cure. Int J Radiat Oncol Biol Phys 1994;28:39–45.
14. Shipley WU, Thames HD, Sandler HM et al. Radiation therapy for clinically localized prostate cancer: a multi-institutional pooled analysis. JAMA 1999;28:1598–1604.
15. Zagars GK, Pollack A, Smith LG. Conventional external-beam radiation therapy alone or with androgen ablation for clinical stage III (T3, Nx/N0, M0) adenocarcinoma of the prostate. Int J Radiat Oncol Biol Phys 1999;44:809–819.
16. Crook JM, Bahadur YA, Bociek RG et al. Radiotherapy for localized prostate carcinoma. The correlation of pretreatment prostate specific antigen and nadir prostate specific antigen with outcome as assessed by systematic biopsy and serum prostate specific antigen. Cancer 1997;79: 328–336.
17. Laverdière J, Gomez JL, Cusan L et al. Beneficial effect of combination hormonal therapy administered prior to and following external beam radiation therapy in localized prostate cancer. Int J Radiat Oncol Biol Phys 1997;37:247–252.
18. Kestin LL, Martinez AA, Stromberg JS et al. Matched-pair analysis of conformal high-dose-rate brachytherapy boost versus external-beam radiation therapy alone for locally advanced prostate cancer. J Clin Oncol 2000;18:2869–2880.
19. Hanks GE, Martz KL, Diamond JJ. The effect of dose on local control of prostate cancer. Int J Radiat Oncol Biol Phys 1988;15:1299–1305.
20. Valicenti R, Lu J, Pilepich M, Asbell S, Grignon D. Survival advantage from higher-dose radiation therapy for clinically localized prostate cancer treated on the Radiation Therapy Oncology Group Trials. J Clin Oncol 2000;18:2740–2746.
21. Leibel SA, Hanks GE, Kramer S. Patterns of care outcomes studies: results of the national practice in adenocarcinoma of the prostate. Int J Radiat Oncol Biol Phys 1984;10:401–409.
22. Smit WGJM, Helle PA, Van Putte WLJ et al. Late radiation damage in prostate cancer patients treated by high dose external radiotherapy in relation to rectal dose. Int J Radiat Oncol Biol Phys 1990;18:23–29.
23. Fuks Z, Leibel SA, Kutcher GE et al. Three dimensional conformal treatment: a new frontier in radiation therapy. In: DeVita VT Jr, Hellman S, Rosenberg SA, eds. Important Advances in Oncology. Philadelphia: Lippincott, 1991:151–172.

24. Leibel, SA, Zelefsky MJ, Kutcher GJ et al. The biological basis and clinical application of three-dimensional conformal external beam radiation therapy in carcinoma of the prostate. Semin Oncol 1994;21:580–597.
25. Munro TR, Gilbert CW. The relation between tumour lethal doses and the radiosensitivity of tumour cells. Br J Radiol 1961;34:246–259.
26. Hendry JH, Moore JV. Is the steepness of dose-incidence curves for tumor control or complications due to variation before or as a result of irradiation? Br J Radiol 1984;57:1045–1046.
27. Thames HD, Schultheiss TE, Hendry JH et al. Can modest escalations of dose be detected as increased tumor control? Int J Radiat Oncol Biol Phys 1994;22:241–246.
28. Bentzen SM. Radiobiological considerations in the design of clinical trials. Radiother Oncol 1994; 32:1–11.
29. Jackson A, Skwarchuk MW, Zelefsky MJ et al. Late rectal bleeding after conformal radiotherapy of prostate cancer: II. Volume effects and dose volume histograms. Int J Radiat Oncol Biol Phys 2001;49:685–698.
30. Hanks GE, Hanlon AL, Pinover WH et al. Dose selection for prostate cancer based on dose comparison and dose response studies. Int J Radiat Oncol Biol Phys 2000;46:823–832.
31. Pollack A, Zagars GK, Smith LG et al. Preliminary results of a randomized radiotherapy dose-escalation study comparing 70 Gy to 78 Gy for prostate cancer. J Clin Oncol 2000;18:3904–3911.
32. Lyons JA, Kupelian PA, Mohan DA et al. Importance of high radiation doses (72 or greater) in the treatment of stage T1–T3 adenocarcinoma of the prostate. Urology 2000;55:85–90.
33. Perez CA, Michalski JM, Purdy JA et al. Three-dimensional conformal or standard irradiation in localized carcinoma of prostate: preliminary results of a nonrandomized comparison. Int J Radiat Oncol Biol Phys 2000;47:629–637.
34. Fiveash JB, Hanks G, Roach M III et al. 3D conformal radiation therapy (3DCRT) for high grade prostate cancer: A multi-institutional review. Int J Radiat Oncol Biol Phys 2000;47:335–342.
35. Mohan R, Barest G, Brewster LJ et al. A comprehensive three-dimensional radiation treatment planning system. Int J Radiat Oncol Biol Phys 1988;15:481–495.
36. Leibel SA, Zelefsky MJ, Kutcher GJ et al. Three-dimensional conformal radiation therapy in localized carcinoma of the prostate: interim report of a phase I dose-escalation study. J Urol 1994; 152:1792–1798.
37. Prescribing, Recording and Reporting Photon Beam Therapy. ICRU report no. 50. Bethesda, MD: International Commission on Radiation Units and Measurements, 1993.
38. LoSasso TJ, Chui C-S, Kutcher GJ et al. The use of multi-leaf collimator for conformal radiotherapy in carcinomas of the prostate and nasopharynx. Int J Radiat Oncol Biol Phys 1993;25:161–170.
39. Ling CC, Burman CM, Chui CS et al. Conformal radiation treatment of prostate cancer using inversely planned intensity-modulated photon beams produced with dynamic multileaf collimation. Int J Radiat Oncol Biol Phys 1996;35:721–730.
40. Burman CM, Chui CS, Kutcher GJ et al. Planning, delivery, and quality assurance of intensity-modulated radiotherapy using dynamic multileaf collimator: a strategy for large-scale implementation for the treatment of carcinoma of the prostate. Int J Radiat Oncol Biol Phys 1997;39:863–873.
41. Spirou SV, Chui C-S. A gradient inverse planning algorithm with dose-volume constraints. Med Phys 1998;25:321–333.
42. Spirou SV, Chui C-S. Generation of arbitrary fluence profiles by dynamic jaws or multileaf collimators. Med Phys 1994;21:1031–1041.
43. Leibel SA, Fuks Z, Zelefsky MJ et al. The treatment of localized prostate cancer with three-dimensional conformal and intensity modulated radiation therapy at the Memorial Sloan-Kettering Cancer Center. In: Purdy J, Grant W III, Palta J et al, eds. 3D Conformal Radiation Therapy and

Intensity Modulated Radiation Therapy in the Next Millennium. Madison, WI: Advanced Medical Publishing (in press).

44. Zelefsky MJ, Fuks Z, Happersett L et al. Clinical experience with intensity modulated radiation therapy (IMRT) in prostate cancer. Radiother Oncol 2000;55:241–249.

45. Zelefsky MJ, Fuks Z, Hunt M et al. High dose radiation delivered by intensity modulated radiotherapy is required for the cure of localized prostate cancer. J Urol (submitted).

46. Zelefsky MJ, Leibel SA, Burman CM et al. Neoadjuvant hormonal therapy improves the therapeutic ratio in patients with bulky prostatic cancer treated with three-dimensional conformal radiation therapy. Int J Radiat Oncol Biol Phys 1994;29:755–761.

47. Lawton CA, Won M, Pilepich MV et al. Long-term treatment sequelae following external beam irradiation for adenocarcinoma of the prostate: analysis of RTOG studies 7506 and 7706. Int J Radiat Oncol Biol Phys 1991;21:935–939.

48. American Society for Therapeutic Radiology and Oncology Consensus Panel. Consensus statement: guidelines for PSA following radiation therapy. Int J Radiat Oncol Biol Phys 1997;37:1035–1041.

49. Hanks GE, Hanlon AL, Pinover WH et al. Survival advantage for prostate cancer patients treated with high-dose three-dimensional conformal radiotherapy. Cancer J Sci Am 1999;5:152–158.

50. Pollack A, Zagars GK. External beam radiotherapy dose-response of prostate cancer. Int J Radiat Oncol Biol Phys 1997;39:1011–1018.

51. Goldenberg SL, Bruchovsky N. Androgen withdrawal therapy: new perspective in the treatment of prostate cancer. In: Raghavan D, Scher HI, Leibel SA, Lange PH. Principles and Practice of Genitourinary Oncology. Philadelphia: Lippincott-Raven, 1997:583–591.

52. Zeitman AL, Prince EA, Nakfoor BM, Park JJ. Androgen deprivation and radiation therapy: sequencing studies using the Shionogi in vivo tumor system. Int J Radiat Oncol Biol Phys 1997;38:1067–1070.

53. Zeitman AL, Nakfoor BM, Prince EA, Gerweck LE. The effect of androgen deprivation and radiation therapy on an androgen-sensitive murine tumor: an in vitro and in vivo study. Cancer J Sci Am 1997;3:31–36.

54. Pollack A, Ashoori F, Sikes C et al. The early supra-additive apoptotic response of R3327-G prostate tumors to androgen ablation and radiation is not sustained with multiple fractions. Int J Radiat Oncol Biol Phys 2000;46:153–158.

55. Forman JD, Kumar R, Haas G et al. Neoadjuvant hormonal downsizing of localized carcinoma of the prostate: effects on the volume of normal tissue irradiation. Cancer Invest 1995;13:8–15.

56. Yang FE, Chen GT, Ray P et al. The potential for normal tissue dose reduction with neoadjuvant hormonal therapy in conformal treatment planning for stage C prostate cancer. Int J Radiat Oncol Biol Phys 1995;33:1009–1017.

57. Pilepich MV, Krall JM, al-Sarraf M et al. Androgen deprivation with radiation therapy compared to radiation therapy alone for locally advanced prostatic carcinoma: a randomized comparative trial of the Radiation Therapy Oncology Group. Urology 1995;45:616–623.

58. Pilepich MV, Winter K, Roach M et al. Phase III Radiation Therapy Oncology Group (RTOG) Trial 86-10 of androgen deprivation before and during radiotherapy in locally advanced carcinoma of the prostate [abst]. Int J Radiat Oncol Biol Phys 1998;42[suppl 1]:177.

59. Pilepich MV, Winter K, Byhardt RW et al. Androgen ablation adjuvant to definitive radiotherapy in carcinoma of the prostate: year 2000 update of RTOG phase III studies 86-10 and 85-31 [abst]. Int J Radiat Oncol Biol Phys 2000;42[suppl]:169.

60. Pilepich MV, Caplan R, Byhardt RW et al. Phase III trial of androgen suppression using goserelin in unfavorable-prognosis carcinoma of the prostate treated with definitive radiotherapy: report of Radiation Therapy Oncology Group protocol 85-31. J Clin Oncol 1997;15:1013–1021.

61. Lawton C, Winter K, Murray K et al. Updated results of the phase III Radiation Therapy Oncology Group (RTOG) Trial 85-31 evaluating the potential benefit of androgen deprivation following standard radiation therapy for unfavorable prognosis carcinoma of the prostate. Int J Radiat Oncol Biol Phys 2001;49:937–946.
62. Hanks GE, Lu JD, Machtay M et al. RTOG Protocol 92-02: a phase III trial of the use of long term androgen suppression following neoadjuvant hormonal cytoreduction and radiotherapy in locally advanced carcinoma of the prostate [abst]. Int J Radiat Oncol Biol Phys 2000;48[suppl]: 112.
63. Bolla M, Gonzalez D, Warde P et al. Improved survival in patients with locally advanced prostate cancer treated with radiotherapy and goserelin. N Engl J Med 1997;337:295–300.
64. Bolla M. Adjuvant hormonal treatment with radiotherapy for locally advanced prostate cancer. Eur Urol 1999;35[suppl 1]:23–26.
65. Zelefsky MJ, Lyass O, Fuks Z et al. Predictors of improved outcome for patients with localized prostate cancer treated with neoadjuvant androgen ablation therapy and three-dimensional conformal radiation therapy. J Clin Oncol 1998;16:3380–3385.
66. Roach M III, Lu J, Pilepich MV et al. Predicting long-term survival, and the need for hormonal therapy: a meta-analysis of RTOG prostate cancer trials. Int J Radiat Oncol Biol Phys 2000;47: 617–627.
67. D'Amico AV, Schultz D, Loffredo M et al. Biochemical outcome following external beam radiation therapy with or without androgen suppression therapy for clinically localized prostate cancer. JAMA 2000;284:1280–1283.
68. Zelefsky MJ, Kelly WK, Scher HI et al. Results of a phase II study using estramustine phosphate and vinblastine in combination with high-dose three-dimensional conformal radiotherapy for patients with locally advanced prostate cancer. J Clin Oncol 2000;18:1936–1941.

Treatment of Prostate Cancer: Brachytherapy

Irving D. Kaplan

Edward J. Holupka

Soon after the discovery of x-rays and the purification of radium in the 1890s, ionizing irradiation was used to treat superficial tumors. Brachytherapy ("close therapy") is the implantation of radioactive sources into or near tumors. The use of brachytherapy for prostate cancer dates back to the early 1900s. In 1911, Pasteur and Degais described the placement of radium-containing needles into the prostatic urethra.[1] The pioneering American urologist H. H. Young[2] at Johns Hopkins Hospital performed transperineal implantation with radium needles, and his results were published in the 1920s. In the 1970s, Whitmore et al[3] at the Memorial Sloan-Kettering Cancer Center began using permanently implanted ^{125}I seeds. Their procedure was performed after surgical lymph node dissection. The exposed prostate receives the implant under direct visualization. Seeds are placed directly into the prostate via needles, without the use of a template or guide.[3] This "free-hand" technique often resulted in suboptimal seed distribution and, consequently, unreliable dosimetry.[4]

In the 1980s, a series of innovations led to a dramatic improvement in the accuracy of source placement and optimization of dosimetry. The use of transrectal ultrasonography permitted the transperineal placement of seeds under ultrasonographic guidance, obviating the need for an open procedure.[5] Development of the serum prostate-specific antigen (PSA) test and the standardization of pathology grading by means of the Gleason scoring system resulted in both early detection of prostate cancer and improved patient selection.

ISOTOPES

Presently, two isotopes are suitable for low-dose permanent seed implantation. Iodine 125 (^{125}I) and palladium 103 (^{103}Pd) emit very soft x-rays of 27 KeV and 21 KeV, respectively. This is in contrast to external-beam irradiation, which delivers 6- to 15-MeV photons, a difference of two orders of magnitude of penetrating energy. The low energy of the seed sources and the associated geometric falloff leads to a steep dose gradient surrounding the implant, which permits easy handling of the seed sources with minimal shielding requirements. The rectum and bladder receive a low dose owing to this rapid falloff. In addition, few irradiation safety issues accrue to the patient.

The main difference between isotopes is their half-lives, the half-life of ^{125}I being 59.6 days and the half-life of ^{103}Pd, 17 days. Implants deliver continuous low-dose irradiation. For example, the typical dose rate at the periphery of an ^{125}I implant is 6 cGy/hour, whereas that for ^{103}Pd is 22 cGy/hour. In contrast, external-beam irradiation delivers a dose rate of 180–200 cGy in 1 minute of treatment. The relationship between dose rate and total dose as they relate to cell killing is complex. Ling[6] argued that the use of ^{103}Pd, with its higher dose rate, is preferable to the use of ^{125}I for high-grade cancers, specifically those prostate tumors with potential doubling times [T(pot)s] of less than 10 days. Dickers et al[7] performed calculations using longer T(pot)s from published studies, ranging from 16 to 67 days. These calculations predicted a theoretic advantage for ^{103}Pd for tumors with a short T(pot); however, the therapeutic gain was minimal. No randomized clinical trials have been undertaken to compare ^{103}Pd to ^{125}I; however, several retrospective series have shown no difference in clinical outcomes with either isotope.[8,9]

Several techniques are employed for implantation of radioactive seeds. The patient is given anesthesia—general, spinal or, more recently, local.[10] Subsequently, the patient is placed in the high dorsal lithotomy position, which permits maximum perineal exposure and minimizes interference of the pubic arch in the trajectory of the transperineal needles. An ultrasonographic probe with both sagittal and transverse imaging capabilities is introduced into the rectum. The transrectal ultrasonographic probe is fixed to a stepper-stabilizer device, thereby permitting accurate imaging of the prostate at distinct and reproducible views. A template with predrilled holes is attached, and the template is calibrated so that the pattern of holes is superimposed accurately over the ultrasonographic images. Needles are inserted through the template into the prostate. A needle can be visualized either in transverse or parasagittal images. The seeds are deployed as the needle is withdrawn.

The method popularized by Blasko et al[11,12] in Seattle requires that the patient undergo a preimplantation planning session in which a transrectal ultrasonographic study is performed in the treatment position. These images are used to calculate a plan for needle and seed placement. Kaplan et al[13] described a method for intraoperative treatment planning that obviates the need for and discomfort of the preplanning transrectal ultrasonography. This intraoperative planning technique has been reported to result in significantly improved posttreatment dosimetry.[13,14] Several algorithms have been developed to optimize implantation preplanning using simulated annealing and a genetic algorithm.[15,16] Such algorithms ensure adequate dose to the gland while minimizing dose to the rectum and urethra.

By use of a nomogram, the method suggested by Stock et al[17-19] determines the number of seeds to be implanted on the basis of the gland size. Rather than by calculating a dosimetric preplan, the seeds are implanted on the basis of empiric implantation rules described by Patterson and Parker[20] in the 1930s. Recently, Koutrouvelis[21] reported using computed tomographic images to guide needles via a retropubic approach. D'Amico et al,[22] in Boston, have used an intraoperative split magnetic resonance imaging device for image-guided implantation.

In permanent brachytherapy, a postimplantation computed tomography scan is used to determine the final position of the implanted seeds in the prostate, for dosimetric calculations. The American Brachytherapy Society has published recommended standards to assess the quality of the implant.[23] The dose delivered to 80% of the prostate (D_{80}) should be at least 80% of the prescribed dose. In addition, the volume of the prostate receiving 100% and 140% of the prescribed dose (D_{100} and D_{140}) should be calculated.[23] Postimplantation dosimetry is complicated by the swelling that invariably occurs after implantation. Such swelling initially separates the seeds, decreasing the dose intensity of the implant. As the edema resolves, the radioactive sources move closer together. The calculated dose that is delivered to the urethra has been shown to increase as much as 30% depending on the time at which the postimplantation computed tomographic scan is obtained.[24-26]

In an effort to improve dosimetry, some investigators routinely place sources outside the gland to increase the dose delivered to the periphery of the prostate. However, the periprostatic tissues are richly vascularized, and seed embolization has been observed in 20% of patients when seeds were placed outside the gland.[27] More recently, seeds have been embedded into suture material to improve seed fixation.[28]

RESULTS OF IMPLANTATION

Defining end points for prostate cancer therapy is problematic. Prostate cancer has a long natural history. Moreover, this disease occurs in an older population in which competing morbidities and mortalities make analysis of outcomes difficult. The possible use of adjuvant androgen ablation further complicates interpretation of results.

The recurrence of disease after irradiation for prostate cancer generally is defined by PSA-based criteria, although this method of defining disease recurrence remains controversial. Some investigators use an absolute PSA level after treatment to characterize relapse,[29] whereas others use a rising PSA to define recurrent disease.[30] The American Society for Therapeutic Radiology and Oncology[30] defines failure for patients treated with external-beam irradiation on the basis of consecutively rising PSA levels, and this definition has been applied to implantation. An absolute threshold level of 0.5 ng/ml or 1.0 ng/ml after treatment has been used as an alternative end point.[31,32] The trauma caused by the implantation procedure and inflammation of the gland as the radiation is delivered causes an increase in the PSA levels within the first 3 months after implantation in approximately 25% of patients.[33] Recently, a temporary spike in the PSA level has been reported to occur up to 2–3 years after implantation in as many as 30% of patients.[34,35] These phenomena have led to difficulty in interpreting changes in the PSA and can cause significant anxiety for patients during follow-up. Consequently, long-term follow-up and monitoring of PSA levels to evaluate long-term trends are necessary to determine treatment efficacy.

PATIENT SELECTION CRITERIA

Retrospective correlation of the results of detailed pathologic analysis of prostatectomy specimens with pretreatment clinical criteria (PSA level, digital examination, and biopsy histology) has defined risk groups for extracapsular disease.[36,37] In the absence of randomized trials of surgery, external-beam irradiation, and brachytherapy for prostate cancer, these risk groups have been analyzed to compare outcomes in patients treated using different modalities.[38,39] Table 14.3.1 summarizes the clinical outcome of permanent implant monotherapy without hormonal adjuvant therapy. It can be seen that low-risk patients—those who present with a PSA level of less than 10 ng/ml, a Gleason score no higher than 6, and minimal or no palpable disease—experience prolonged freedom from relapse (based on a PSA-defined end point). In contrast, patients who are in the intermediate- or high-risk groups have worse PSA-defined outcomes.[39–46]

Many patients with more advanced disease are treated with combined therapy. External-beam irradiation is used to treat the prostate and any microscopic extracapsular disease in the periprostatic tissues. A brachytherapy implant is used as a dose boost prior to or after external-beam irradiation, typically to a dose of 41–45 Gy delivered to the prostate and periprostatic tissues, which compares to 67–72 Gy with external-beam monotherapy. The implant boost dose is 60%–70% of the prescribed dose provided by implantation monotherapy. Table 14.3.2 summarizes series that employed external-beam irradiation and an implant boost.[34,40,47–49] No randomized trials have been performed to assess external-beam irradiation with an implant boost as compared to permanent implant monotherapy. Brachytherapy alone and external-beam irradiation with an implant

TABLE 14.3.1 Clinical Outcome of Permanent-Implant Monotherapy Without Adjuvant Hormonal Therapy

Study	Isotope	Patient Characteristics	Freedom-from-Relapse Rate (%)	No. of Years
Kaye 1995[43]	125I	Tumor < 2 cm and Gleason ≤ 7	90	5
Zelefsky 1999[41]	125I	PSA < 10 and Gleason ≤ 6	82	5
Storey 1999[44]	125I	PSA < 10	76	5
Sharkey 1998[45]	103Pd	Stage T1 or T2	83	5
Beyer 1997[46]	125I	Stage T1	94	5
Beyer 1997[46]	125I	Stage T2c	34	5
Ragde 1998[40]	125I	PSA > 10	60	10
Storey 1999[44]	125I	PSA > 10	51	5
Brachman 2000[39]	125I, 103Pd	PSA 10.0–20.0	53	5

PSA, prostate-specific antigen.

TABLE 14.3.2 Clinical Outcome of External-Beam Irradiation with Implant Boost

Study	Isotope	Patient Characteristics	Freedom-from-Relapse Rate (%)	No. of Years
Potters 1999[9]	125I	PSA < 10 and Gleason ≤ 6; stage ≤ T2b	92	5
	103Pd			
Singh 2000[48]	103Pd	PSA > 10 or Gleason ≥ 7 (or both)	80	3
Sylvester 2000[49]	103Pd	PSA > 10, Gleason ≥ 7, and T2c–T3a (two of three)	58	5
	125I			
Critz 2000[34]	125I	PSA 4.1–10.0	93	5
Critz 2000[34]	125I	PSA 10.1–20.0	75	5
Ragde 1998[40]	125I	PSA > 10.0	75	10

PSA, prostate-specific antigen.

boost have been compared after patients were classified into risk groups on the basis of pretreatment prognostic factors (pretreatment PSA level, biopsy Gleason sum, and clinical stage). Blasko et al[47] and Grado et al[50] did not find either treatment superior in a multivariate analysis.

Brachytherapy as a treatment modality has been criticized because it is a relatively new procedure. As can be seen in Tables 14.3.1 and 14.3.2, long-term follow-up is not yet available from most series. However, the Seattle group reports results for up to 12 years. Using the strict American Society for Therapeutic Radiology and Oncology criteria for PSA failure (three consecutively rising PSA values), 75% of the failures occur within the first 5 years of treatment, 25% in posttreatment years 5–10, and 0% in posttreatment years 10–20.[40] These data suggest that the durability of brachytherapy response is similar to the response to external-beam irradiation.

TOXICITY

Three types of toxicities can be observed after brachytherapy. Urinary and rectal symptoms may be observed both acutely and chronically, and sexual functioning may be altered, significantly affecting a patient's quality of life. Rectal toxicity can be minor (e.g., a change in bowel habits) or more significant (e.g., rectal bleeding requiring medical or surgical intervention). Significant rectal toxicity after seed implantation is unusual. Merrick et al[51] recently reported that fewer than 20% of patients undergoing brachytherapy reported minor bowel dysfunction after treatment. Similarly, Gelblum and Potters[52] reported that rectal symptoms were minor and tended to peak at 8 months after therapy. In their series of 825 patients, no surgical interventions or blood transfusions were required for rectal toxicities. The rate of more significant complications, such as bleeding, has been reported to be 1%–4%.[41] The colostomy rate after implantation in a study of Medicare claims was 0.3%.[53]

The risk of rectal complications is correlated to the rectal dose and the length of rectum receiving a high dose.[54] Merrick et al[55] reported that rectal complications are more common if the rectal wall receives 85% or more of the prescribed dose. Because external-beam irradiation delivers more dose to the rectum, rectal toxicity is more likely if patients receive combined external-beam and implant therapy.

The rapid falloff of dose from the radioactive seeds leads to a steep dose gradient outside the prostatic implant. Because the urethra runs through the center of the prostate, the prostatic urethra cannot be protected as is the rectum and, therefore, receives a high dose of radiation. To reduce the dose to the center of the gland and the urethra, implantations are performed using a peripheral loading technique, whereby a greater density of sources is placed in the periphery of the gland. This mode of placement leads to a more homogeneous dose throughout the prostate and can eliminate "hot spots" on the urethra.

Urinary symptoms may be minor irritative symptoms (e.g., urgency and dysuria) or more significant effects (e.g., outlet obstruction requiring catheterization). The most commonly used self-reporting scoring tool by which to measure urinary symptoms is the International Prostate Symptom Score (I-PSS).[56] The risk of posttreatment urinary toxicity is related to both the dose delivered to the urethra and the patient's preimplantation urinary function.[54] Pretreatment urinary symptoms are a strong predictor of postimplantation symptoms. Terk et al[57] reported that patients with a preimplantation I-PSS exceeding 20 demonstrated a 29% risk of experiencing postimplantation urinary retention, as compared to only a 2% risk when the pretreatment I-PSS was less than 2. The change in the I-PSS peaked early after implantation.[58,59] Pre- and posttreatment use of an α-blocker reduces urinary symptoms.[59] Patient urinary function is optimized with the use of α-blockers or antibiotics prior to the performance of any assessment for a person's appropriateness for implantation.

Significant urinary toxicity is unusual yet still more common than is rectal complication after implantation. Individual series report prolonged catheterization and the need for subsequent transurethral resection of the prostate (TURP) in 1%–5% of patients after implantation.[52-61] Benoit et al[53] reported a 6.6% rate of incontinence after brachytherapy in a study of Medicare claims. TURP is generally avoided owing to a risk of incontinence after implantation. Initially, a history of prior TURP was reported to be a contraindication for implantation. Grimm et al[62] reported that significant urinary morbidity occurred in 24% of patients after brachytherapy if prior TURP had been performed. More recently, several authors report that implantation can be safely performed in patients who have undergone TURP[63,64] or who have a history of clinical or pathologically confirmed chronic prostatitis.[65]

Potency can be significantly affected by prostate cancer treatment, and this often is a critical factor in a patient's decision-making process as he chooses among treatment modalities. Sanchez-Ortiz et al[66] report on a retrospective study using a validated questionnaire. At 2 years after implantation, 25% of patients studied reported complete dysfunction and 26% erectile dysfunction.[66] Age at time of treatment is an important factor in posttreatment potency rate. The mean age at implantation in this series was 69. These results are slightly superior to those reported after conformal external-beam irradiation.[67]

Conformal external-beam irradiation is a process by which a relatively low dose of radiation is delivered to the periprostatic tissues, specifically the neurovascular bundle (NVB), with brachytherapy. These nerves are crucial for the maintenance of potency. Implantation has the theoretic advantages of delivering a lower radiation dose to the NVB and, subsequently, offering a higher rate of potency sparing as compared to external-beam irradiation. DiBase calculated dose to the NVBs. The dose ranged from 130% to 226% of the prescription dose for ^{103}Pd and from 140% to 225% for ^{125}I. An excessive dose to the NVB is an important factor in early postimplantation impotence.[68] In contrast, external-beam irradiation delivers significant amounts of radiation to the NVBs. The rate of potency after combined external-beam irradiation and implant boost is inferior to the potency sparing of brachytherapy alone.[69] Sildenafil citrate is effective in 80% for the treatment of erectile dysfunction after brachytherapy. This efficacy rate is similar to that reported after other treatments for prostate cancer.[42]

Prostate brachytherapy is an appropriate treatment modality for the properly selected patient. This modality delivers a very high dose of irradiation to the prostate while minimizing dose to the rectum. This leads to long-term, durable, PSA-defined control that is comparable to prostatectomy or external-beam irradiation. Toxicities are generally well tolerated but should not be understated.

REFERENCES

1. Pasteur O. Traitement du cancer de la prostate par le radium. Rev de Mal de la Nutrition 1911: 363–365.
2. Young HH. Technique of radium treatment of cancer of the prostate and seminal vesicles. Surg Gynecol Obstet 1922;34:93–98.
3. Whitmore WF, Hilaris B, Grabstald H. Retropubic implantation of iodine-125 in the treatment of prostatic cancer. J Urol 1972;108:918–920.
4. D'Amico AV, Coleman CN. Role of interstitial radiotherapy in the management of clinically organ-confined prostate cancer: the jury is still out. J Clin Oncol 1996;14:304–315.
5. Holm HH, Jaal N, Pedersen JF et al. Transperineal seed implantation in prostatic cancer guided by transrectal ultrasonography. J Urol 1983;130:283–286.
6. Ling CC. Permanent implants using Au-198, ^{103}Pd and ^{125}I: radiobiological considerations based on the linear quadratic model. Int J Radiat Oncol Biol Phys 1992;23:81–87.
7. Dickers AP, Lin CC, Leeper DB, Waterman FM. Isotope selection for permanent prostate implants? An evaluation of ^{103}Pd versus ^{125}I based on radiobiological effectiveness and dosimetry. Semin Urol Oncol 2000;18:152–159.
8. Cha CM, Potters L, Ashley R et al. Isotope selection for patients undergoing prostate brachytherapy. Int J Radiat Oncol Biol Phys 1999;45:391–395.
9. Potters L, Cha C, Oshinsk G et al. Risk profiles to predict PSA relapse-free survival for patients undergoing permanent prostate brachytherapy. Cancer J Sci Am 1999;5:301–305.
10. Smathers S, Wallner K, Simpson C, Roof J. Patient perception of local anesthesia for prostate brachytherapy. Semin Urol Oncol 2000;18:142–146.
11. Blasko JC, Ragde H, Grimm PD. Transperineal ultrasound-guided implantation of the prostate: morbidity and complications. Scand J Urol Nephrol Suppl 1991;137:113–118.
12. Blasko JC, Grimm PD, Ragde H. Brachytherapy and organ preservation in the management of carcinoma of the prostate. Semin Radiat Oncol 1993;3:240–249.
13. Kaplan ID, Holupka EJ, Meskell P et al. Intraoperative planning for radioactive seed implant therapy for prostate cancer. Urology 2000;56:492–495.
14. Gewanter RM, Wuu C, Laguna JL et al. Intraoperative preplanning for transperineal ultrasound-guided permanent prostate brachytherapy. Int J Radiat Oncol Biol Phys 2000;48:377–380.
15. Wilkinson DA, Lee EJ, Ciezka JP et al. Dosimetric comparison of pre-planned and/or planned prostate seed brachytherapy. Int J Radiat Oncol Biol Phys 2000;48:1241–1244.

16. Zelefsky MJ, Yamada Y, Cohen G et al. Postimplantation dosimetric analysis of permanent transperineal implantation improved dose distribution: improved dose distribution with an intraoperative computer-optimized conformal planning technique. Int J Radiat Oncol Biol Phys 2000;48: 601–608.

17. Stock RG, Stone NN, Wesson MF, DeWyngaert JK. A modified technique allowing interactive ultrasound-guided three-dimensional transperineal prostate implantation. Int J Radiat Oncol Biol Phys 1995;32:219–225.

18. Messing EM, Zhang JB, Rubens DJ et al. Intraoperative optimized inverse planning for prostate brachytherapy: early experience. Int J Radiat Oncol Biol Phys 2000;44:801–808.

19. Anderson LL. Spacing nomographs for interstitial implants of ^{125}I seeds. Med Phys 1976;3:48.

20. Patterson R, Parker HM, Spiers FW. A system for cylindrical distribution of radium. Br J Radiol 1936;9:487.

21. Koutrouvelis PG. Three-dimensional stereotactic posterior ischiorectal space computerized tomography guided brachytherapy of prostate cancer: a preliminary report. J Urol 1998;159:142–145.

22. D'Amico AV, Cormack R, Tenpany CM et al. Real-time magnetic resonance image-guided interstitial brachytherapy in the treatment of select patients with clinically localized prostate cancer. Int J Radiat Oncol Biol Phys 1998;42:507–515.

23. Nag S, Beyer D, Friedland J et al. American Brachytherapy Society (ABS) recommendations for transperineal permanent brachytherapy of prostate cancer. Int J Radiat Oncol Biol Phys 1999;44: 789–799.

24. Waterman FM, Yue N, Corn BW, Dicker AP. Edema associated with ^{125}I or [103]Pd prostate brachytherapy and its impact on post-implant dosimetry: an analysis based on serial CT acquisition. Int J Radiat Oncol Biol Phys 1998;41:1069–1077.

25. Prestidge BR. Radioisotopic implantation for carcinoma of the prostate: does it work better than it used to? Semin Radiat Oncol 1998;8:124–131.

26. Waterman FM, Dicker AP. The impact of postimplantation edema on the urethral dose in prostate brachytherapy. Int J Radiat Oncol Biol Phys 2000;47:661–664.

27. Dafoe-Lambie JC, Abel LJ, Blatt HJ Radioactive seed embolization to the lung following prostate brachytherapy. W V Med J 2000;96:357–360.

28. Merrick GS, Butler WM, Dorsey AT et al. Seed fixity in prostate/periprostatic regions following brachytherapy. Int J Radiat Oncol Biol Phys 2000;46:215–220.

29. Critz FA, Levinson AK, William WH et al. Simultaneous radiotherapy for prostate cancer: [125]I prostate implant followed by external-beam radiation. Cancer J Sci Am 1998;4:359–363.

30. American Society for Therapeutic Radiology and Oncology Consensus Panel. Consensus statement: guidelines for PSA following radiation therapy. Int J Radiat Oncol Biol Phys 1997;37:1035–1041.

31. Borghede G, Aldenborg F, Wurzinger E et al. Analysis of the local control in lymph-node staged localized prostate cancer treated by external beam radiotherapy, assessed by digital rectal examination, serum prostate-specific antigen and biopsy. Br J Urol 1997;80:247–255.

32. Critz FA, Levinson AK, Williams WH et al. Prostate specific antigen nadir achieved by men apparently cured of prostate cancer by radiotherapy. J Urol 1999;161:1199–1203.

33. Ianuzzi CM, Stock RG, Stone NN. PSA kinetics following ^{125}I radioactive seed implantation in the treatment of T_1–T_2 prostate cancer. Radiat Oncol Invest 1999;7:30–35.

34. Critz FA, Williams WH, Benton JB et al. Prostate specific antigen bounce after radioactive seed implantation followed by external beam radiation for prostate cancer. J Urol 2000;163:1085–1089.

35. Cavanaugh W, Blasko JC, Grimm PD, Sylvester JE. Transient elevation of serum prostate-specific antigen following (125)I/(103)Pd brachytherapy for localized prostate cancer. Semin Urol Oncol 2000;18:160–165.

36. Blute M, Bergtralh EJ, Partin AW et al. Validation of Partin tables for predicting pathological stage of clinically localized prostate cancer. J Urol 2000;164:1591–1595.
37. D'Amico AV, Whittington R, Malkowicz SB et al. Pretreatment nomogram for prostate-specific antigen recurrence after radical prostatectomy or external beam radiation therapy for localized prostate cancer. J Clin Oncol 1999;17:168–172.
38. D'Amico AV, Whittington R, Malkowicz SB et al. Biochemical outcome after radical prostatectomy, external beam or interstitial radiation therapy for clinically localized prostate cancer. JAMA 1998; 28:969–974.
39. Brachman DG, Thomas T, Hilbe J, Beyer DC. Failure-free survival following brachytherapy or external beam irradiation alone for T1-2 prostate tumors in 2222 patients: results from a single practice. Int J Radiat Oncol Biol Phys 2000;48:111–117.
40. Ragde H, Korb LJ, Elgamal AA et al. Modern prostate brachytherapy. Prostate specific antigen results in 219 patients with up to 12 years of observed follow-up. Cancer 2000;89:135–141.
41. Zelefsky MJ, Wallner KE, Ling CC et al. Comparison of the 5-year outcome and morbidity of three-dimensional conformal radiotherapy versus transperineal permanent iodine-125. J Clin Oncol 1999;17:517–522.
42. Merrick GS, Butler WM, Lief JH et al. Efficacy of sildenafil citrate in prostate brachytherapy patients with erectile dysfunction. Urology 1999;53:1112–1116.
43. Kaye KW, Olson DJ, Payne T. Detailed preliminary analysis of 125-iodine implantation for localized prostate cancer using percutaneous approach. J Urol 1995;153:1020–1025.
44. Storey MR, Landgren RC, Cottone JL et al. Transperineal ^{125}iodine implantation for treatment of clinically localized prostate cancer: 5-year tumor control and morbidity. Int J Radiat Oncol Biol Phys 1999;43:565–570.
45. Sharkey J, Chovnick SD, Behar RJ et al. Outpatient ultrasound-guided palladium-103 brachytherapy for localized adenocarcinoma of the prostate: a preliminary report of 434 patients. Urology 1999;51:796–803.
46. Beyer DC, Priestly JB Jr. Biochemical disease-free survival following ^{125}I prostate implantation. Int J Radiat Oncol Biol Phys 1997;37:559–563.
47. Blasko JC, Grimm PD, Sylvester JE, Cavanagh W. The role of external beam radiotherapy with ^{125}I/^{103}Pd brachytherapy for prostate carcinoma. Radiother Oncol 2000;57:273–278.
48. Singh A, Zelefsky MJ, Raben A et al. Combined 3-dimensional conformal radiotherapy and transperineal ^{103}Pd permanent implantation for patients with intermediate and unfavorable risk prostate cancer. Int J Cancer 2000;20:275–280.
49. Sylvester J, Blasko JC, Grimm PD et al. Short-course androgen ablation combined with external-beam radiation therapy and low-dose-rate permanent brachytherapy in early-stage prostate cancer: a matched subset analysis. Mol Urol 2000;4:155–160.
50. Grado GL, Larson TR, Balch C et al. Actuarial disease-free survival after prostate cancer brachytherapy using interactive techniques with biplane ultrasound and fluoroscopic guidance. Int J Radiat Oncol Biol Phys 1998;42:289–298.
51. Merrick GS, Butler WM, Dorsey AT et al. Rectal function following prostate brachytherapy. Int J Radiat Oncol Biol Phys 2000;48:667–674.
52. Gelblum DY, Potters L. Rectal complications associated with transperineal interstitial brachytherapy for prostate cancer. Int J Radiat Oncol Biol Phys 2000;48:119–124.
53. Benoit RM, Naslund MS, Cohen JK. Complications after prostate brachytherapy in the Medicare population. Urology 2000;55:91–96.
54. Wallner K, Roy J, Atarnison L. Dosimetry guidelines to minimize urethral and rectal morbidity following transperineal ^{125}I prostate brachytherapy. Int J Radiat Oncol Biol Phys 1995;32:465–471.

55. Merrick GS, Butler WM, Dorsey AT, Lief JH. Potential role of various dosimetric quality indicators in prostate brachytherapy. Int J Radiat Oncol Biol Phys 1999;44:717–724.
56. Van Venrooij GE, Boon TA, de Geir RP. International prostate symptom score and quality of life assessment versus urodynamic parameters in men with benign prostatic hyperplasia symptoms. J Urol 1995;153:1516–1519.
57. Terk MD, Stock RG, Stone NN. Identification of patients at increased risk for prolonged urinary retention following radioactive seed implantation of the prostate. J Urol 1998;160:1379–1382.
58. Lee WR, McQuellon, McCullough DL. A prospective analysis of patient-reported quality of life after prostate brachytherapy. Semin Urol Oncol 2000;18:147–151.
59. Merrick GS, Butler WM, Lief JH, Dorsey AT. Temporal resolution of urinary morbidity following prostate brachytherapy. Int J Radiat Oncol Biol Phys 2000;47:121–128.
60. Peschel RE, Chen Z, Roberts K, Nath R. Long-term complications with prostate implants: iodine-125 vs. palladium-103. Radiat Oncol Invest 1999;7:278–288.
61. Gelblum DY, Potters L, Ashley R et al. Urinary morbidity following ultrasound-guided transperineal prostate seed implantation. Int J Radiat Oncol Biol Phys 1999;45:59–67.
62. Grimm PD, Blasko JC, Ragde H et al. Does brachytherapy have a role in the treatment of prostate cancer? Hematol Oncol Clin North Am 1996;10:653–673.
63. Stone NN, Ratnow ER, Stock RG. Prior transurethral resection does not increase morbidity following real-time ultrasound prostate seed implantation. Tech Urol 2000;6:123–127.
64. Wallner K, Lee H, Wasserman S, Dattoli M. Low risk of urinary incontinence following prostate brachytherapy in patients with prior transurethral prostate resection. Int J Radiat Oncol Biol Phys 1997;37:565–569.
65. Aggarwal S, Wallner K, True LD et al. Prostate brachytherapy in patients with prior evidence of prostatitis. Int J Radiat Oncol Biol Phys 2000;45;867–869.
66. Sanchez-Ortiz RF, Broderick GA, Rovner ES et al. Erectile function and quality of life after interstitial radiation therapy for prostate cancer. Int J Impot Res 2000;12:S18–24.
67. Wilder RB, Chou RH, Ryu JK et al. Potency preservation after three-dimensional conformal radiotherapy for prostate cancer: preliminary results. Am J Clin Oncol 2000:23:330–333.
68. DiBiase SJ, Wallner K, Tralins K, Sutlief S. Brachytherapy radiation doses to neurovascular bundles. Int J Radiat Oncol Biol Phys 2000;46:1301–1307.
69. Zeitlin SI, Sherman J, Raboy A et al. High-dose combination radiotherapy for the treatment of localized prostate cancer. J Urol 1998;160:91–95.

Indexes

SUBJECT INDEX

A

Ablation
    androgen, adjuvant prostate cancer treatment, 335–346
    radiofrequency, for liver metastases, 258–277
Acute
    dysesthesias of the hand and feet, 139–167
    graft-versus-host disease, 228–257
    inflammation of lung tissue, 91–116
    leukemia
        B-cell, 191–203
        invariably fatal, 191–203
        lymphoblastic, 1–15, 117–138, 191–203, 228–257
        lymphocytic 117–138, 191–203, 228–257
        lymphoid, 228–257
        myeloblastic, 117–138, 228–257
        myelocytic, 228–257
        myeloid, 72–90, 228–257
    morbidity, prostate cancer, 278–312
    rectal and urinary symptoms following prostate cancer brachytherapy, 335–346
ADCC, *See* Antibody-dependent cell-mediated cytotoxicity, 204–227
Adjuvant(s) cancer therapy, *See also* Neoadjuvant
    colorectal, advanced, trials in combination with 5-fluorouracil/leucovorin, 139–167
    prostate
        androgen
            ablation, 335–346
            deprivation, 313–334
        hormonal therapy, 278–312, 335–346
    non-Hodgkin's Lymphoma, low grade, rituximab for, 191–203
Age factors determining prostatectomy, 278–312
Akt/protein kinase B apoptosis regulation, 72–90
Alkylating drugs, treatment for cervical cancer, 168–190
ALL, *See* Acute lymphocytic leukemia
Allogeneic hematopoietic stem cell transplantation, 228–257
Allografting, cancer treatment, 228–257
Allo-HSCT *See* Allogeneic hematopoietic stem cell transplantation, 228–257
AML *See* Acute myeloblastic leukemia
Amplification, rolling circle, 46–71
Amyloidosis, anecdotal activity, 117–138

Androgen deprivation therapy for prostate cancer, 278–312, 313–334, 335–346
Angiogenesis, tumor, 117–138
Anthracyclines/radiation combination for cervical cancer treatment, 168–190
Antibody(ies)
    -dependent cell mediated cytotoxicity, 204–227
    therapy for B-cell non-Hodgkin's lymphoma, 204–227
Antigen(s) (Ag)
    CD20, 204–227
    cellular, recognition for cancer diagnosis, 16–28
    -nonspecific innate/specific adaptive immunities, 29–45
    onconeural, 29–45
    prostate specific, detection by immunohistochemistry/immunofluorescence, 46–71
    target for graft-versus-tumor response, 228–257
Anti-tumor
    activity against cervical cancer, 168–190
    immunity, 29–45
    remission response, chimerism conversion timing and, 228–257
Apoptosis
    B-cell non-Hodgkin's lymphoma, 204–227
    cancer cell therapy response, 72–90
    cervical carcinoma, 168–190
    chronic myelogenous leukemia, 191–203
    direct anti-tumor effect of thalidomide, 117–138
    DNA repair and, 91–116
    induction, cervical carcinoma, 228–257
    tumor cell, 228–257
Autosomal gene for lung cancer predisposition, 91–116

B

Basal cell carcinomas, 91–116
Basic fibroblast growth factor, 117–138
B-cell lymphoma
    diffuse large, 46–71
    non-Hodgkin's, 204–227
Bcr-Abl kinase activity, 191–203
bFGF, *See* Basic fibroblast growth factor, 117–138
Biomarkers, RCA/HRCA-based, utility in specific cancers, 46–71
Biopsy(ies)
    neoadjuvant androgen deprivation impact on, in prostate cancer treatment, 313–334
    specimens, Gleason score identification, 278–312
    Gleason score identification in, 278–312
Bipartite probes, point mutations in genomic DNA, 46–71
Bleomycin use in cervical cancer use, 168–190
Brachytherapy for prostate cancer, 278–312, 335–346
Breast carcinoma, global expression of tumor analysis for, 16–28

C

Cancer *See also Specific Cancers*
    detection technology in the field of DNA amplification, 46–71

gene expression profiling, 1–15
microheterogeneity in tissue, 46–71
molecular diagnostics, 16–28
mutations analysis, 46–71
therapy
   B-cell non-Hodgkin's lymphoma, 204–227
   cervical, 168–190
   cisplatin, 168–190
   colorectal, 139–167, 191–203
   disruption, 72–90
   immuno-adoptive cellular, 228–257
   kinase Bcr-Abl for chronic myelogenous leukemia, 191–203
   mitochondria targeting for, 72–90
   ovarian, 72–90
   prostate
      adjuvant hormonal, 278–312, 335–346
      androgen deprivation, 278–312, 313–334, 335–346
      mono-, permanent seed implantation, 335–346
      radical prostatectomy to control, 278–312
   thalidomide, multiple myeloma, 117–138
   Th1/Th2 and regulatory T cells, 29–45
vaccine development, 29–45
Carboplatin for epithelial malignancies, 139–167
Carcinogenesis
   possible gene involvement, 72–90
   tobacco, genetic susceptibility, 91–116
Carcinoma
   basal cell, 91–116
   breast, global expression of tumor analysis for, 16–28
   cervical, apoptosis induction, 168–190
   hepatocellular control rate following radiofrequency ablation, 258–277
   renal cell, thalidomide therapy for, 117–138
   squamous cell, metastatic, head/neck, 117–138
CD20 antigen, 204–227
CDC, See Complement-dependent cytotoxicity, 204–227
cDNA, See complementary deoxyribonucleic acid) microarrays, 1–15
Cell(s)
   basal, carcinoma, 91–116
   circulating tumor, analysis, 46–71
   cycle arrest regulation, gene-induced, 72–90
   dendritic, and cancer immunization, 29–45
   effector, and their cytokines, 228–257
   metastatic squamous, head/neck, 117–138
   renal, carcinoma, 117–138
   stem, allogeneic hematopoietic transplantation, 228–257
   tumor
      apoptosis, 228–257
      growth decrease in B-cell non-Hodgkin's lymphoma, 204–227
Cellular
   antigen recognition for cancer diagnosis, 16–28
   immunotherapy, adoptive, 228–257

Cerebellar degeneration, paraneoplastic, 29–45
Cervical
   cancer
      chemoradiation, 168–190
      cisplatin chemotherapy, 168–190
      taxanes, 168–190
   carcinoma, apoptosis induction, 168–190
CGH, *See* Comparative genomic hybridization, 46–71
Chemoradiation for cervical cancer, 168–190
Chemotherapy
   cisplatin-based
      for cervical cancer, post- and preoperative, 168–190
      + 5-fluorouracil, cervical cancer treatment, 168–190
      for ovarian cancer, 72–90
   combination for cancer therapy, 117–138
   response/resistance, 72–90
   /rituximab combined therapy for B-cell non-Hodgkin's lymphoma, 204–227
   /therapy, adjuvant, for colorectal cancer, 139–167
Chimeric mouse/human monoclonal antibody, 204–227
Chimerism conversion timing and anti-tumor complete remission response, 228–257
Chronic
   graft-versus-host disease, 228–257
   leukemia
      lymphatic, 228–257
      myelogenous, 191–203
   rectal and urinary symptoms following prostate cancer brachytherapy, 335–346
Cisplatin
   -based chemotherapy
      cervical cancer, 168–190
      ovarian cancer, 72–90
   /carboplatin, testes cancer treatment, 139–167
   with/without thalidomide in refractory, multiple myeloma and post-transplant relapse, 117–138
Cisplatin + 5-fluorouracil cervical cancer chemotherapy, 168–190
CLL, *See* Chronic lymphatic lymphoma, 228–257
CML, *See* Chronic myelogenous lymphoma, 228–257
Colorectal cancer
   liver metastases from, 258–277
   oxaliplatin treatment, 139–167
Comorbidity factors determining prostatectomy, 278–312
Comparative genomic hybridization, 46–71
Complement-dependent cytotoxicity, 204–227
Complementary deoxyribonucleic acid microarrays, 1–15
Computed tomography scan following RFA, 258–277
CT, *See* Computed tomography, 258–277
Cyclophosphamide response decrease in Myc-induced lymphoma in mouse model, 72–90
Cystoprostatectomy series for incidentally detected cancers, 278–312
Cytokine(s)
   effector cells, 228–257
   /rituximab combined therapy for B-cell non-Hodgkin's lymphoma, 204–227
Cytometry, flow, 46–71

Cytotoxic/non-cytotoxic drugs for cervical cancer treatment, 168–190
Cytotoxicity
   complement-dependent, 204–277
   radiation/oxygenation relationship, 168–190

D

Dendritic cell(s)
   and cancer immunization, 29–45
   subsets, 29–45
Deoxyribonucleic acid
   adducts, platinum, 139–167
   amplification, 46–71
   damage
      induces cell cycle arrest or apoptosis regulation, 72–90
         repair, 91–116
   fragmentation in B-cell non-Hodgkin's lymphoma, 204–227
   microarrays, gene analysis using, 1–15
   probes, 16–28, 46–71
   repair systems, 91–116
   synthesis inhibition, 313–334
Desorption ionization, matrix-assisted, 1–15, 16–28
Dexamethasone
   (plus fludarabine and mitotoxantrone) for indolent lymphoma, 204–227
   (plus thalidomide) for multiple myeloma therapy, 117–138
DHQ, *See* Digital hybridization quantitation, 46–71
Diagnostics, molecular, of cancer, 16–28
Diet
   /lung cancer relationship, 91–116
   /metabolic enzyme activity induction relationship, 91–116
Diffuse large B-cell lymphoma, 46–71
Difluorodeoxycytidine, antitumor activity against cervical cancer, 168–190
Digital hybridization quantitation, 46–71
DLBCL, *See* Diffuse large B-cell lymphoma, 46–71
DLI, *See* Donor leukocyte infusion, 228–257
DNA, *See* deoxyribonucleic acid
Donor leukocyte infusion, 228–257

E

Emesis resultant from platinums use against cervical cancer, 168–190
Endothelial growth factor, 1–15
Enzymes, metabolic, dietary factors inducing activity, 91–116
Epidemiology of tobacco carcinogenesis, 91–116
Epithelial malignancies, 139–167
Erectile function, post-radical prostatectomy, 278–312
European Organization for Research and Treatment of Cancer (EORTC), 313–334
External beam irradiation
   /brachytherapy response similarities, 335–346
   therapy for prostate cancer, 278–312, 313–334

F

FADD, *See* Fas-associated death domain protein, 72–90
Fas-associated death domain protein, 72–90
FDA, *See* Food and Drug Administration
FIGO staging of carcinoma of the cervix uteri, 168–190
FISH, *See* Fluorescent in situ hybridization, 16–28, 46–71
5-fluorouracil
    cervical cancer control use, 168–190
    /leucovorin combination for advanced colon cancer, 139–167
    /methotrexate, tumor resistance to, 72–90
5FU, *See* 5-fluorouracil
Flow cytometry, RCA, potential application, 46–71
Fludarabine, mitotoxantrone and dexamethasone for indolent lymphoma, 204–227
Fluorescent in situ hybridization, 16–28, 46–71
Fluoropyramidines use against cervical cancer, 168–190
FND, *See* Fludarabine, mitotoxantrone, dexamethasone
Follicular lymphoma, chromosomal translocation, 72–90
Food and Drug Administration
    approval
        for cisplatin and carboplatin, 139–167
        for rituximab, B-cell non-Hodgkin's lymphoma therapy, 204–227
    applications, new drug, for thalidomide use in advanced malignancies, 117–138

G

Gastrointestinal malignancies, 258–277
GBM, *See* Glioblastoma multiforme, 117–138
Gemcitabine (difluorodeoxycytidine), antitumor activity against cervical cancer, 168–190
Gender differences in lung cancer susceptibility, 91–116
Gene(s)
    analysis using microarrays, 1–15
    autosomal, for lung cancer predisposition, 91–116
    cell cycle arrest or apoptosis regulation, 72–90
    DNA repair, 91–116
    expression, cancer profiling, 1–15
    alterations in tumor DNA, 16–28
    predisposition of lung cancer, 91–116
    susceptibility to tobacco carcinogenesis, 91–116
Generator, radiofrequency, 258–277
Genome DNA, point mutations in, 46–71
Genomic hybridization, comparative, 46–71
Gleason score identification in biopsy specimens, 278–312
Glioblastoma multiforme, thalidomide therapy for, 117–138
Glutathione S-transferases, 91–116
GOG, *See* Gynecologic Oncology Group, 168–190
Graft-versus-host disease, 228–257
Graft-versus-tumor reactions, 228–257
GVHD, *See* Graft-versus-host disease, 228–257
GVT, *See* Graft-versus-tumor, 228–257

Gynecologic Oncology Group, 168–190

H

Head/neck squamous cell carcinoma, metastatic, 117–138
Health factors determining prostatectomy, 278–312
Hematologic
  miscellaneous malignancies, thalidomide therapy for, 117–138
  tumors, PCR use in minimal residual disease, 46–71
Hematopoietic stem cell transplantation, allogeneic, 228–257
Hemoglobin level, predictor of pelvic recurrence from cervical cancer, 168–190
Hepatic resection, 258–277
Hepatocellular carcinoma
  control rate following radiofrequency ablation, 258–277
  thalidomide therapy for, 117–138
Heterozygosity loss, 16–28, 46–71
Hormonal therapy/adjuvant therapy for prostate cancer, 278–312, 313–334
HRCA, See Hyperbranched rolling circle amplification, 46–71
HSCT, See Hematopoietic stem cell transplantation, 228–257
Hybridization, fluorescent, in situ, 46–71
Hyperbranched rolling circle amplification, 46–71
Hysterectomy, radical, 168–190

I

IAP, See Inhibitor of apoptosis protein, 72–90
Ifosfamide and alkylating drugs in combination against cervical cancer, 168–190
IGF, See Insulin-like growth factor, 72–90
Immune mediated anti-tumor effects, 204–227
Immunization strategies using dendritic cells, 29–45
Immunofluorescence analysis for specific antigen detection, 46–71
Immunohistochemistry analysis for specific antigen analysis, 46–71
Immunotherapy, adoptive cellular, 228–257
Implantation, permanent seed, for prostate cancer, 335–346
IMRT, See Intensity modulated radiation therapy, 313–334
Incontinence, urinary, post-radical prostatectomy, 278–312
Inheritance, Mendelian codominant, of autosomal gene for lung cancer
      predisposition, 91–116
Inhibitor of apoptosis protein, 72–90
Insulin-like growth factor, 72–90
Intensity modulated radiation therapy, 313–334
Interferon plus dexamethasone for stage IV indolent lymphoma, 191–203
Interferon-γ, anti-tumor immunity and, 29–45
Interleukin-2 producing Th1 cells, anti-tumor immunity and, 29–45
Interleukin-4 producing Th2 cells, nonproductive responses to anti-tumor
      immunity and, 29–45
Interleukin-10 producing Th2 cells, nonproductive responses to anti-tumor
      immunity and, 29–45
Irradiation therapy, external beam, for prostate cancer, 278–312, 313–334
Isotopes suitable for low dose permanent seed implantation, 335–346

K

Kinase Bcr-Abl therapy for chronic myelogenous leukemia, 191–203

L

Laser(s)
  capture microdissection, 1–15, 16–28
  ultraviolet, 1–15
LCM, *See* Laser capture microdissection, 1–15, 16–28
Leucovorin plus oxaliplatin for advanced colorectal cancer, 139–167
Leucovorin/5-fluorouracil, adjuvant cancer therapy, 139–167
Leukemia
  acute
    lymphocytic, 191–203, 228–257
    lymphoid, 228–257
    myeloid, 228–257
    myeloblastic, thalidomide therapy for, 117–138
  chronic
    myelogenous, 191–203
  global expression of tumor analysis for, 16–28
Leukemic recurrence after allo-HSCT, 228–257
Leukocyte infusion, donor, 228–257
Liver metastases, local recurrence after RFA, 258–277
LOH, *See* Loss of Heterozygosity, 16–28, 46–71
Loss of Heterozygosity, 16–28, 46–71
Lung cancer/diet relationship, 91–116
Lymphocytic leukemia
  acute, 117–138, 191–203, 228–257
  chronic, 117–138, 228–257
Lymphoid leukemia, acute, 228–257
Lymphoma
  B-cell non-Hodgkin's, 204–227
  diffuse large B-cell, 46–71
  follicular, chromosomal translocation, 72–90
  global expression of tumor analysis for, 16–28
  indolent, 204–227
  Myc-induced, 72–90
Lysis, complement mediated, 204–227

M

Macroglobulinemia, Waldenström's, 117–138
Magnetic resonance imaging following radiofrequency ablation, 258–277
MALDI, *See* Matrix-assisted laser desorption ionization, 1–15
Malignancies
  CD20 positive, 204–227
  epithelial, cisplatin and carboplatin use for, 139–167
  hematologic, thalidomide therapy for, 117–138
  solid, 228–257

Subject Index

Markers
  molecular, used in cancer diagnosis, 16–28
  RCA/HRCA-based, utility in specific cancers, 46–71
Matrix-assisted laser desorption ionization, 1–15
MDS, myelodysplasia, thalidomide therapy, 117–138
Mendelian codominant inheritance of autosomal gene for lung cancer predisposition, 91–116
Metabolic
  enzme activity/diet factors induction relationship, 91–116
  polymorphisms, 91–116
Metastases, liver, radiofrequency ablation for, 258–277
Metastatic squamous cell carcinoma, head/neck, 117–138
Methotrexate/5 fluorouracil tumor resistance, 72–90
Microarray-based technologies in cancer detection, 46–71
Microarrays
  DNA, 1–15
  tissue, 16–28
Microdissected tissue samples, 1–15
Microdissection
  human tissue for molecular analysis, 16–28
  laser capture, 1–15
Microheterogeneity, cancer, in tissue, 46–71
Minimal residual disease, 46–71
Mismatch repair, DNA capacity for, 91–116
Mitochondria targeting for therapy, 72–90
Mitomycin C, treatment for cervical cancer, 168–190
Mitotoxantrone for indolent lymphoma (with fludarabine and dexamethasone), 204–227
MM, *See* Multiple myeloma
MMR, *See* Mismatch repair, 91–116
Molecular
  diagnostics of cancer, 16–28
  markers used in cancer diagnosis, 16–28
Monoclonal antibodies, 204–227
Monotherapy, permanent seed implant for prostate cancer, 335–346
Morbidity, acute, prostate cancer, 228–257
MRD, *See* Minimal residual disease, 46–71
MRI, *See* Magnetic resonance imaging, 158–177
Multiple
  drug resistance (MDR), 46–71
  myeloma (MM)
    curative potential of allo-HCTSCT, 12
    dexamethasone/thalidomide therapy for refractory, advanced, post-transplant, 117–138
Mutagen sensitivity assay, 91–116
Mutations, point, detection in genomic DNA, 46–71
Myc-induced lymphoma in mouse model, 72–90
Myeloblastic leukemia, acute, thalidomide therapy, 117–138
Myelodysplasia, thalidomide therapy, 117–138
Myelofibrosis, idiopathic, anecdotal activity, 117–138
Myelogenous leukemia, chronic, 191–203
Myeloid leukemia, acute, 228–257

Myeloma, multiple
  curative potential of allo-HSCT, 228–257
  thalidomide therapy for, 117–138

N

National Cancer Institute cervical cancer standard treatments, 168–190
Neck/head metastatic squamous cell carcinoma, 117–138
Neoadjuvant chemotherapy, See also Adjuvant therapy
  for cervical cancer, 168–190
  for prostate cancer, 313–334
NER, See Nucleotide excision repair, 91–116
Neurologic disorders, paraneoplastic, 29–45
NHL, See Non-Hodgkin's lymphoma, B-cell, 204–227
Non-Hodgkin's lymphoma, B-cell, 204–227
Non-myeloablative preparative regimen for graft–versus–donor response, 228–257
Nucleotide
  excision repair (NER), 91–116
  polymorphisms, single, analysis of, 46–71
Nutrition, 91–116

O

Oligonucleotide arrays, 1–15
Onconeural antigens, 29–45
Ovarian cancer, cisplatin-based chemotherapy, 72–90
Oxaliplatin treatment for colorectal cancer, 139–167
Oxygenation/radiation cytotoxicity relationship, 168–190

P

Paclitaxel for advanced cervical cancer, 168–190
Padlock probes, cancer mutations analysis with, 46–71
Paraneoplastic neurologic disorders, 29–45
PCR, See Polymerase chain reaction
PDGF, See Platelet-derived growth factor, 72–90
Pelvic recurrence of cervical cancer, hemoglobin level predictor, 168–190
PET, See Positron emission tomography, 335–346
p53 mutation in mouse model of Myc-induced lymphoma, 72–90
p14ARF mutation in mouse model of Myc-induced lymphoma, 72–90
Pharmacokinetics
  of oxaliplatin, 139–167
  /trials of ST1571 for chronic myelogenous leukemia, 191–203
Plasmacytoid dendritic cells, 29–45
Platelet-derived growth factor, 72–90
Platinums
  cervical cancer use, 168–190
  DNA adducts, 139–167
Point mutations detection in genomic DNA, 46–71

Polymerase chain reaction
  Bcl-2 translocation by, 204–227
  cDNA probe amplification, 1–15
  diagnosis
    minimal residual disease in hematologic tumors, 46–71
    molecular impact on, 16–28
Polymorphisms
  in DNA repair genes, 91–116
  single nucleotide, analysis, 46–71
Positron emission tomography following RFA, 258–277
Probes
  DNA
    amplification, 46–71
    bipartite, point mutations in genomic, 46–71
    in situ hybridization with, 16–28
    padlock, cancer mutations analysis with, 46–71
Prognostic factors, pathologic, in radical prostatectomy, 278–312
Prostate
  -associated membrane antigen, 46–71
  cancer therapy
    androgen deprivation 313–334
    brachytherapy, 335–346
    external beam, 313–334
  -specific antigen relapse-free survival, 313–334
  surgery, 278–312
Prostatectomy, radical, 278–312
Protein(s)
  altered, detection in cancer, 46–71
  analysis with immuno-rolling circle amplification application, 46–71
  Fas-associated death domain, 72–90
  human tissue, 1–15
  inhibitor of apoptosis, 72–90
  kinase B, 72–90
  myeloma, response, 117–138
  specific cellular differentiation, 16–28
  tumor necrosis factor receptor-associated death domain, 72–90
Proteomic analysis of human tissue, 16–28
Prostate-specific antigen
  detection with immuno-rolling circle amplification, 46–71
  -free survival, 278–312
PSA, See Prostate-specific antigen
PSMA, See Prostate-associated membrane antigen, 46–71
PTEN/Akt disruption in tumors, 72–90

R

Radiation
  cytotoxicity/oxygenation relationship, 168–190
  external beam, 335–346
  conventional, limitations, 313–334
  intensity modulated, for prostate cancer, 313–334
  3-D conformal, 313–334

Radiation Therapy Oncology Group, 313–334
Radical prostatectomy, 278–312
Radioactive seed implants for prostate cancer, 278–312
Radiofrequency ablation for liver metastases, 258–277
Radiosensitizers for cervical cancer treatment, 168–190
Radiotherapy *See also* Brachytherapy
   external beam for prostate cancer, 278–312, 313–334, 335–346
RCA *See* Rolling circle amplification, 46–71
Recurrence of liver metastases post-RFA, 258–277
Refractory myeloma, thalidomide therapy for, 117–138
Relapse-free survival, prostate cancer, 313–334
RFA *See* Radiofrequency ablation, 258–277
Renal
   cell carcinoma, thalidomide therapy for, 117–138
   toxicity resultant from platinum's use against cervical cancer, 168–190
Reverse transcription-polymerase chain reaction for altered RNA molecules' detection, 46–71
RNA
   molecules, altered detection with RT-PCR, 46–71
   probes, 16–28
   tumor cell–derived, 29–45
Ribonucleic acid, *See* RNA
Rituximab antibody therapy for B-cell non-Hodgkin's lymphoma, 204–227
Rolling circle amplification, 46–71
RT-PCR, *See* Reverse transcription-polymerase chain reaction

S

Seed implantation for prostate cancer, 278–312, 335–346
SELDI, *See* Surface-enhanced laser desorption, 1–15
Serum prostate-specific antigen, 278–312
Solid malignancies, thalidomide therapy for, 117–138, 228–257
Somatic mutation analysis on DNA, 46–71
Spectrometry, mass, 1–15
Squamous cell carcinoma, metastatic head/neck, 117–138
Stem cell, allogeneic hematopoietic transplantation, 228–257
ST1571 for chronic myelogenous leukemia, pharmacokinetics and trials, 191–203
Surface-enhanced laser desorption ionization mass spectrometry, 1–15
Surgery, prostate cancer, 278–312

T

T cells, regulatory, Th1/Th2 and, 29–45
Taxanes in advanced cervical cancer, 168–190
Testes cancer treatment, 139–167
Thalidomide for multiple myeloma therapy, 117–138
Therapy
   apoptotic mechanism in B-cell non-Hodgkin's lymphoma, 204–227
   cancer, disruption of, 72–90
   cervical cancer, 168–190

cisplatin, 168–190
colorectal cancer, 139–167, 191–203
immuno-adoptive cellular, 228–257
kinase Bcr-Abl for chronic myelogenous leukemia, 191–203
mitochondria targeting for, 72–90
ovarian cancer, 72–90
prostate cancer
    androgen deprivation, 278–312, 313–334, 335–346
    hormonal, 258–277-1, 335–346
    mono-, permanent seed implantation, 335–346
thalidomide
    direct anti-tumor effect, 117–138
    multiple myeloma, 117–138
Th1/Th2 and regulatory T cells, 29–45
3D-CRT, See Three-dimensional conformal radiation, 313–334
Three-dimensional conformal radiation therapy (3D-CRT), 313–334
Tissue(s)
    cancer, microheterogeneity in, 46–71
    human
        microarrays (TMA), 16–28
        proteins in, 1–15
        proteomic analysis, 16–28
        samples for molecular analysis, 1–15, 16–28
TNFR, See Tumor necrosis factor receptor associated death domain, 72–90
Tobacco carcinogenesis, genetic susceptibility to, 91–116
Tomography
    computed, 258–277
    positron emission, 258–277
Topoisomerase 1 inhibitors, 168–190
Toxicity
    after brachytherapy for prostate cancer, 335–346
    of 3D–conformal radiation therapy and IMRT, 313–334
TRADD, See Tumor necrosis factor receptor-associated death domain, 72–90
TRAIL, See Tumor necrosis factor–related apoptosis inducing ligand, 72–90
Transplantation, allogeneic hematopoietic stem cell, 228–257
Trials
    oxaliplatin for advanced colorectal cancer, See also Colorectal cancer, 139–167
    rituximab, selected single agent NHL, 204–227
Tumor(s)
    analysis, global expression, for lymphoma, 16–28
    angiogenesis, 117–138
    associated antigens, 29–45
    cell
        apoptosis, 228–257
        circulating, analysis, 46–71
        -derived RNA, 29–45
        growth decrease in B-cell NHL, 204–227
    classification system enhancement, 1–15
    decreased response to cyclophosphamide, 72–90
    DNA, genetic alterations, 16–28
    hematologic, PCR use in MRD in hematologic tumors, 46–71

immunity, 29–45
necrosis factor
  receptor associated death domain, 72–90
  -related apoptosis inducing ligand, 72–90
PCR use in MRD, 46–71
proliferation rate, 46–71
PTEN/Akt disruption in, 72–90
resistance to 5-fluorouracil/methotrexate, 72–90
solid, thalidomide therapy for, 117–138
vaccines development, 29–45
Tumor necrosis factor-related apoptosis inducing ligand, 72–90
Tumor necrosis factor receptor associated death domain, 72–90
Tyrosine kinase inhibitors for chronic myelogenous leukemia, 191–203

U

Ultraviolet lasers, 1–15
Urinary incontinence, post-radical prostatectomy, 278–312

V

Vaccine development, cancer, 29–45
Vascular endothelial growth factor, 1–15, 117–138
VEGF, See Vascular endothelial growth factor, 1–15, 117–138
Vinca alkaloids, treatment for cervical cancer, 168–190

W

Waldenstrom's macroglobulinemia, 117–138

INDEX OF TABLES

Table 1.1: Commercial Sources for Microarrays, 2
Table 1.2: Information for Microarray Preparation and Analysis, 3
Table 2.1: Diagnostic Methods to Analyze Structural DNA Alterations, 20
Table 3.1: Antigen Delivery Systems, 37–38
Table 6.1: Human DNA Repair Pathways, 93
Table 7.1: Phase II Study of Thalidomide, 119
Table 7.2: Thalidomide in Advanced Myeloma, 120
Table 7.3: Myeloma Protein Response and Associated Laboratory Change, 121
Table 7.4: Prognostic Variables with Thalidomide, 122
Table 7.5: Higher Thalidomide Dose Benefits Patients with High-Risk Disease, 124
Table 7.6: Thalidomide in Multiple Myeloma, 126–128
Table 7.7: Efficacy of Total Therapy II, 130
Table 8.1: Phase I Studies with Oxaliplatin Alone, 148
Table 8.2: Phase II with Oxaliplatin Alone in Patients with Advanced Colorectal Cancer, 149
Table 8.3: Grade III and IV Toxicities (%) Associated with Two Regimens Incorporating Single Agent Oxaliplatin in Patients with Advanced Colorectal Cancer, 150

Table 8.4: Phase II Oxaliplatin with Fluorouracil/Leucovorin in Patients with Advanced Colorectal Cancer, 152–155
Table 8.5: Grade 3–4 Toxicities Associated with 5-fluorouracil/Leucovorin Plus Oxaliplatin, 157
Table 8.6: Phase III 5-fluorouracil/Leucovorin in Patients with Advanced Colorectal Cancer, 161
Table 9.1: Chemoradiation Versus Radiation Trials (National Cancer Institute Clinical Alert, 169
Table 9.2: International Federation of Gynecology and Obstetrics Staging of Carcinoma of the Cervix Uteri, 171
Table 9.3: Relationship Between Local Control and Five-Year Survival, 172
Table 9.4: Four-Year Actuarial Outcome by Total Treatment Time, 173
Table 9.5: Prospective Randomized Trials of Sequential Chemotherapy Prior to Radiation Versus Radiation, 175
Table 9.6: Risk Factors for Determining Need for Postoperative Pelvic Radiation Therapy After Radical Hysterectomy with Negative Pelvic Lymph Nodes, 182
Table 11.1: CD20 Antigen Characteristics, 205
Table 11.2: Rituximab Chimeric anti-CD20 Antibody Characteristics, 207
Table 11.3: Selected Single-Agent Rituximab NHL Trials, 213
Table 11.4: Selected Chemoimmunotherapy Combination NHL Trials with Rituximab, 219
Table 12.1: GVHD is Associated with a Reduced Relative Risk (RR) of Leukemic Relapse After Allogeneic SCT, 232
Table 12.2: Graft-versus-tumor Effect of Donor Leukocyte Infusion, 235
Table 13.1: Liver Metastases from Colorectal Cancer: Patient Survival, 259
Table 13.2: Complications of Radiofrequency Ablation, 268
Table 13.3: RFA for Liver Metastases: Collected Review, 271
Table 13.4: RF Ablation of Liver Metastases: Predictors of Local Failure, 272
Table 14.1.1: Clinical and Incidental Detection of Cancers, 280
Table 14.1.2: Survival Rates for Conservatively Managed and Surgically Managed Cancers, 283
Table 14.1.3: Probability of Dying from Prostate Cancer Managed Conservatively According to Biopsy Tumor Grade, 283
Table 14.1.4: Actuarial (PSA-based) 5-Year Nonprogression Rates After Radical Prostatectomy for Clinical Stage T1–2NXNO Prostate Cancer, 285
Table 14.1.5: Predicted Probability of Each Pathologic Stage Based on Preoperative Serum Prostate Specific Antigen (PSA) Level, Clinical Stage, and Gleason Grade in the Biopsy Specimen, 290
Table 14.1.6: Actuarial 5-Year Progression-free Probability Rates After Radical Retropubic Prostatectomy, 292
Table 14.1.7: Multivariate Analysis of Risk of Progression, 293
Table 14.1.8: Incidence of Incontinence After Radical Prostatectomy, 295
Table 14.1.9: Probability of Recovery of Potency by 24 and 36 Months Based on a Combination of Preoperative and Postoperative Parameters, 301
Table 14.1.10: Positive Margin Rates, 306
Table 14.1.11: PSA-free Survival, 307
Table 14.2.1: Characteristics of 1100 Stage T1c–T3 Prostate Cancer Patients Treated with 3D-CRT and IMRT, 319
Table 14.2.2: Local Failure According to Prognostic Risk Group and Dose Assessed by Biopsies in 252 Patients at $\geq$ 2.5 Years After 3D-CRT and IMRT, 324
Table 14.2.3: Five-Year Outcomes of Randomized Trials Testing the Effect of Androgen Deprivation Combined with Radiation Therapy, 326

Table 14.2.4: Impact of Neoadjuvant Androgen Deprivation on Local Control Assessed by Biopsies in 252 Patients at $\geq$ 2.5 Years After 3D–CRT and IMRT, 328

Table 14.3.1: Clinical Outcome of Permanent-Implant Monotherapy Without Adjuvant Hormonal Therapy, 339

Table 14.3.2: Clinical Outcome of External Beam Irradiation with Implant Boost, 340